The Lower Extremity and Spine
in Sports Medicine

The Lower Extremity and Spine
in Sports Medicine

Edited by

James A. Nicholas, M.D.

Director, Department of Orthopaedic Surgery and the
Institute of Sports Medicine and Athletic Trauma, Lenox Hill
Hospital; Professor of Clinical Orthopaedic Surgery, New York
Medical College; Adjunct Professor of Physical Education, New
York University; Consultant in Orthopaedic Surgery, Hospital
for Special Surgery; Team Physician, New York Jets;
Orthopaedic consultant, New York Cosmos, New York
Rangers, and New York Knickerbockers, New York, New York;
and Keller Army Hospital, West Point, New York

Elliott B. Hershman, M.D.

Assistant Adjunct Orthopaedic Surgeon, Consultant, Institute
for Sports Medicine and Athletic Trauma, Lenox Hill Hospital,
New York, New York

with **2,077** illustrations and **4** color plates

The C. V. Mosby Company

St. Louis • Toronto • Princeton   1986

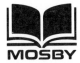

MOSBY

A TRADITION OF PUBLISHING EXCELLENCE

Acquisition Editor: Eugenia A. Klein
Assistant Editor: Jean Carey-Brendle
Manuscript Editors: Timothy O'Brien and Suzanne Seeley
Designer: Nancy Steinmeyer
Cover design: John R. Rokusek
Production: Jeanne A. Gulledge

The C. V. Mosby Company
11830 Westline Industrial Drive, St. Louis, Missouri 63146

Library of Congress Cataloging in Publication Data
Main entry under title:

The Lower extremity and spine in sports medicine.

　　Includes bibliographies and index.
　　　1. Extremities, Lower—Wounds and injuries.
2. Spine—Wounds and injuries.　　3. Sports—Accidents
and injuries.　　I. Nicholas, James A., 1921-
II. Hershman, Elliott B. [DNLM:　1. Athletic injuries.
2. Leg Injuries.　　3. Spinal Injuries.　WE 850 L917]
RD560.L69　1986　　　617′.58044　　　　85-25909
ISBN 0-8016-3616-7 (set)

C/MV/MV　9　8　7　6　5　4　3　2　1　　　03/B/327

CONTRIBUTORS

Wayne H. Akeson, M.D.

Professor and Head, Division of Orthopaedics
and Rehabilitation,
University of California, San Diego,
La Jolla, California

David Amiel, Dip. Ing.

Division of Orthopaedics and Rehabilitation,
University of California, San Diego,
La Jolla, California

**Steven Paul Arnoczky, D.V.M., Dip.
A.C.V.S.**

Director, Laboratory of Comparative
Orthopaedics,
The Hospital for Special Surgery;
Associate Professor of Surgery (Orthopaedic),
Cornell University Medical College,
New York, New York

Richard A. Boiardo, M.D.

Fellow, Southwestern Orthopaedic Medical
Group,
Inglewood, California, in affiliation with
Centenila Hospital

Arthur L. Boland, Jr.

Clinical Assistant Professor of Orthopedic
Surgery,
Harvard Medical School;
Orthopedic Surgeon,
Brigham and Women's Hospital,
Boston, Massachusetts

John Boyle, M.D.

Research and Clinical Fellow,
Department of Orthopaedic Surgery,
Massachusetts General Hospital,
Boston, Massachusetts

Clive E. Brewster, M.S., R.P.T.

Director of Physical Therapy,
Department of Physical Therapy,
Southwestern Orthopaedic Medical Group,
Inc.,
Inglewood, California

David M. Brody, M.D.

Associate Clinical Professor of Orthopaedic
Surgery and Consultant to The Runner's
Clinic,
George Washington University,
Washington, D.C.

**T. Pepper Burruss, A.T.C., R.P.T.,
E.M.T.**

Assistant Athletic Trainer,
New York Jets Football Club,
New York, New York

Jerome V. Ciullo, M.D.

Former Memorial Hospital Sports Medicine
Fellow;
Assistant Professor, Department of
Orthopaedic Surgery,
Director of Sports Medicine and Teams
Physician,
Wayne State University;
Medical Director, Institute for Sports
Medicine and Human Performance,
Harper Hospital, Detroit, Michigan;
Team Physician, Michigan Panthers Football
Club

Kenneth E. DeHaven, M.D.

Professor of Orthopaedics and Head,
Section of Athletic Medicine.
University of Rochester School of Medicine,
Rochester, New York

Vincent J. DiStefano, M.D.

Clinical Assistant Professor of Orthopaedic
    Surgery,
Department of Orthopaedic Surgery,
University of Pennsylvania;
Team Physician, Philadelphia Eagles,
Philadelphia, Pennsylvania

David J. Drez, Jr., M.D.

Clinical Professor of Orthopaedics,
Louisiana State University Medical School,
New Orleans, Louisiana;
Team Physician, McNeese State University,
Lake Charles, Louisiana

Howard J. Ellfeldt, M.D.

Clinical Assistant Professor,
Department of Surgery, University of Kansas
    School of Medicine,
Kansas City, Kansas;
Team Physician, Kansas City Chiefs and
    Kansas City Kings,
Kansas City, Missouri

Joseph F. Fetto, M.D.

Associate Clinical Professor, Department of
    Orthopaedics,
New York University Medical Center;
Team Physician, U.S. Judo Federation,
New York University Intercollegiate Athletics,
New York, New York

James M. Fox, M.D.

Medical Director,
Center for Disorders of the Knee,
Van Nuys, California

Victor H. Frankel, M.D., Ph.D.

Chairman, Department of Orthopaedic
    Surgery,
Hospital for Joint Diseases, Orthopaedic
    Institute;
Lecturer, Mount Sinai School of Medicine,
New York, New York

Marc J. Friedman, M.D.

Clinical Instructor, Department of
    Orthopaedics,
University of California, Los Angeles,
Los Angeles, California

William E. Garrett, Jr., M.D., Ph.D.

Assistant Professor, Department of
    Orthopaedic Surgery and Anatomy,
Duke University,
Durham, North Carolina

Gilbert Gleim, Ph.D.

Research Coordinator, Institute of Sports
    Medicine and Athletic Trauma,
Lenox Hill Hospital;
Adjunct Assistant Professor,
New York University,
New York, New York

James M. Glick, M.D.

Associate Clinical Professor, Department of
    Orthopedic Surgery,
University of California,
San Francisco;
Team Physician, San Francisco State
    University;
Chief, Department of Orthopaedics,
Mount Zion Hospital,
San Francisco, California

Karl R. Glick, Jr.

Mid-America Center for Sports Medicine,
Wichita, Kansas

Douglas L. Gollehon, M.D.

Cincinnati Sportsmedicine and Orthopaedic
    Center,
Cincinnati, Ohio

Charles E. Henning, M.D.

Associate Clinical Professor, University of
    Kansas School of Medicine;
Mid-America Center for Sports Medicine,
Wichita, Kansas

Jack H. Henry, M.D.

Private Practice, Orthopaedic Surgery and
    Athletic Medicine;
Team Physician, San Antonio Spurs,
San Antonio, Texas

Letha Y. Hunter, Ph.D., M.D.

Clinical Instructor, Orthopaedic Surgery,
Emory University School of Medicine;
Staff, Peachtree Orthopaedic Clinic,
Atlanta, Georgia

Douglas W. Jackson, M.D.

Director, Southern California Center for
　Sports Medicine,
Long Beach, California

Donald C. Jones, M.D.

Team Physician, University of Oregon;
Private Practice, Orthopaedic and Fracture
　Clinic,
Eugene, Oregon

Lawrence I. Karlin, M.D.

Assistant Professor of Orthopaedic Surgery,
Tufts University School of Medicine,
Boston, Massachusetts

Mary A. Lynch, M.D.

Mid-America Center for Sports Medicine,
Wichita, Kansas

Anthony V. Maddalo, M.D.

Chief Resident, Department of Orthopaedic
　Surgery,
Lenox Hill Hospital,
New York, New York

Roger A. Mann, M.D.

Associate Clinical Professor, Department of
　Orthopaedic Surgery,
University of California School of Medicine,
San Francisco, California

Michael Marino, R.P.T.

Research Associate, Institute of Sports
　Medicine and Athletic Trauma,
Department of Orthopaedic Surgery,
Lenox Hill Hospital,
New York, New York

Lyle J. Micheli, M.D.

Director, Division of Sports Medicine,
Boston Children's Hospital,
Boston, Massachusetts;
Associate Professor of Orthopaedic Surgery,
Harvard Medical School,
Cambridge, Massachusetts

David L. Milbauer, M.D.

Department of Diagnostic Radiology,
Yale University School of Medicine,
New Haven, Connecticut;
Formerly Department of Diagnostic Radiology,
Lenox Hill Hospital,
New York, New York

Matthew C. Morrissey, M.A., R.P.T.

Assistant Director of Physical Therapy,
Coordinator of Physical Therapy Research,
Department of Physical Therapy,
Southwestern Orthopaedic Medical Group,
　Inc.,
Inglewood, California

James A. Nicholas, M.D.

Director, Department of Orthopaedic Surgery,
Institute of Sports Medicine and Athletic
　Trauma,
Lenox Hill Hospital;
Professor of Clinical Orthopaedic Surgery,
New York Medical College;
Associate Clinical Professor of Surgery
　(Orthopaedics),
Cornell University Medical College;
Adjunct Professor of Physical Education,
New York University;
Team Physician, New York Jets;
Orthopaedic Consultant, New York Cosmos,
　New York Rangers, and New York
　Knickerbockers,
New York, New York

Barton Nisonson, M.D.

Section Chief, Division of Arthroscopy,
Department of Orthopaedic Surgery,
Lenox Hill Hospital;
Associate Orthopaedic Surgeon,
New York Jets;
Associate Team Physician,
New York Rangers

Patrick F. O'Leary, M.D.

Chief, Section of Spinal Surgery,
Department of Orthopaedics,
Lenox Hill Hospital;
Assistant Clinical Professor, Department of
　Orthopaedic Surgery,
Mount Sinai School of Medicine,
The City University of New York;
Attending Surgeon, Department of
　Orthopaedic Surgery,
The Hospital for Joint Diseases Orthopaedic
　Institute,
New York, New York

**Shashikant A. Patel, M.B., F.R.C.S.,
　F.R.C.R., M.D.**

Associate Radiologist, Department of
　Radiology,
Lenox Hill Hospital,
New York, New York

Lars Peterson, M.D.

Associate Professor of Orthopaedic Surgery,
University of Goteborg,
Goteborg, Sweden

Robert C. Reese, Jr., A.T.C.

Head Athletic Trainer, New York Jets,
New York, New York

G. James Sammarco, M.D., F.A.C.S.

Associate Clinical Professor, Department of
   Orthopaedics,
University of Cincinnati,
Cincinnati, Ohio

Thomas G. Sampson, M.D.

Assistant Clinical Professor, Department of
   Orthopedics,
University of California,
San Francisco;
Assistant Team Physician,
San Francisco State University,
San Francisco, California

Frank S. Santopietro, D.P.M.

Chief Podiatrist, Sports Medicine Division,
Boston Children's Hospital,
Boston, Massachusetts

Steven G. Scott, D.O.

Assistant Professor of Physical Medicine and
   Rehabilitation,
Mayo Medical School;
Consultant, Department of Physical Medicine
   and Rehabilitation,
Mayo Clinic and Mayo Foundation,
Rochester, Minnesota

Clarence L. Shields, Jr., M.D.

Assistant Clinical Professor, Department of
   Orthopaedics,
University of Southern California;
Team Physician, Los Angeles Rams,
Los Angeles, California

Franklin H. Sim, M.D.

Professor of Orthopedic Surgery,
Mayo Medical School;
Consultant, Department of Orthopedics,
Mayo Clinic and Mayo Foundation,
Rochester, Minnesota

Kenneth M. Singer, M.D.

Clinical Instructor of Surgery, Division of
   Orthopaedic Surgery and Rehabilitation,
University of Oregon Health Sciences Center;
Associate Team Physician,
University of Oregon;
Private Practice, Orthopaedic and Fracture
   Clinic,
Eugene, Oregon

Roger Sohn, M.D.

Fellow in Sports Medicine, Sports Medicine
   Division,
Boston Children's Hospital,
Boston, Massachusetts

Anthony J. Spinella, M.D.

Associate Orthopaedic Surgeon,
St. Francis Hospital;
Clinical Instructor, Department of
   Orthopaedics,
University of Connecticut School of Medicine;
Associate Team Physician, Hartford Whalers,
Hartford, Connecticut

J.R. Steadman, M.D.

Assistant Clinical Professor, Department of
   Orthopaedic Surgery, University of
   California, Davis, and University of Nevada,
   Reno;
Chairman, Medical Group of the U.S. Ski
   Team

Alan M. Strizak, M.D.

Assistant Clinical Professor, Department of
   Orthopaedic Surgery,
Harbor-University of California at Los Angeles
   Medical Center,
Los Angeles, California;
Team Physician, Cerritos College,
Long Beach, California;
Medical Director, STAAR Institute,
Fountain Valley, California

Albert J. Stroberg

Assistant Clinical Professor, Department of
   Orthopaedic Surgery,
Harbor-UCLA Medical Center,
Los Angeles, California

Peter A. Torzilli, Ph.D.

Associate Professor of Applied Biomechanics,
Department of Surgery (Orthopaedics),
Cornell University Medical College;
Associate Scientist, Department of
  Biomechanics,
  Hospital for Special Surgery,
  New York, New York

Vincent J. Turco, M.D.

Attending Orthopaedist, St. Francis Hospital,
Hartford, Connecticut;
Team Physician, Hartford Whalers;
Assistant Clinical Professor of Orthopaedics,
University of Connecticut School of Medicine,
Hartford, Connecticut

John F. Waller, Jr., M.D.

Adjunct, Department of Orthopaedic Surgery,
Lenox Hill Hospital,
New York, New York

Russell F. Warren, M.D.

Associate Professor of Orthopaedic Surgery,
Cornell University Medical Center;
Director, Sports Medicine Service,
Director, Shoulder Service,
Hospital for Special Surgery;
Team Physician, New York Giants,
New York, New York

Thomas L. Wickiewicz, M.D.

Assistant Orthopaedic Surgeon,
Hospital for Special Surgery;
Assistant Professor of Clinical Surgery,
Cornell University Medical College,
New York, New York

Savio L-Y. Woo, Ph.D.

Professor in Residence,
Division of Orthopaedics and Rehabilitation,
University of California, San Diego,
La Jolla, California

John L. Xethalis, M.D.

Adjunct, Department of Orthopaedic Surgery,
Lenox Hill Hospital;
Team Physician, New York Cosmos Soccer
  Club,
New York, New York

John G. Yost, Jr., M.D.

Assistant Team Physician, Kansas City Kings
  Basketball Club,
Kansas City, Missouri

Paul M. Zabetakis, M.D., F.A.C.P.

Associate Chief, Nephrology-Hypertension
  Department of Medicine,
Lenox Hill Hospital,
New York, New York;
Research Physician, Institute of Sports
  Medicine and Athletic Trauma,
Lenox Hill Hospital,
New York, New York;
Assistant Professor of Clinical Medicine,
New York Medical College,
Valhalla, New York

Bertram Zarins, M.D.

Assistant Clinical Professor of Orthopaedic
  Surgery,
Harvard Medical School;
Chief, Sports Medicine Unit,
Massachusetts General Hospital;
Team Physician, Boston Bruins and New
  England Patriots,
Boston, Massachusetts

FOREWORD

Over the past 20 years I have been privileged to participate with, listen to, and engage in discussions about many aspects of sports medicine with Dr. Nicholas. A recurring theme in many of these encounters was his belief that to focus only on the area of injury and its treatment was to lose sight of the broader aspects of rehabilitation. Alteration of function to parts both proximally and distally occurs. Secondary effects occur to the cardiorespiratory system and the neurovascular system. The psychological manifestations of injury as perceived by the patient play a part in the response of the athlete to treatment and his or her rehabilitation. Anatomy, physiology, kinematics, and the biomechanics of injury are all integrally related in the consideration of specific injuries. This intertwining of all of these aspects, not only in the broad sense but also in the narrow confines of a specific athlete, has been conceptualized by Dr. Nicholas as "linkage."

This multidisciplinary approach to sports injury, as promulgated by Dr. Nicholas, was manifested into one of the first facilities to evaluate, treat, and rehabilitate all aspects of sports injury: the Institute of Sports Medicine and Athletic Trauma, of which Dr. Nicholas is the founder and director. This advocacy of total conceptualization is depicted in his seven "P's" of athletic activity: Performer, Performance, Pathology, Prescription, Practitioner, Practice, and Prevention.

Comprehensive care of the athlete involves all of these and is closely associated with the underlying theme of this text—"linkage" of basic science, other disciplines of medicine, and alteration of function of other parts not directly related to the injury.

The section on basic science and that on principles of rehabilitation, reconditioning, and training are the first parts of this book. This emphasizes their importance as the groundwork for the understanding, treatment, and rehabilitation of specific injuries. Subsequent chapters in the clinical sections are also introduced with basic science material germane to that particular anatomic area. Review of the Table of Contents reflects the detailed discussion provided with each.

Dr. Nicholas' insistence on the importance of the various levers, torques, and forces generated by body motion and their relationship to functional rehabilitation has engendered an awareness of them by all who follow his teaching. Those who have contributed their expertise to this text have been encouraged by the editors to be mindful of the diction of "total body linkage."

The challenge of producing yet another book on sports medicine has been met by providing a fresh outlook and a broader interpretation of injury to the athlete. The various types of treatment—both nonoperative and operative—are presented. The pros and cons of various surgical techniques are given, but more importantly, the nonoperative treatment is emphasized, and justifiably so. When a surgical procedure is not appropriate, treatment is often more casual and carried out in a less than enthusiastic manner. The editors have required detailed and explicit steps and goals in nonoperative care and rehabilitation from the authors and have provided boxed summary material for ready reference to such treatment.

It is the intent of the editors to provide information not only to the orthopedic surgeon but to the entire sports medicine community. The perception of an understanding of the basic science of athletic performance and injury, the multidisciplined approach to treatment and rehabilitation of the entire athlete, and an awareness of total body involvement in injury as well as performance is the thrust that the editors hope to communicate to the reader. If this hope becomes a reality, the editors should be well satisfied that proper attention has been given to the entire "linkage mechanism" that is the human body in action.

Robert L. Larson, M.D.

PREFACE

Within the last two decades, sports medicine has emerged to become a rapidly expanding, multilayered discipline. The increased participation in athletics by millions of individuals, coupled with demand for knowledge about prevention, care, and treatment of athletic injuries, led to the development of the Institute of Sports Medicine and Athletic Trauma (IS-MAT), a special section of the Department of Orthopaedic Surgery at Lenox Hill Hospital in New York City. Indeed, ISMAT was the first hospital-based sports medicine institute of its type in the country. The Institute is currently a national center devoted to research, education, and clinical service, supported in part by an endowment fund.

The exponential growth and explosion of interest has contributed to the development of the sports medicine physician. Although a number of medical specialities are involved in the care of the athlete, the orthopaedic surgeon is at the core of sports medicine because of the fundamental importance of the musculoskeletal system in athletic endeavors. The role of the sports medicine physician is clear: to provide scientifically based intervention to all athletes, male or female, young or old, novice or professional, that will enable individuals to participate to their fullest potential so as to enjoy recreation and enhance physical fitness and ability. This should include disabled persons who wish to indulge in recreational activities.

We feel that the musculoskeletal system is of primary importance in the acquisition of fitness by an individual. It provides part of the fuel system as well as the motors, levers, and joints that move the body through space. For this reason, injuries to this finely coordinated and conditioned system demand a special emphasis, with rehabilitation being an integral part of treatment. The economy of motion and efficiency in overcoming inertia decide, to a large extent, the impact of sports on the ability of the individual to train and enjoy sports without danger.

The human musculoskeletal system is highly integrated, and its malfunctioning parts are inextricably related to the whole spectrum which comprises the integrated human system. The brain can be likened to a giant emotional computer, the heart to a pump, the kidneys to a waste system, and the musculoskeletal system to a leverage system, which overcomes inertia when we move about. Sports medicine must therefore emphasize how injury and pathology affect the body, encompassing areas such as anatomy, biochemistry, biomechanics, histopathology, pharmacology, and physiology.

With this in mind, this text has been written to emphasize the complex interrelationship between various parts of the musculoskeletal system, as well as the physiologic and psychologic implications of musculoskeletal injury. Every substantial injury to the body leaves a residual effect. Subsequently, the ability to meet maximal demands of sport at a later date, perhaps even years later, may be compromised. Musculoskeletal derangement, pathology, or physiologic malfunction can occur far from the site of the initial injury. Tunnel vision of a malfunctioning part must not occur. To exclude the implications of such a pathologic condition on the rest of the body may lead to further defects in the musculoskeletal system. Interrelationships between body segments and systems are emphasized by the concepts inherent in the linkage system. Throughout the text, the reader should relate each joint and its injury in relation to the linkage system. Assessment and treatment of the entire proximal and distal links of the spine and lower extremity then must always be kept in mind in treating athletic injuries.

We have attempted to relate clinical situations to some basic scientific knowledge. Hence significant sections of the text have been devoted to the basic sciences. Coupling basic science with clinical experience yields basic patterns of intervention firmly grounded on scientific inquiry, an approach now possible in sports medicine as a result of the excellent research being done in the basic sciences.

The text has been written by a talented cadre of health care professionals who are heavily involved or interested in the care of athletes. Our aim is to have them describe their opinions as to the mechanisms of injuries in the lower extremity and in the spine, their recognition, treatment, and rehabilitation, and how they may be prevented. Because of this comprehensive approach, we have limited the text to the lower extremity and entire spine to allow complete discussion of the areas covered. We have also included a number of chapters on some sports-specific injuries, which will enable the reader to consider injuries directly in light of the demands of specific sports. Moreover, the skeletally immature athlete is considered in a separate section of the text, because treatment of these individuals is significantly different from their adult counterparts. Because of the rapidly changing nature of the way upper extremity work is being done, such as diagnostic and surgical arthroscopy of the shoulder, elbow,

and hand, the use of scanning techniques, and the early, less-defined studies of upper body training on the entire linkage system, we thought it wise to defer the upper extremity volume until more clinical material becomes readily available.

We think that the young field of sports medicine will continue to advance with the assistance of computerized study into the linkage phenomena. In particular, it is important that we recognize and understand the relationship of motions used in various sports and how these motions are directly related to the causes of injury, and the subsequent effects of recurring injury on the body. We do not believe in any "average individual," and we are confident that future research will substantiate this premise. With time, the concept of profiling—the interrelationship between physical and psychologic attributes of athletes and the demands of sport—will be better understood by those professionals responsible for the prevention, diagnosis, and treatment of injuries. Exercise programs will then be specifically adapted to each athlete's profile, pathology, and performance demands.

Although this text has been written primarily for practicing orthopaedic surgeons, orthopaedic residents, and sports medicine specialists, it is also intended for allied health professionals, including the athletic trainer, health and physical educator, exercise physiologist, physical therapist, and others who are part of the sports medicine team. Understanding the mechanisms of injuries in sports, the diagnosis, treatment, and rehabilitation of injuries, and the subsequent course of an individual following an injury is an immense task, but a great challenge. This book will hopefully integrate the multidisciplinary concepts of sports medicine and provide the reader with an understanding of the importance of the musculoskeletal system and the concept of linkage.

James A. Nicholas
Elliott B. Hershman

ACKNOWLEDGMENTS

Our thanks and deepest appreciation:

To each of the contributing authors, who found time, when there was none available, to write complete and superbly written chapters.

To Phil Rosenthal, Assistant Director of the Institute of Sports Medicine and Athletic Trauma, who coordinated countless aspects of this text, always with infinite attention to detail and an ever present smile.

To Debra Elaine Ryals, for her energetic and gracious assistance throughout the publication process.

To Rose Marie Spitaleri, Clifford Goldthwaite, Roberta Coulter, and Mary Ellen Latella of the Lenox Hill Hospital Department of Medical Photography, for the seemingly endless hours of work devoted to producing many of the fine photographs used throughout the text.

To our typists, Margaret Unser-Schutz and Patricia Guardala for all their efforts.

To our editors at the C.V. Mosby Company, Eugenia A. Klein, Jean Carey-Brendle, and Timothy O'Brien, for their faith, support, and thoughtful guidance.

And to our biggest supporters, Kiki, Philip, Stephen, and Nicole, and Susan, who make everything in life possible and worthwhile.

James A. Nicholas
Elliott B. Hershman

CONTENTS

---

part three Regional considerations

Basic science of athletic injuries

Cartilage and ligament: physiology and repair processes

Wayne H. Akeson

David Amiel

Savio L-Y. Woo

The purpose of this chapter is to summarize existing knowledge of the physiology and repair processes of synovial joints. This subject has ramifications of such breadth that we have narrowed the focus on two subjects of practical and timely importance in sports medicine, the physiology and repair processes of cartilage and ligament. Readers interested in additional detail, including historical aspects, are referred to other review papers recently published.[18,65,74,76]

■ ARTICULAR CARTILAGE

Articular cartilage is a paradigm of functional efficiency. This efficiency is derived from design features that are marveled at by those attempting to design substitutes for diseased joints. The superior lubricating efficiency of articular cartilage in its synovial environment is well known to students of this subject. This efficiency is of a magnitude superior to the best lubrication mechanisms known to modern engineers; it is far superior even to ice skates on ice, for example.

The functional efficiency of articular cartilage is maintained throughout life in most humans. This achievement is remarkable, because the tissue is only a few millimeters thick and has extremely limited repair capability. No mechanical device known to man is expected to last 80 years; indeed, most automobile graveyards are filled with hulks scarcely one

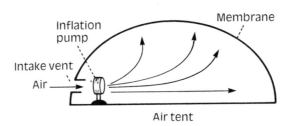

Air tent articular cartilage
analogy

Fig. 1-1 ■ Air tent articular cartilage analogy. It is conceptually useful to think of cartilage as a pressurized structure such as exemplified by an air tent. This system requires a pump, which must be working constantly to maintain inflation of system because of leaks through fabric. In the case of cartilage, the surface membrane is a fine collagen fibril network concentrated at the surface. The inflation pump is proteoglycan molecules, and the inflation medium is an ultrafiltrate of synovial fluid. In cartilage, of course, there is no single intake vent for inflation medium to enter; rather, the fluid that inflates tissues enters through the same fabric pores at the surface from which it exits when compressed (see text).

tenth that age. The reasons for the spectacular success and survival of articular cartilage are found in the precise morphologic, biomechanical, biologic, and biophysical interactions of this unique tissue.

Function-form relationships of articular cartilage

It is useful to consider the question, what is the purpose of articular cartilage? Intuitive responses are not particularly helpful. It has been clearly shown by Radin,[92] for example, that articular cartilage does not serve as the major shock absorber of the synovial joint complex. That role is assumed by the cancellous bone that is subadjacent to the subchondral plate. Rather, cartilage serves to prevent osseous high points from contacting one another during the excursions of normal movement. Because of the complex geometry necessary for bone structures to achieve the functional requirements of synovial joints, complete congruity of the bone surfaces cannot be achieved. For this reason, a fluid-filled capsule between the bone surfaces will permit the disparate geometries to accommodate to each other by fluid flow. Because of the joint

capsule, there is no contact between bony asperities, wear is minimized, and durable function is ensured.

Before the details of morphology and biochemistry of the articular cartilage matrix are reviewed, it will be helpful to consider a simple scheme that describes the interrelationship of these elements. A useful analogy for articular cartilage is the air tent used as a cover for recreational areas such as swimming pools and tennis courts or as a temporary cover for exhibitions (Fig 1-1). The requirements for the tent are a membrane (fabric cover), an inflation medium (air), and an energy source to keep the membrane inflated (fan). These elements are interrelated, and a deficiency in any of them will result in failure of the system, the collapse of the tent. If the fabric has a tear or an air leak occurs for which the pump is not able to compensate, the tent will collapse. If the pump fails, the tent will also gradually collapse as pressurized air leaks through the pores of the fabric.

There is a fabriclike structure at the cartilage surface that consists of fine collagen fibrils packed tightly in a matted pattern. This is much different from the pattern seen in the deeper layers, where

5

Chapter 1
Cartilage and ligament:
physiology and repair processes

fibers become thicker, the orientation becomes vertical, and the spaces between the fibers increase. The surface "fabric" of cartilage has tiny pores that permit fluid and small molecules access to and egress from the tissue but block movement of large molecules. The inflation medium in articular cartilage is fluid rather than air. The cartilage fluid is in equilibrium with the synovial fluid, which in turn is essentially an ultrafiltrate of plasma. The fluid in articular cartilage is significantly pressurized. Calculations by Ogston[83] led him to conclude that articular cartilage is inflated to "motor tyre pressure."

The pump for this pressurized system is not intuitively obvious, but its presence has been established beyond doubt by modern techniques of rheology and biophysics. The pump for the articular cartilage system is chiefly the proteoglycan and proteoglycan aggregate molecules, large macromolecules trapped within the articular cartilage fibrillar matrix as a result of their large size and volume. They are much too large to move between the fibrils of collagen and much, much too large to exit through the small pores in the matted, capsulelike surface of the articular cartilage. Side-arm branches of these molecules contain many negative surface charges that repel each other, causing the molecules to attempt to unwind and enlarge their domain within the cartilage. In addition, the protein polysaccharides have a large number of hydroxyl groups, which attract water molecules through a phenomenon called **hydrogen bonding.** These reactions collectively cause fluid to be pulled into articular cartilage through the matrix pores and cause the collagen matrix of the system to be expanded. This tendency to imbibe water creates a swelling pressure within the enclosed cartilage space. The collagen fibers are therefore placed under tension as the fluid pressure rises. In this manner the collagen and "fabric" is inflated, and the cartilage is pressurized. The equilibrium state reached is a balance that can be up-

set by external applied pressure. If the external pressure exceeds the internal pressure, fluid will be caused to flow outward until a new equilibrium is reached. This fluid movement will be of great interest to us later in this chapter, as it explains the mechanism of several indispensible elements of the articular cartilage system, such as lubrication, load-bearing, and nutrition.

The collagen matrix of cartilage, the proteoglycan, and proteoglycan aggregate and the movement of fluid within cartilage will be described in greater detail with respect to morphologic, biochemical, metabolic, and functional aspects.

Articular cartilage morphology

The details of form of the articular cartilage fabric are well suited to the functional requirements of synovial joints. The pressurized interstitial fluid is constrained from expansion by the "armor plate" layer of matted fine fibrils at the surface and by the firm anchoring of deeper collagen fibers into the calcified cartilage layer and the subchondral bone layer.

The collagen pattern at the cartilage surface is morphologically quite different from the pattern in deeper layers. Benninghoff[19] described an arcade pattern of articular cartilage collagen organization in 1925 (Fig. 1-2). This pattern has been subsequently challenged with respect to the precise accuracy of the proposed scheme.[60] However, with respect to functional understanding, the concept is useful and substantially correct. Certainly the surface fiber characteristics differ from those of fibers in deeper layers. The surface collagen fibrils are smaller (30 to 32 nm in diameter) and more closely packed in the middle and deeper layers.[122] The heterogeneity of concentration of the principal cartilage constituents—collagen and proteoglycan—by dry weight is seen in Fig. 1-3. The collagen concentration is greatest at the surface, where the small fibrils are compacted tangential to the surface. This arrangement creates an effec-

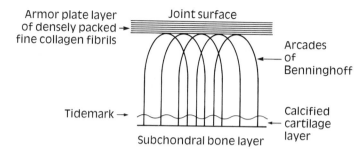

Fig. 1-2 ■ Schematic diagram of collagen fibril orientation within articular cartilage. Fibrils are tightly packed near the articular surface in tangential layer that has been termed the "armor plate" layer. Fibrils in the deeper layers become progressively larger as they progress toward the subchondral bone layer. Fibrils are also more widely spaced in deeper layers of cartilage. The change in orientation from tangential to perpendicular in deeper layers creates a pattern which Benninghoff[7] termed an "arcade." Although this is an idealized conception and fibrils of cartilage are not so precisely ordered, the concept is still useful in visualizing the fundamental interaction of cartilage with other constituents of cartilage. Collagen fibrils anchor into the subchondral bone layer after traversing the calcified cartilage, which is demarcated by a change in staining properties termed "tidemark line." Anchoring of these fibrils into bone is analogous to continuation of ligamentous attachments into bone termed "Sharpey's fibrils."

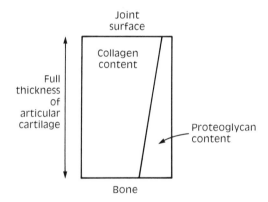

Fig. 1-3 ■ Relative amounts of collagen and proteoglycan in cartilage. Collagen is the predominant organic constituent by weight in articular cartilage and is most concentrated at surface layer. In contrast, proteoglycan is most concentrated in deeper layers. The functional importance of the two constituents is more equal than these percentages might suggest, both constituents being essential for normal cartilage function.

tive pore size, which has been calculated by McCutchen[68] to be about 6 nm. The largest molecule that can traverse a pore of this dimension is hemoglobin. Therefore the surface pores readily admit most of the synovial fluid molecules, which are essentially an ultrafiltrate of plasma. Small ions and glucose, for example, easily traverse these pores, but larger molecules such as proteins and hyaluronic acid do not enter cartilalge in significant amounts under normal conditions. Exter-

nally synthesized proteolytic enzymes would also be excluded, an important matrix protective factor.

Collagen fibers in the intermediate layers no longer are oriented principally tangential to the surface but are obliquely or randomly directed. They are larger than the surface fibrils, most ranging between 40 and 100 nm.[122] The deepest fibrils are the largest in cartilage. They are perpendicularly disposed relative to the joint surface. They perforate the calcified basal

7

Chapter 1
Cartilage and ligament:
physiology and repair processes

layers of cartilage through the tidemark regions and eventually enter the subchondral bone layer, where they are firmly attached, much as in the case of Sharpey's fibers of cortical bone.

This anatomic arrangement is the key to the secure structural anchorage of cartilage to the bone that it overlies. The surface collagen fibrils possess characteristics that create the necessary functional barrier to fluid movement. However, this movement is rate limited by the small pore size of the collagen meshwork of the cartilage surface, an important factor that prevents all the fluid from being expressed, as, for example, when an individual stands for hours at a time.

The surface pattern of the collagen framework described has been implicitly recognized for decades by the term "armor plate layer," referring to the tough, resilient cartilage surface. It has been well demonstrated clinically that **loss of the densely packed collagen mat at the surface of cartilage in weight-bearing regions is the prelude to fibrillation, thinning, and ensuing degenerative arthritis.** This seems completely logical, as the coarse, widely spaced fibrils oriented principally vertically in deeper layers are poorly suited to constraining the swelling forces generated by the matrix proteoglycans. The term "fibrillation" describes the tendency of these fibrils to be split vertically all the way to their subchondral attachment, much as wood splits along the grain of its fibers. The villuslike strands are prone to tear off at the base when mechanically loaded and exposed to shear stresses. It is clear that the "armor plate" term applied well to the normal surface mat of collagen fibrils, but that loss of this layer no longer permits the cartilage to function as a pressurized unit suited to weight bearing.

Evidence of the fibril pattern of collagen derives from several types of observation, including routine histology, transmission electron microscopy, scanning electron microscopy, and the demonstration of Hultkranz lines.[50] The latter are typically observed on the surface of cartilage and are analogous to the Langer's lines of skin.[56] The Hultkranz lines become visible when the surface of cartilage is pricked with a pin that is circular in cross-section. The defect so created is emphasized by coating the cartilage with India ink and then wiping it dry. Hultkranz noted many years ago that the puncture holes appeared as slits rather than round holes. Furthermore, the slits have an axis that is generally perpendicular to the principal axis of movement of the joint. Hultkranz lines are therefore different for each joint of the body. Mechanical tensile tests have shown that the Hultkranz lines indicate the preferred orientation of the collagen fibrils at the surface of the joint, because the specimens are found to be strongest when the long axis of the specimen is parallel to the Hultkranz lines. Bullough and Goodfellow[23] have shown this characteristic of joint surfaces very elegantly. Electron microscopy has also been used to show a preferred orientation of these fibrils at the surface and to characterize the dimensions of the fibrils at different depths from the surface.[23,122]

Routine histology does not show the collagen fibrils of cartilage well, because they tend to be masked by the abundant proteoglycan that is intertwined within the fibril network. Proteoglycan contains dense electronegative charges that are responsible for many of the observed staining characteristics of cartilage, such as metachromasia. However, the collagen fibril pattern can be inferred by viewing sections with polarized light, since a fibrillar pattern of preferred orientation will alter the polarized light characteristically. A key paper by Bullough and Goodfellow on cartilage fibril patterns describes the interpretation of this type of photomicrograph.[23]

Collagen chemistry

Collagen is the key protein for the achievement of stability of the musculoskeletal system. It provides the mechanical properties that impart the "connect" function to connective tissue. It constitutes 65% to 80% of the mass by dry weight of such specialized connective tissues as tendon, ligament, skin, and joint capsule, as well as cartilage.

The key to the tensile force–resisting properties of cartilage derives from the precise molecular configuration of the collagen molecules. This molecule is one of the largest in the body, forming a rod-like structure whose dimensions are 300 nm in length and 1.5 nm in diameter. These rods are termed "tropocollagen." They are assembled in a three-dimensional array in the extracellular environment, being somehow influenced by environmental stresses and additional biologic factors, the details of whose nature are as yet unclear. The sum of the extracellular influences somehow affects the orientation and size of fibrils that are assembled from the tropocollagen units. The assembly is typically patterned in a quarter stagger (Fig. 1-4), which is seen as a 64 nm subbonding on transmission electron micrographs. A small gap that exists between the head to tail linear assembly of the tropocollagen units may be of functional importance in bone with respect to nucleation of apatite crystals in the process of matrix mineralization of osteoid.[41]

The individual tropocollagen units are made up of three chains that are synthesized independently intracellularly in the manner of other proteins (Fig. 1-4). The length of the messenger RNA molecule required for the synthesis is extraordinary, as each chain contains about 1000 amino acids. Most of the chains (called alpha chains) are precisely ordered with a general sequence of glycine-proline-hydroxyproline, glycine-proline-x-, or glycine-x-proline, where x is another amino acid.[66] The higher percentages of the amino acids glycine, proline, and hydroxyproline are unique to collagen. Glycine is the smallest amino acid and permits the close packing necessary for the assembly of the three alpha chains into tropocollagen. Proline and hydroxyproline are cyclic amino acids whose structure presumably

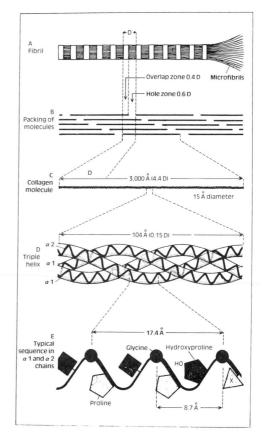

Fig. 1-4 ■ Relationship between single strand protein of alpha chain to triple helix, collagen molecule, and fully developed fibril. The characteristic feature of a collagen molecule is its rigid, very long, narrow, rodlike structure, which is created by tight winding of three alpha chains into a triple helix termed "tropocollagen."

Reprinted, by permission of The New England Journal of Medicine, **301**:13, 1979.

imparts rigidity to the final triple helix configuration. Further details of the collagen molecular arrangements are presented in recent reviews.[55,66,70,79,104] Collagen undergoes numerous modifications following ribosomal assembly that are initiated by intracellular or extracellular enzymes. Examples of these processes include hydroxylation of proline or lysine and glycosylation of lysine. These modifications are termed "secondary features," as distinguished from the direct-coded structure (Fig 1-5).

9

Chapter 1
Cartilage and ligament:
physiology and repair processes

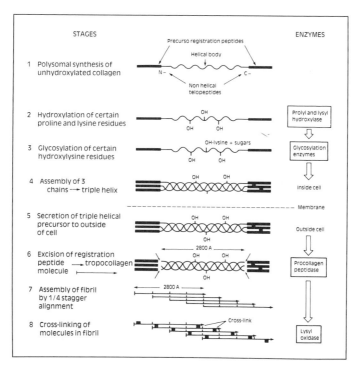

Fig. 1-5 ■ Enzymatic stages in the maturation of collagen. Several enzymatic steps are necessary for creation of the final collagen molecule and its maturation into collagen fibril. These enzymatic steps take place partly within the cell and partly outside the cell. Even those steps which occur inside the cell are posttranslational, that is, they are not directly under genetic control. However, they are very essential for proper development of the final structure. Defects in many steps have been identified in a variety of heritable disorders of connective tissues. Final aggregation of collagen into a structure that becomes cross-linked is essential to produce the requisite tensile stress-resistant properties characteristic of mature connective tissue.
From Levene, C.I.: J. Clin. Pathol. (Suppl.) **12**:82, 1978.

The assembly of the three alpha chains into tropocollagen is facilitated by a group of amino acids at the end of each alpha chain that are called **registration peptides.** The triple helix and its registration peptide are larger than the tropocollagen molecule and is termed "procollagen." Once the assembly of the triple helix is completed, the registration peptides are no longer useful and are cleaved by an enzyme, procollagen peptidase, as the procollagen passes through the cellular membrane into the extracellular space.

The alpha chains are not identical among species or within a single species. Early data on mammalian skin collagen showed two types of alpha chain, $\alpha 1$ and $\alpha 2$, present in a ratio of 2:1. Three types of alpha chains were identified in codfish skin collagen, $\alpha 1$, $\alpha 2$, and $\alpha 3$.[88] Many studies on typing of collagen soon followed. Miller and Matakus[71] were the first to show that cartilage possesses a collagen different in composition from that in most fibrous connective tissue. This collagen contains a different type of $\alpha 1$ chain, which they termed $\alpha 1$, Type II. The collagen in most cartilage consists of three such identical chains, and the abbreviated nomenclature now used is ($\alpha 1$ {II})$_3$, or Type II collagen.

A summary of the makeup and distribution of major collagen types accepted at present is given in Table 1-1. A large num-

Table 1-1 ■ Structurally and genetically distinct collagens

Type	Tissue distribution	Molecular form	Chemical characteristics
I	Bone, tendon, skin, dentin, ligament fascia, artery, and uterus	$\{\alpha 1(1)\}_2 \alpha 2$	Hybrid composed of two kinds of chains; low in hydroxylsine and glycosylated hydroxylsine
II	Hyaline cartilage	$\{\alpha 1(II)\}_3$	Relatively high in hydroxylsine and glycosylated hydroxylsine
III	Skin, artery, and uterus	$\{\alpha 1(III)\}_3$	High in hydroxyproline and low in hydroxylysine; contains interchain disulfide bonds
IV	Basement membranes	$\{\alpha 1(IV)\}_3$	High in hydroxylysine and glycosylated hydroxylysine; may contain large globular regions
V	Basement membranes and perhaps other tissues	αA and αB	Similar to Type IV

ber of "minor" collagens have also been discovered but their functional importance is presently unresolved.[80]

Collagen cross-links. Stabilization of collagen occurs extracellularly after assembly into the quarter stagger arrays that make up filaments, fibrils, and fibers. The stabilization and ultimate tensile strength of the structure are thought to result mainly from the development of intramolecular and intermolecular cross-links. The former occur between alpha chains of the same tropocollagen molecule, the latter between adjacent tropocollagen molecules. The cross-links result from enzyme-mediated reactions involving mainly lysine and hydroxylysine. The lysine and hydroxylysine molecules have secondary amine groups on terminal projections extending laterally from the alpha chain; these are available for cross-linking reaction. The initial reaction in this process is the oxidative deamination of the terminal amine to an aldehyde by the enzyme lysyl oxidase (Fig. 1-6). These reactions have general similarity to the reactions that stabilize elastin. The resulting allysyl residues condense with one another to form an aldol condensation product[89] characteristic of intramolecular cross-links[34,52] (Fig. 1-7). Intermolecular cross-links characteristically form the re-

action of allysine with lysine or hydroxylysine to form a Schiff base (delta semialdehyde) (see Fig. 1-7). These aldolcondensation and Schiff base–reaction products possess double bonds that apparently are reduced to more stable forms in vivo with the passage of time. Most studies on cross-linking of collagen in the past decade have used the presence of the double bond of the unsaturated compound to label the "reducible" cross-links with tritium. Typically this has been done by reducing the aldol condensation product or delta-semialdehyde with tritium-labeled sodium borohydride. The reduced product is thereby labeled with tritium and can be detected following acid hydrolysis and column chromatography using separation systems similar to those used in amino acid analysis. The details of the bifunctional, trifunctional, or quadrifunctional cross-links so detected are beyond the scope of this chapter, but are presented in several reviews.[38,104,106]

The significance of the Type II collagen to cartilage is not yet known. The principal differences between this collagen and the more common Type I found in fibrous connective tissue consist of the number hydroxylysine molecules present and the presence of a small number of residues of cysteine. Table 1-1 summa-

11

Chapter 1
Cartilage and ligament:
physiology and repair processes

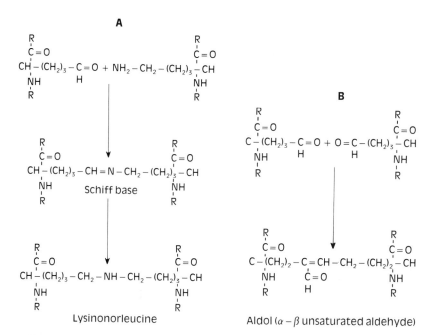

Fig. 1-6 ■ The reaction that precedes formation of collagen cross-links illustrated in Fig. 1-5 is given here in more detail. The enzyme lysyl oxidase is required for cleavage of terminal (secondary) amino group of lysine and formation of an aldehyde. The aldehyde, in turn, reacts with another lysine or lysine-derived aldehyde to form a cross-link. (See Fig. 1-7.)

Fig. 1-7 ■ **A,** Schiff base reaction occurring between lysine-derived aldehyde and unmodified amino group. This reaction is responsible for intermolecular cross-link formation involving either lysine or hydroxylysine. **B,** Aldol condensation reaction involving lysine-derived aldehydes located near N-terminal of molecule. This aldol condensation is responsible for formation of intramolecular cross-link.

rizes the principal differences between Type I and Type II collagen.

The fundamental process of formation of collagen by the chondroblasts and chondrocytes is apparently nearly identical to the process of synthesis by the fibroblast and fibrocyte. The steps in synthesis are outlined in Fig. 1-5. The several post-translational transformations are notable. The collagen turnover in cartilage proceeds at a rate not unlike that seen in connective tissue of the fibrous type. Since significant synthesis occurs in adult cartilage, it is clear that control processes for spatial orientation of the product are crucial.

It is notable that attempts to achieve cartilage repair, as in surgical arthroplasty, are seldom completely satisfactory clinically. This is probably because the collagen architecture of the arthroplasty surface is disordered, and the surface of the arthroplasty lacks the membranelike characteristics of the surface layer of articular cartilage. Details of the repair process are described later in this chapter.

Proteoglycans. The proteoglycans of articular cartilage serve as the "pump" of the highly pressurized cartilage system.

The characteristics of the proteoglycan molecules that permit this crucial function include their very large size and hence their immobility within the collagen fibril meshwork, their densely concentrated, fixed negative charges, and their large number of hydroxyl groups. These characteristics collectively serve to attract water and small ions into the cartilage. The sum of this attraction is termed "swelling pressure" and consists of osmotic forces, ionic forces, and Donnan forces. The purpose of this section is to briefly describe the chemical structure of the functionally vital proteoglycan and its aggregate and to illustrate the manner in which the functional role derives from the chemical structure.

The extraordinary size of the proteoglycan aggregate molecules of articular cartilage is achieved by supraassembly of

these different types of linear chain molecular species: (1) sulfated glycosaminoglycans, (2) the core protein, and (3) hyaluronic acid, a nonsulfated proteoglycan.

Glycosaminoglycans. The terminology for the glycosaminoglycans has undergone complete change in recent years. A review of the modifications in terminology is offered in a recent review by Mathews.[67] The earlier term applied to this group of molecules was "acid mucopolysaccharides." The more precise chemical term "glycosaminoglycans" has been accepted as preferable, although references are still occasionally found to the older term. Furthermore, there is not complete unanimity with respect to this terminology, and the term "polyanionic glycans" is also applied to these molecules.[19] The "acid" part of the earlier term refers to the large number of carboxyl and sulfate groups, which possess negative charges and confer many predictable characteristics in chemical and staining reactions to the tissue. The prefix "muco-" refers to the gross physical characteristics of this molecular class, members of which are typically quite viscous and gel-like. Finally, the "polysaccharide" part of the term refers to the chemical structure of the molecule. It is made of many hexose units assembled linearly into long chains in a manner roughly analogous to the assembly of glucose into glycogen, but in this case the chains are unbranched.

The glycosaminoglycans are covalently bound to core protein in a pattern that locates keratan sulfate side arms preferentially close to the linkage region to hyaluronate. Therefore a keratan sulfate–rich region exists in the protein polysaccharide, as illustrated in Fig. 1-8, which therefore contains little chondroitin sulfate. The keratan sulfate molecules are characteristically of lower molecular weight than the chondroitin sulfate chains, as indicated by diagrammatic representation Fig. 1-8.

Proteoglycan aggregate. The ability of proteoglycan to aggregate further by com-

13

Chapter 1
Cartilage and ligament:
physiology and repair processes

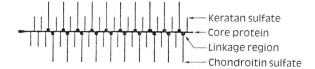

Fig. 1-8 ■ Proteoglycan. This diagram of a proteoglycan molecule demonstrates the method of aggregation of chondroitin-4-sulfate, chondroitin-6-sulfate, and keratan sulfate to core protein. Linkage regions indicated are composed of highly specific molecular configurations (see text). The attachment site of core protein to hyaluronic acid, at which an aggregate is created, is seen at far left of diagram. There is typically a high concentration of keratan sulfate, a shorter-chain glycosaminoglycan, near the attachment site of core protein to hyaluronic acid, symbolized by shorter side arms in that location.

From Rosenberg, L.: Structure of cartilage proteoglycan. In Simon, W.H., ed.: The human joint in health and disease, Philadelphia, 1978, University of Pennsylvania Press.

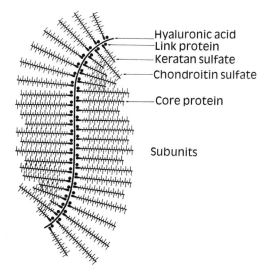

Fig. 1-9 ■ Pattern of aggregate formed by a complex of proteoglycan and hyaluronic acid. The aggregate is stabilized in part by a glycopeptide called link protein at the junction site. The spectacular augmentation in molecular weight of approximately 50,000 daltons to that of proteoglycan, reaching millions of daltons, and the further increase to a structure with molecular weight of many millions of daltons by aggregate formation with hyaluronic acid, are well illustrated by this diagram.

From Rosenberg, L.: Structure of cartilage proteoglycan. In Simon, W.H., ed.: The human joint in health and disease, Philadelphia, 1978, University of Pennsylvania Press.

bining with hyaluronic acid was described by Hardingham and Muir[45], who elaborated on the dissociation and association experiments of Sajdera and Hascall[100] to establish the mechanism of formation of aggregate (Fig. 1-9). It has since been demonstrated that the formation of proteoglycan aggregate is facilitated and stabilized by a small protein termed "link protein."[43,47,49] Much attention has been given recently to the degree of proteoglycan aggregate formation in various tissues and in various pathologic conditions. Clearly, the ability of the proteoglycan molecule to form aggregates of even greater molecular size amplifies its physiologic functional properties as the "pump" of the system. This is true because the aggregate formed will create even greater fixation of the proteoglycan molecules, locking them more securely within the interstices of the collagen framework of the tissue, ensuring fixation of the negative charges and assuring the cartilage of an adequate swelling pressure to maintain expansion of that matrix.

Nature of aggregate linkage. As distinguished from the covalent linkage of glycosaminoglycans to core protein in proteoglycan subunit (PGS), the linkage of PGS to hyaluronate is noncovalent. The linkage is facilitated and strengthened by a low molecular weight protein termed "link protein." The linkage can occur without the presence of link protein, but the latter has been found in all cartilages so far examined.[97] The noncovalent linkage of PGS and hyaluronate can be dissociated by concentrated solutions of guanidinium hydrochloride, calcium chloride, or magnesium chloride.[100] The dissociated components can be reassociated by the reduction of the concentration of the dissociative solvents. This process has been the key technique in unraveling the chemical structure of PGS and aggregate and in understanding the nature of their association as well as the role of link protein. Recently it has been shown that link protein consists of more than one molecular species.[105] Two link proteins that differ in molecular weight and chemical composition have been characterized. Under denaturing conditions, the molecular weights of the link proteins were found to be 44,000 and 48,000 daltons, based on the determinations by sodium dodecyl sulfate polyacrylamide gel electrophoresis (SDS-PAGE). The major structural difference between the two forms of link proteins is in their carbohydrate content and oligosaccharide structure.

Articular cartilage interstitial fluid

As noted in the air tent analogy described earlier, the inflation medium of articular cartilage is synovial fluid. This is essentially an ultrafiltrate of plasma along with hyaluronic acid. Hyaluronic acid molecules are too large to enter cartilage through its 6 nm diameter surface pores, but most of the remaining ions and molecules of normal synovial fluid, such as water, sodium, potassium, and glucose, are sufficiently small to pass easily through these pores. Movement of fluid into and out of cartilage occurs to some extent by diffusion, but as will be noted in the discussion on cartilage nutrition, diffusion does not seem adequate in and of itself to provide for cartilage health. Most of the fluid of articular cartilage is water, of course. The percentage of water in cartilage ranges from over 60% to nearly 80%[30,63] The water is bound by a variety of weak forces, such as hydrogen bonding to proteoglycan and collagen or simple hydration shell formation, but it is sufficiently mobile that clearance studies indicate essential equivalence in behavior between labeled water and urea.[51] Urea is uncharged and not subject to hydrogen bonding, so the equivalence of movement of water and urea molecules suggests that the binding forces holding water are extremely weak and that molecular exchange occurs readily.

Mankin and Thrasher[63] performed additional experiments that appeared to demonstrate that a small fraction, about 6%, of the water of articular cartilage is not easily exchangeable. After equilibration with tritiated water for 20 days then drying with mild to severe methods, a small percentage of water remained in cartilage. Net flow into and out of cartilage is induced by the normal weight-bearing function of synovial joints. Maroudas[64] has calculated that, for normal articular cartilage the sum of swelling pressures is greatly exceeded (10 times) by loading conditions such as walking. The implication of this fact would seem to be that cartilage would be rapidly and completely compressed under loading conditions, much as a wet sponge is compressed by a weight. However, the rate of fluid movement permitted by the small surface-pore size and the cartilage microarchitecture is sufficiently slow that cartilage is only partially compressed even after loading for hours. The elegant experiments of Linn and Sokoloff illustrate this point well.[59] Subsequent experiments by Linn using an animal joint demonstrated the processes of fluid movement in cartilage more directly.[58] The device constructed for this experiment was termed an "arthrotrypsometer" (Fig. 1-10). By developing the necessary design criteria, it was possible to vary loading conditions as to amplitude of load and stationary vs. cyclic conditions. The joint was immersed in synovial fluid during testing. Deformation vs. time is seen to be greater for stationary than for

15

Chapter 1
Cartilage and ligament:
physiology and repair processes

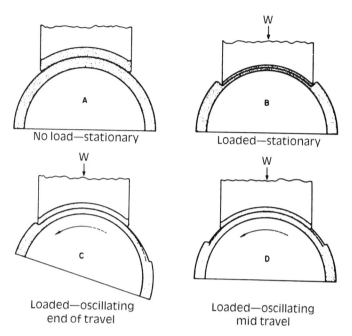

Fig. 1-10 ■ The effect of loading an articular cartilage. A stationary load, as illustrated in example *B,* shows significant cartilage compression after a period of time. However, when oscillation occurs using the same loading condition, the compressive effect for a given time is considerably less. Since cartilage is unloaded a portion of the time, it resorbs some of the fluid that had been expressed during loading.
From Linn, F.C.: J. Bone Joint Surg. **49A:**1079, 1967.

cyclic loads. The explanation for this observation is that in the cyclic condition, partial recovery occurs because of swelling pressure in pulling fluid back into cartilage during the phase of the cycle when the cartilage is unloaded. This unparalleled system of load bearing by articular cartilage is dependent for its effectiveness on functional integrity and detailed interaction of each of the architectural, biomechanical, and biochemical elements within the system.

The fluid movement that occurs during the loading process described appears to be important for lubrication of the joint surfaces as well as for load carriage. On the basis of calculations obtained from complex mathematical models, Mow has proposed that fluid is expressed out of cartilage in front of the advancing contact surface of cartilage.[72] This process provides a fluid film that minimizes cartilage-to-cartilage contact, thus also minimizing wear. Indeed, if this analysis is correct, then humans walk on water!

Nutrition

Fluid movement is necessary not only for load carriage and lubrication but also for nutrition of the chondrocytes. Students of articular cartilage generally agree that in the adult very little of the chondrocytic nutritional requirement is satisfied from subchondral vessels of bone. Rather, cartilage nutrition is derived almost entirely from synovial fluid.[61] The pumping action of fluid into and out of cartilage during loading and unloading appears to be a key to this process. Joints that are immobilized suffer relatively quickly in a number of important respects. The metabolic activity of cells appears affected, as a loss of proteoglycan and an increase in water content are soon observed.[4] The normal white, glistening appearance of the cartilage changes to a dull, bluish color, and the cartilage thickness is reduced. How much of this process is caused by nutritional deficiency and how much by an upset in the stress-dependent metabolic homeostasis is not yet clear. The process is of sufficient significance, in any case, that it adds weight to the arguments for early mobilization of injured extremities.

Articular cartilage metabolism

It should come as no surprise that this highly specialized, functionally complex tissue should be active metabolically. The specialized functional structures of cartilage, the collagen fabric and the proteoglycan pump, require constant maintenance and renewal. The protein synthesis necessary to maintain these elements requires much the same complex synthetic apparatus as that present in other cells of the body. Indeed, one is struck more by the metabolic similarities than the dissimilarities of chondrocytes as compared with other mammalian cell types.

However, early anatomists and physiologists tended toward the view that articular cartilage had an insignificant metabolic rate. This was reinforced by histologic studies showing the avascular nature of the tissue and its sparse cellular population. In addition, early metabolic experiments seemed to support this concept.[25] However, corrections for cell density expressing metabolic activity in relation to cellular volume altered that perception.[98] By most measures of cellular activity, cartilage cells are nearly equally active metabolically to other cell types from relatively avascular tissue sources.[62]

Some distinctive metabolic features of chrondocytes can be discerned with modern metabolic pathway analysis. Chondrocytes use anaerobic pathways for the most part,[25,117] a choice well suited to the relative isolation of the cells, their lack of cell-to-cell contact, and their remote situation from capillary beds. Mankin and co-workers[62] used autoradiographic techniques to demonstrate that ^{3}H-cytidine is incorporated into cells and that the messenger RNA inhibitor actinomycin D inhibited this incorporation dramatically. This evidence was adduced to show another similarity of chondrocytes to the general pattern of mammalian cellular metabolism.

Proteoglycan aggregation and collagen cross-linking both occur outside the cell. In this respect the chondrocyte is able to avoid a very troublesome problem, that of exporting and properly locating molecules much too large to diffuse through cartilage matrix. As it is, proteoglycan and procollagen are among the largest molecules mammalian cells are called on to synthesize. Each chain of procollagen has over 1000 amino acids, for example. The messenger RNA is therefore necessarily one of the largest in the cellular protein synthetic apparatus. The schemata for synthesis of collagen and proteoglycan are summarized in Fig. 1-5 and Fig. 1-11. Each of these pathways is intricate. The general mode of synthesis for the proteoglycans involves primary formation of the protein core followed by addition of polysaccharide elements. This is thought to result from a stepwise glycosyl transfer from nucleotide sugars, beginning with transfer to a specific monosaccharide, xylose, to a specific amino acid sequence of the protein. Usually this sequence includes serine or threonine. Chain growth of the polysaccharide then occurs through a series of glycosyl transfer steps in which sugars are transferred to the nonreducing terminal monosaccharide of the lengthening polysaccharide side chain. Studies of the subcellular localization of biosynthesis of cartilage proteoglycans show that the enzymes catalyzing the transfer of the three sugars adjacent to the carbohydrate-protein linkage are found in highest concentration in the rough endoplasmic reticulum. Polymerizing enzymes necessary for the formation of disaccharide-repeating units are more uniformly distributed between rough and and smooth subcellular membrane fractions. It is as yet uncertain

17

Chapter 1
Cartilage and ligament:
physiology and repair processes

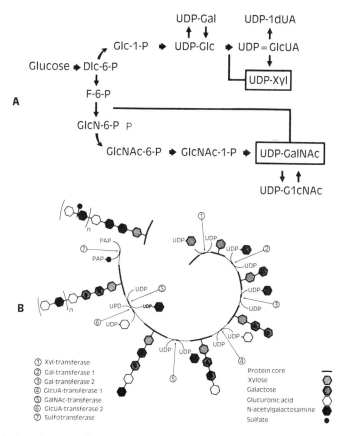

Fig. 1-11 ■ Proteoglycan synthesis. **A,** Pathways taken by uridine nucleotide sugars involved in mucopolysaccharide synthesis. **B,** Pathway of biosynthesis of a typical glycosaminoglycan, chondroitin-4-sulfate.

From Dorfman A., Matlon, R.: The mucopolysaccharidoses. In Stanbury, J.B., et al.: The metabolic basis of inherited disease, ed. 3, New York, 1972, McGraw-Hill Book Co.

whether the monosaccharide transfers occur exclusively one by one to the growing polysaccharide chain or whether part of the process might take place by assembly of an oligosaccharide chain on a lipid intermediate before transfer to the proteoglycan molecule in a manner analogous to certain synthetic steps that occur in glycoprotein synthesis. It is clear that the enzymes involved in these steps are highly specific. For example, the steps involved in the assembly of chondroitin sulfate shown in Fig. 1-11 require six specific enzymes. Further details of collagen and proteoglycan synthesis are beyond the scope of this chapter, and the interested reader is referred to more detailed reviews on the subject.[75,90,91,95]

Repair

Considering the anatomic, biochemical, and biophysical complexity of articular cartilage, it comes as no surprise that attempts at repair are frustrated. A cellular response is observed after partial thickness defects are created, but complete restitution of the surface does not follow. Typically cartilage cells form clusters, called clones, that metabolize collagen and proteoglycan at a more rapid rate than normal. However, the products of synthesis are not assembled into the fabric and ground substance of normal cartilage matrix. Rather, they diffuse away, leaving a matrix that is mechanically soft, highly hydrated (swollen), and deficient in the proteoglycans required to maintain fixed charge density—one of the keys to normal cartilage function.

Likewise, full-thickness defects do not heal effectively. Several yeas ago, we demonstrated in a cup arthroplasty model the sequence of events of repair. Exposure of primitive marrow elements by removal of cartilage and the subchondral plate allows the proliferation of a soft vascular surface covering, which matures into a coarse fibrous structure and gradually undergoes metaplasia to fibrocartilage. It is not usually possible for the entire surface to survive because of mechanical factors that place the soft, early cellular response at risk. Incomplete healing was characteristic of the animal models[5] and was also commonly observed after cup arthroplasty in humans in the decades before total hip replacement.

Similarly, craterlike defects of articular cartilage do not undergo satisfactory spontaneous healing. Large animal studies have shown limits to the size of defects that can be expected to heal. In femoral condyles of horses $\frac{1}{8}$-inch drill-holes were observed to heal effectively; whether this was by cellular response or by collapse of the drill-hole walls toward the defect could not be clearly ascertained.[28] Salter and colleagues have shown effective healing responses of similar sized defects in small animals, and the healing response was facilitated by continuous passive motion (CPM).[102]

However, defects greater than $\frac{1}{8}$ inch are beyond the capacity of effective response by the cells of the subchondral bone. Larger defects become partially filled with fibrocartilage, but the response never reaches the normal joint surface and does not articulate with the opposing cartilage. There appear to be limits in terms of absolute defect geometry that can be met by the healing response of subchondral bone cells. One has reason for optimism about repair potential of fracture lines through cartilage, so long as congruity of joint surfaces are restored and the defect is less than $\frac{1}{8}$ inch. How-

ever, the typical defect seen in osteochondritis dissecans will not fill in to the extent required for a stable joint interface.

The marvel of articular cartilage function and durability can be understood by the analysis of its complex form and composition. However, it is the complexity of this form and function that defeats biologic attempts at repair. The biologic response takes the form of scar; a random, coarse fibrous response not suited to load bearing. It seems unlikely that biologic keys will be found soon to alter this response. **It is therefore incumbent on the orthopaedist to preserve cartilage at all costs.** It is a precious, unique, and so far irreplaceable tissue.

■ LIGAMENT FORM, COMPOSITION, AND FUNCTION

One of the greatest challenges to modern orthopaedic surgery is the problem of ligament healing, and of the innumerable ligaments susceptible to common injury, those of the knee dominate most discussion of healing deficiency. To be sure, each synovial joint has a pattern of ligament injuries and occasional joint instabilities secondary to incomplete healing or residual ligament laxity. However, the impact of disability from ligament injury in individuals of all age groups most frequently affects the knee. The wide range of motion of the knee, its lack of osseous stability, and its weight-bearing function provide the need for ligament integrity for most ambulatory activities. Many key questions remain to be answered about knee ligament disability, not the least of which are elementary questions of natural history following ligament injury resulting in instability. The combined approach of basic and clinical sciences using multidisciplinary techniques will hopefully answer these questions in the next decade. The following review briefly summarizes the basic information accumulated on normal ligament properties and ligament healing.

Morphology

Grossly, ligaments belong to a family of dense regular connective tissues (including tendons, fasciae, and aponeuroses) with closely packed parallel collagenous bundles that have a characteristic shining white appearance.[20] Microscopically, these tissues contain a meshwork of interlacing fibers, flattened cells, and ground substance (including water). Polarized light and specialized stains have been used to differentiate and isolate the fibrous elements (collagen, elastin, and reticulin) and to distinguish ground substance and fibroblasts in the interfibrillar spaces (Fig. 1-12).

Ultrastructural methods have been used to define detailed hierarchies of arrangement down to microfibril size in tendons.[14] Presumably, similar arrangements are present in ligaments. Fasciae and aponeuroses are arranged regularly in multi-

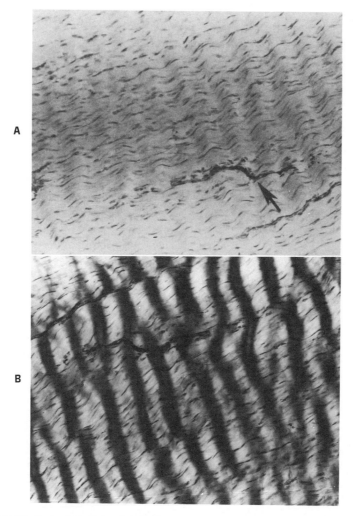

Fig. 1-12 ■ **A,** Normal medial collateral ligament injected with India ink. Note longitudinal orientation of matrix and infrequent vessels *(arrow)* seen under low power magnification. **B,** Section of normal medial collateral ligament under polarizing light demonstrates undulating pattern of matrix (crimp).

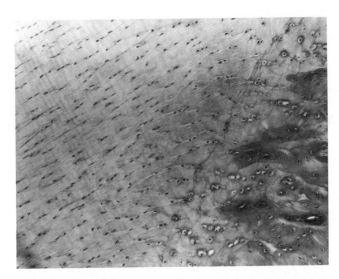

Fig. 1-13 ■ Insertion of normal anterior cruciate ligament demonstrates progression from normal ligament *(left)* through fibrocartilage and mineralized fibrocartilage to bone *(right)*. Note line separating fibrocartilage and mineralized fibrocartilage passing obliquely through this specimen *(arrow)*.

ple sheets, or lamellae, which may or may not have similar orientation. Tendons and ligaments, on the other hand, are regularly arranged, with bundles of fibers oriented in the direction of "functional need."

Insertions

The insertions of ligaments and tendons progress from fibril to fibrocartilage (usually less than 0.6 mm) to mineralized fibrocartilage (less than 0.4 mm) and finally to bone[29,57] (Fig. 1-13). Transmission electron microscopy shows two types of collagen fiber insertions into bone. The more common type crosses the mineralization front described, and the second, less common type inserts directly into bone in relation to the periosteum.[29,57,81] Combinations of these insertion patterns serve to dissipate force and minimize insertional failures. Mechanical loading within the functional range is important in maintaining the functional integrity of the insertion sites.[82,108]

Blood supply

Ligaments normally receive blood vessels from periarticular arterial plexuses,

from which numerous offsets also supply synovium and loose areolar tissue in the region. Intraligamentous vessels are relatively sparse, implying that at least some degree of diffusion is necessary for midsubstance cellular nutrition. Insertion sites are nearly avascular in a number of ligaments, and tenuous vascular connections are easily damaged.[84] Lymphatic vessels form a plexus in the subintima of the synovium and drain along blood vessels to regional lymph nodes.[120] The details of blood supply to each joint, however, are both complex and variable and must be studied individually (e.g., in the knee joint).[103]

Biomechanics

Being a composite material, ligament demonstrates complex static and rheologic behavior similar to that of the other connective tissues.[35,36] When a bone-ligament-bone complex is subjected to tensile testing, a typical load-deformation curve (as shown in Fig. 1-14) is obtained. This curve begins with a concave upward slope (the "toe" region, a region that corresponds to low in vivo forces applied during clinical tests such as the stress test

21

Chapter 1
Cartilage and ligament:
physiology and repair processes

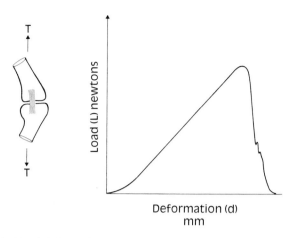

Fig. 1-14 ■ A typical load-deformation curve obtained from tensile testing of a bone-ligament complex.

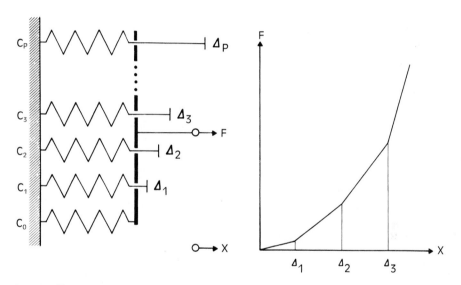

Fig. 1-15 ■ A model of nonlinear elasticity demonstrates different components coming into action at different stages of deformation, resulting in a nonlinear load deformation curve.
Reprinted with permission from *Journal of Biomechanics,* **2,** Frisen, et al.: Rheological analysis of soft collagenous tissue: theoretical considerations. Copyright 1969, Pergamon Press, Ltd.

for ligament laxity). The wavy collagen fibers are straightened as load is applied. With further loading, which corresponds to moderate to high in vivo forces corresponding to strenuous activities (such as sports activities), the slope of the curve increases and becomes linear. The ligament remains elastic. At the higher end of the functional loading region, microfailure of collagen fibers occurs, and with further load application, there is progressive failure of collagen fibers. Eventually, a major-

ity of the collagen fibers are disrupted, and the ligament becomes discontinuous or is pulled out at its insertion site. Large joint displacements occur at this point because the ligaments are no longer capable of their tethering function.

The nonlinearity of the load-deformation curve can be easily demonstrated by means of mechanical analogs (Fig. 1-15). The fibers are represented by a parallel array of springs with different initial

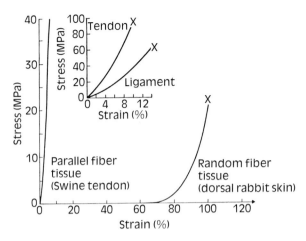

Fig. 1-16 ■ Typical stress-strain curves for various soft tissues showing a wide spectrum of mechanical properties.

lengths. As a ligament is stretched, there is a recruitment process in which the components (springs) are coming into the action at different stages of deformation, thus resulting in nonlinear elastic properties.

The load-deformation curves obtained from tensile testing of the bone-ligament complex represent what we call "structural properties." Structural properties are products of (1) geometric properties, that is, the cross-sectional area, length, and shape, as well as the complex variation of the ligament substance and its insertion to bones, and (2) mechanical (material) properties of the ligament, that is stress-strain curves that are dependent on the organization of collagen fibers as well as on the percentages of its biochemical constituents (i.e., contents of water, collagen, and ground substances). With improved experimental methodology, we are now able to measure the mechanical properties of ligament substance simultaneously with the structural properties of the ligament-bone complex.

Stress-strain curves (mechanical properties) of a wide range of soft tissues—ranging from parallel fibered tissues, such as digital tendons, to random-fibered tissue, such as the dorsal skin of the rabbit—have been obtained (Fig. 1-16). It can

be seen that organization and initial waviness of the collagen fibers contribute significantly to the differences in the mechanical properties of various soft tissues. Even for the parallel-fibered tissues, that is, between ligaments and tendons, we can discern significantly different mechanical properties. However, the overall stiffness characteristics of the densely packed and parallel-fibered ligaments suggest that ligaments are well suited for their functions, that is, offering early and increasing resistance to tensile loading within a relatively narrow range of joint displacement.

It should be noted that the mechanical properties of ligaments are quite sensitive to other factors, such as **age** and **temperature** environment. For example, our laboratory has demonstrated that the mechanical properties of ligament substance of mature animals were superior to those

---

**FACTORS AFFECTING MECHANICAL
PROPERTIES OF LIGAMENTS**

Age
Temperature
Skeletal Maturity
Sex
Body Weight
Local Conditions, e.g., drug administration

23

Chapter 1
Cartilage and ligament:
physiology and repair processes

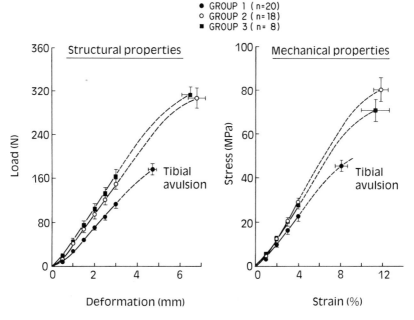

Fig. 1-17 ■ Tensile properties of rabbit medial collateral ligament.

of the immature animals. Also, there are significant differences in the structural properties of the bone-ligament complex between young and mature animals. (Fig. 1-17). It appears that the major changes in these properties occur during the closing of the animals' epiphyses and also at the ligament insertion to bone (Fig. 1-17). Also, we have demonstrated significant changes in tissue behavior with respect to temperature.[127] The tissue, in general, softens with increased temperature in a linear fashion. Recently, we have included lower temperature studies (i.e., from 6° C) and have found a logarithmic relationship between tissue stiffness and temperature. Although peripheral joints are probably maintained near the core temperature under normal circumstances, many alterations in ligament tissue temperature can occur. **Superficial wrapping, heat, or ice,** for example, **may significantly alter joint temperature and therefore the mechanical properties of the ligament.** Similarly, in pathologic conditions such as trauma, infection, or inflammation, joint temperature can be considerably altered,

which alters the knee-ligament biomechanics. Additional variables, including sex, body weight, and local conditions such as drug administration, can also significantly alter the ligament biomechanics and will undoubtedly be evaluated in the future.

Ligaments exhibit significant time- and history-dependent viscoelastic properties. In-depth discussion of viscoelasticity is beyond the scope of this chapter, and interested readers are referred to Woo.[125] However, several behavioral phenomena and the associated terminologies should be introduced here. For example, **hysteresis** is a representation of the different paths of stress-strain curves when a ligament is subjected to a cycle of loading and unloading. The area of hysteresis loop is a measure of loss of energy. Ligaments also **creep** and **stress relax.** When a ligament is subjected to a quick stretch of fixed amount and the stretch is held constant, the corresponding tensile load on the ligament will gradually decrease (stress relax) with time. As shown in Fig. 1-18, the stress relaxation curve of medial collateral ligament is linearly related to the loga-

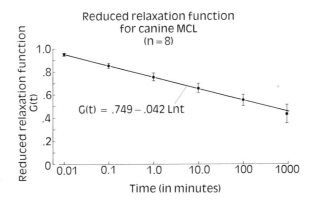

Fig. 1-18 ■ Stress relaxation (decreasing stress with time under constant deformation): a schematic form with typical stress-relaxation curve for medial collateral ligament.
From Woo, S. L-Y., Gomez, M.A., and Akeson, W.H.: J. Biomech. Eng. **103**:293, 1981. Courtesy American Society of Mechanical Engineers.

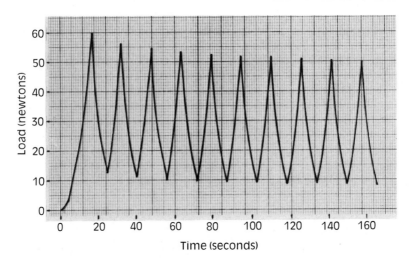

Fig. 1-19 ■ Cyclic loading of medial collateral ligament with strains between 1.6% and 2.4% and strain rate of 0.1% per second. Note decreasing peak loads as cyclic softening occurs.
Reprinted with permission from *Biorheology*, **19**, Woo, S.L-Y.: Mechanical properties of tendons and ligaments. Copyright 1982, Pergamon Press, Ltd.

rithm of time. Stress relaxation of ligaments also exists during cyclic loading and unloading. When a ligament is cycled between two levels of strain, there is stress relaxation both at the peak strain level and at the valley strain level (Fig. 1-19).

Interestingly, there is little strain rate sensitivity for ligaments. One finds practically no difference in the stress-strain behavior of the same ligament tested at three decades using identical same strain

rates (Fig. 1-20). This is in contrast to bone, in which strain rate sensitivity is significant.

The viscoelastic behavior for ligaments, especially cyclic relaxation, can be used to explain in vivo conditions. Clinically, temporary "softening" and increases of excursion in exercised joints have been noted (cyclic relaxation behavior). Further, the differences in strain rate effects on ligaments and bone can be suitably used to clarify the change in failure modes of

29

Chapter 1
Cartilage and ligament:
physiology and repair processes

tion. This results in strain properties that are different than at slow rates. In the latter case, water displacement is greater because force is applied more slowly, therefore allowing greater ligament strain.

Ligament structural-functional relationships

Ligaments function to stabilize joints in concert with architectural features of osseous stability and the kinetic features of musculotendinous stability. In pathologic states of joint instability, the analysis of the defect must obviously include all factors, and frequently a multiplicity of such factors must be recognized and corrected to achieve normal joint function. Neural mechanisms are important in the static-kinetic interplay, and normally these mechanisms protect static stabilizers by superimposing dynamic resistance to displacement forces.

Relationship of structure and function

As with all dynamic physiologic systems, there are functional adaptations to such variables as age, temperature, and sex, even though collagen turnover in ligaments is slow. Extrapolations from animal investigations suggest that **maximal-tensile resistance of ligaments is reached at skeletal maturity, the time of maximal probable need.** Epiphyseal plate closure (the "weak link" in the skeletally immature) and peak physical activity potential at maturity coincide with this event. The mechanism of adaptation may well involve changes in the content and organization of ligament substance secondary to any number of extraligamentous parameters (e.g., sex, hormones, or activity).

The fact that ligaments are dynamic structures requires particular emphasis. Both stress and stress deprivation have been shown to have considerable impact on the structure-function relationship and will be considered in a separate section to follow. This in turn will form the background for a discussion of ligament healing with and without stress application.

Stress and motion effects on ligament

Every change in the form and function of a bone, or of its function alone, is followed by certain definite changes in its internal architecture and equally definite secondary alterations in its mathematic laws.[123]

It is our view that Wolff's law, quoted previously, should not be restricted to bone but should include a more generalized statement of connective tissue adaptation to applied stresses. Wilhelm Roux, a German anatomist and embryologist, may have recognized this deficiency when he published his law of functional adaptation. He stated that "an organ will adapt itself structurally to an alteration, quantitative or qualitative, of function."[99] Unfortunately, his work did not receive widespread recognition in orthopaedic literature. Both Wolff and Roux would probably not be surprised to learn that ligaments are morphologically, biochemically, and biomechanically sensitive to both stress and stress deprivation. This sensitivity appears to fall within a spectrum of situations spanning from stress deprivation (immobilization) to "normal" stress (arbitrarily defined as activities of daily living) to stress application (exercise).

■ STRESS DEPRIVATION (IMMOBILIZATION)
Morphology

The effects of stress deprivation on synovial joints are profound. Intraarticular changes include the following: (1) time-dependent proliferation of fibrofatty synovial connective tissue to the point of

---

**INTRAARTICULAR EFFECTS
OF IMMOBILIZATION**

Proliferation of fatty tissue
Obliteration of joint space
Pressure necrosis of articular cartilage
Extension of marrow space into subchondral plate
Cartilage erosion and ulceration in noncontact areas
Adhesions to articular cartilage
Articular cartilage tears at site of adhesions

obliterating the joint space,[101,107] (2) cartilage necrosis from pressure effects in contact areas,[101,116] (3) breach of the subchondral plate by mesenchymal marrow tissue,[32,33] (4) cartilage erosion and ulceration in noncontact areas,[33] and (5) adhesions with tears of articular cartilage at the point of adhesion attachment.[32,33,44]

Both intraarticular and extraarticular ligaments and periarticular connective tissues are also profoundly affected by immobilization. Gross inspection reveals them to be less glistening in gross appearance and more "woody" on palpation or dissection. Histologically there is a pattern of increased randomness compared with longitudinal sections of controls stained with hematoxylin and eosin. Loss of parallelism of collagen fibers in cruciate ligaments has been observed in an animal model after 9 weeks of immobilization.[3] The pattern of cellular alignment was distorted, presenting a more random matrix organization. Tipton et al.[113] reported that "intercellular collagen fiber bundles" may be decreased in thickness and number as the result of immobilization (atrophy of collagen).

Electron microscopy has confirmed increased cellularity in capsular structures that are stress deprived.[9] This increased population of cells contains increased cytoplasm and prominent secretory endoplasmic reticulum that are consistent with an increased metabolic state. However, metamorphosis of these proliferative cells to so-called myofibroblasts, which are active in the contractile function of granulation tissue, is apparently not a factor in this hypermetabolic contracture process.[37]

Biomechanics

Increased knee joint stiffness after immobilization has been demonstrated using an apparatus called an arthrograph.[128] This apparatus measures the severity of contracture formation in the form of a torque-angular deformation diagram. Quantitative indexes that have been used

during cycling are the amount of torque required to initially extend the knee to a specific joint angle and the area of hysteresis, which measures the energy requirement for bending (Fig. 1-26).

Increases in knee joint stiffness demonstrated by this method have been attributed to a number of changes in the joint tissues (e.g., adhesions, pannus, and decreased lubricity). These changes probably include restricted extensibility of loose periarticular collagen weave by fixed contact at strategic sites. It is hypothesized that newly produced random collagen formation is responsible for these interfibrillar contacts, thus restricting normal fiber sliding and motion (Fig. 1-27).

Ligament substance, however, is uniquely affected by immobility. Rather than becoming relatively more stiff in tension, as may be postulated from increased joint bending energy and tissue "binding," ligaments become less stiff after several weeks of stress deprivation.[81,114, 128] The ultimate load, linear stiffness, and energy-absorbing capacity of a bone–medial collateral ligament–bone preparation are reduced to about one third of normal (Fig. 1-28).

BIOMECHANICAL EFFECTS OF IMMOBILIZATION ON LIGAMENT

↓ Strength
↓ Lineal stiffness
↓ Energy absorbing capacity

To determine whether such quantitative reductions are caused by cross-sectional atrophy[126] and/or alteration in tissue mechanical properties, a specialized video dimensional analyzer system was used to obtain a stress-strain relationship of normal and immobilized lateral collateral ligaments (Fig. 1-29). The diminished slope of the stress-strain curve seen in the immobilized ligaments would suggest some compromise in the mechanical properties of the ligament substance. Despite the

31

Chapter 1
Cartilage and ligament:
physiology and repair processes

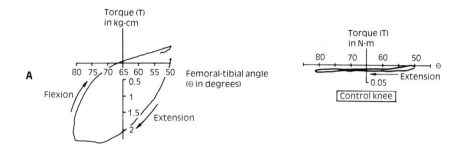

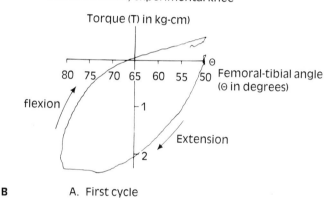

Rabbit No. 32—nine weeks
immobilization, experimental knee

A. First cycle

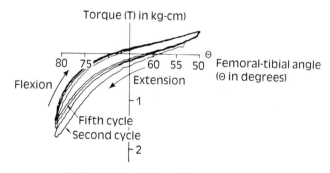

B. Second to fifth cycles

Fig. 1-26 ■ **A,** Diagram comparing typical torque-angular deformation diagram of first cycle of extension-flexion of rabbit knees with 9 weeks of immobilization *(left)* versus contralateral nonimmobilized control *(right)*. Area of each test represents the energy required to bend joint (immobilized joint showing contracture formation). **B,** X-Y recording of torque-angular deformation diagram of experimental contracture rabbit knee showing differences between the first and each successive cycles (energy of bending decreases successively).
From Woo, S.L-Y., et al.: Arthritis Rheum. **18:**257, 1975.

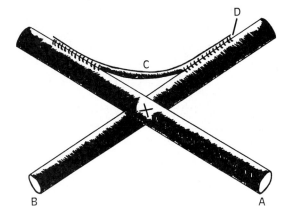

Fig. 1-27 ■ Possible mechanism of intercept binding of two crossing collagen fibrils *(A* and *B)* to newly synthesized fibril *(C)* that is cross-linked at contact points *(D)*.

Reprinted with permission from *Biorheology,* **17,** Akeson, W.H., Amiel, D., and Woo, S.L-Y.: Immobility effects on synovial joints: the pathomechanics of joint contracture. Copyright 1980, Pergamon Press, Ltd.

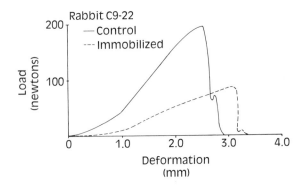

Fig. 1-28 ■ Typical load-deformation curves of lateral collateral ligaments from normal and immobilized knees of the same rabbit.

From Amiel, D., et al.: Acta Orthop. Scand. **53:**325, 1982. © 1982 Munksgaard International Publishers Ltd., Copenhagen, Denmark.

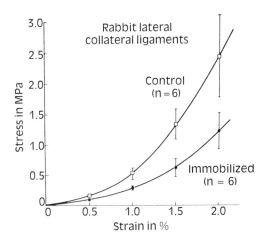

Fig. 1-29 ■ Stress-strain relationship of normal and immobilized rabbit lateral collateral ligaments.

From Amiel, D., et al.: Acta Orthop. Scand. **53:**325, 1982. © 1982 Munksgaard International Publishers Ltd., Copenhagen, Denmark.

33

Chapter 1
Cartilage and ligament:
physiology and repair processes

**MICROSCOPIC EFFECTS OF
IMMOBILIZATION ON LIGAMENT**

Loss of parallelism of collagen fibers
Distorted cellular alignment
Increased randomness of matrix organization

---

possiblity of intercept binding (stiffening) in more randomly distributed and newly produced collagen, qualitative "softening" of the ligament substance predominates.

In addition to these changes in ligament substance compliance, immobilization significantly decreases the strength of the bone-ligament-bone apparatus.[81,82,109-112,114,128] This strength decrease is caused by changes in both the ligament substance itself and its bony insertion sites. After 8 weeks of immobilization in the primate, for example, Noyes and co-workers[81,82] demonstrated that there is a 39% decrease in maximal failure load of the anterior cruciate ligament complex. A portion of these losses was attributed to insertional cortical atrophy with resulting avulsion. Laros et al.[57] documented osteoclastic periosteal resorption around ligament insertion sites and noted that it was anatomically specific (more at tibiofibular insertions than femoral insertions). They speculated that periosteal proximity to in-

sertion sites may partially determine the site specificity of resorption around the ligaments. (The broad tibial insertion of the collateral ligaments is contiguous with periosteum, whereas the femoral insertion is not.) They also showed that even partial immobilization (restricted activity) has similar deleterious effects on insertion sites, raising serious doubt about the validity of using cage activity "controls" in animal model testing.

It is also important to note that recovery of these mechanical alterations after immobilization is a very slow process. **It may take a ligament several months to regain normal compliance and normal tensile failure load after being immobilized for only 8 weeks.**[82] Insertion site recovery may be even slower, consistent with the chronic processes of bone metabolism (Fig. 1-30).[126] More detailed experimental data are required on the recovery process, since the concept has obvious implications for rehabilitation programs and should be placed on a firm scientific foundation.

Biochemical changes

There are a number of significant biochemical changes in periarticular connective tissue consequent to stress deprivation. These include decreased water

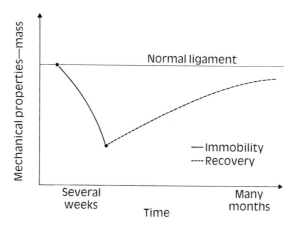

Fig. 1-30 ■ Schematic representation of early degradation in the properties of immobilized ligament, possibly requiring many months for recovery toward normal values.

content,[111,112] decreased total glycosaminoglycans,[2,6] increased collagen turnover,[11,22,86] and parallel increases in certain types of collagen cross-linking associated with increased synthesis.[7]

There is only a small alteration in the total collagen content and no change in the collagen type present in the immobilized tissues.[10,53,114] A qualitative change of collagen is indicated, however, by the dramatic alteration in collagen cross-links, which is consistent with the reduced stiffness observed mechanically. These cross-link changes include significant increases in the reducible intermolecular cross-links DHLNL, HLNL, and HHMD.[7]

To resolve previous debates on the subject, chronic labeling studies have addressed the question of collagen metabolism in stress-deprived connective tissues more specifically.[11,48,53,54] It now appears that immobility causes significantly increased metabolic turnover of collagen with both increased synthesis and degradation.[11] Slightly more degradation, combined with losses of water and GAGs, probably contributes to the decrease in weight-length ratios of the ligaments and to a net decrease in mass.[11,40,111] These changes may well be ligament specific, and it has been suggested that cruciate ligaments are particularly susceptible in this regard.

Duration of immobilization is a significant factor in the magnitude of at least some of these changes. For example, one model has shown no change in ground substance at 6 weeks,[113] whereas significant decreases were noted at 9 weeks in another[2,6] Of course, this may also be a reflection of such variables as species specificity, position of the limb, or rigidity of fixation. It appears that at least 12 weeks of immobility are necessary before the reduction in ligament mass is detectable.[11] Metabolic changes and cross-link alterations probably occur relatively early but require time to become detectable with available techniques.

Recovery from stress deprivation

Diarthrodial joints are profoundly affected by stress deprivation. Although there is variation in tissue response, all tissues of the joint are affected. The ligament complex (bone-ligament-bone) undergoes morphologic, biomechanical, and biochemical changes. Recovery from these changes is slow and presumably is dependent on a number of factors other than reinstitution of exercise (e.g., species, age, sex, specific ligament hormones, and periosteal proximity). Stress deprivation causes both qualitative and quantitative alterations in ligament substance that appear to progress exponentially through the first 12 weeks of immobility, resulting in rapid and severe deterioration in mechanical properties. Recovery from at least some of these effects may be linear; rather than mirroring the extremely rapid onset, recovery is probably prolonged, especially with respect to insertion site integrity.

Ligaments demonstrate a unique response in the process of joint contracture. Although restrictive properties of the contracture itself and certain of the biochemical parameters of the loose periarticular connective tissues may recover in only a few weeks, ligaments are much more chronically affected.[8] Ligament substance properties appear to recover more rapidly than insertion site properties. Joint reconditioning and overall rehabilitation must obviously be planned with these ligament changes in mind.

■ STRESS APPLICATION (EXERCISE)

The effects of exercise on ligaments have only recently been investigated. These investigations have yielded somewhat confusing and apparently contradictory results.* Reasons for discrepancies may include the use of various animal models, inadequate intergroup matching of important variables, different experi-

---

*References 1, 26, 94, 114, 118, 124, 130, and 131.

35

Chapter 1
Cartilage and ligament:
physiology and repair processes

mental procedures, and inconsistent definition of both controls and "exercised" animals. Despite these drawbacks, including inconsistent physiologic proof of exercise effectiveness in other systems (for example, body weights, heart rates, serum cholesterol levels, adipocyte diameters, enzyme activities, and muscle weights[114,118]), a review of results is presented here to summarize the current controversies and thereby provide adequate background for their further investigation.

Morphology

Exercise does not cause persistent gross changes in the appearance of ligament substance itself. There is a suggestion of decreased water content, with a duller appearance and a slight loss of fiber waviness evident acutely after exercise.[121] Increases in ligament mass may occur with certain long-term exercise programs, with increases in both cross-sectional area and weight having been reported.[114] Microscopically, this increased mass has been suggested to be the result of fiber bundle hypertrophy (with increased collagen found between cell bodies) as opposed to cellular hyperplasia.[113,114]

As noted previously, insertions of ligaments are particularly stress sensitive, and morphologic reversal of stress deprivation changes in subperiosteal insertions resulting from exercise have been recognized.[57,81,82] Although these changes are difficult to quantitate and may be specific to individual ligaments, a spectrum of effects paralleling the spectrum of activity from immobilized to exercised can probably be found. The use of cage activity animals as "normal" controls has been questioned,[57,114] particularly in a comparative study with exercise, and must be carefully considered when evaluating previous results.

Biomechanics

According to a number of investigators, several properties of bone-ligament com-

plexes are affected by exercise. These changes must be qualified as either transitory or persistent, with the latter being of primary concern to possible lasting improvement of qualities for clinical purposes. Although not definitely established, it would appear that persistent changes in ligament complexes do occur as a result of exercise. Although the mechanisms of these changes are unknown, either direct stress application to substance or insertions or secondary hormonal and nutritional differences may be responsible.[26,112, 114]

As noted previously, the majority of mechanical tests to failure have been conducted on bone-ligament-bone preparations. Failure strengths therefore are usually an index of the weakest link in that system, and, at low loading rates, most commonly involve the insertions. The absolute separation force[131] of these complexes in various models is usually increased by exercise.*

Such results have been obtained for medial collateral,[109,129] lateral collateral,[131] and anterior cruciate knee preparations.[81,82] Most authors have attributed this improvement to pure insertional change rather than to differences in ligament substance itself. It may be a combined effect, however, as evidence of midsubstance effects of exercise also exists.[26]

Although some investigators have reported elastic stiffness of ligaments to be either significantly increased,[26, 109] or slightly increased [129] as a result of exercise, others have noted the opposite, demonstrating chronically decreased postexercise stiffness (increased compliance)[82,113] (Fig. 1-31). Still others have reported no significant change in stiffness in response to exercise.[21,94] These discrepancies are probably multifactorial and may include evidence that male animals are more affected than females, that certain species are more affected than oth-

---

*References 1, 26, 113, 114, 119, and 130.

Part one
Basic science of
athletic injuries

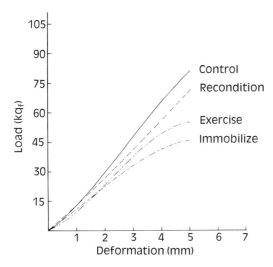

Fig. 1-31 ■ Load-deformation curves of anterior cruciate ligaments subjected to various activity protocols.

From Noyes, F.R., et al.: J. Bone Joint Surg. **56A:**1406, 1974.

ers, and that training protocols are different.[26,94,114]

Exercise recovery from immobilization (reconditioning) must be regarded as a slightly different situation. Exercise effects may be more pronounced and therefore less controversial in aiding the "return toward normal" of biomechanical properties.[82]

Although immobilization effects (predominantly degradative) may be dramatic and exponential with time, exercise effects are probably more gradual in onset and effectiveness in both conditioning and reconditioning situations. Once established, however, both immobilization and exercise effects are probably long lasting.

Biochemical changes

The biochemical changes of ligaments in response to exercise have not been completely elucidated. Collagen content (per unit mass) may be increased,[110] but this has not been a consistent finding. Other studies have noted no change in collagen, water, or glycosaminoglycan content as a result of exercise.[129]

To our knowledge, other biochemical

parameters such as collagen cross-links and collagen metabolism have not yet been studied in exercised ligaments. Collagen turnover in exercised tendons is apparently increased[48]; a similar effect may be expected in ligament, but it remains to be demonstrated.

Systemic biochemical mediation of changing ligament properties has been suggested, with exogenous testosterone and thyroxine in some way increasing ligament complex strength.[26,114] Although these effects may be insertional (on bone), the possibilities of synergistic action of movement and hormonal influence on ligament substance must be considered.[112]

Summary of effects

Ligament complexes seem to be influenced both qualitatively and quantitatively by exercise through mechanisms that are as yet undefined. Changes are subtle, demonstrating minimal gross alteration.

Ligaments increase slightly in mass by fiber bundle hypertrophy, which may be caused by increased collagen production. When compared with normal ligaments, those that have undergone training do not show any other biochemical changes. A ligament recovering from immobilization, however, *does* respond to exercise, probably approaching "normal" biochemical values more quickly than without exercise. At best, however, the recovery is extremely slow by comparison with the rapid onset of stress deprivation effects.

Exercise apparently persistently alters several mechanical properties of bone-ligament bone complexes through action on both bony insertions and ligament substance itself. These alterations are once again more dramatic in postimmobilization recovery of properties than in exercise of "normal" ligaments.

Exercise effects on ligament may be variable, depending on age, sex, species, nutrition, hormones, type of exercise, and perhaps the specific ligament involved. Further elucidation of these and other variables that may mediate exercise phe-

37

Chapter 1
Cartilage and ligament:
physiology and repair processes

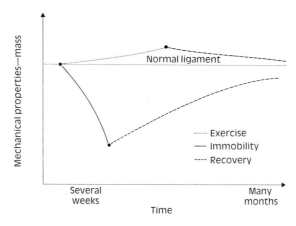

Fig. 1-32 ■ Schematic representation of exercise and immobilization effects and recovery on ligament properties. Note general patterns of deviation from "normal." (Generalization of this formulation remains largely speculative at this time.)

nomena is certainly indicated. If plotted on a time line, the trend of stress- and motion-related soft tissue homeostasis is clearly not a mirror image of that for immobility (Fig. 1-32).

The time necessary for exercise to produce an effect on normal ligament is prolonged. However, it would appear that exercise is beneficial in accelerating the reconditioning of ligaments after stress deprivation. More experimental work is required to determine the parameters of the exercise "dose-response" curve and optimize rehabilitation protocols following ligament injury.

REFERENCES

1. Adams, A.: Effect of exercise upon ligament strength, Res. Q. **37:**163, 1966.
2. Akeson W.H., Amiel, D., and LaViolette, D.: The connective tissue response to immobility: a study of chondroitin-4 and -6 sulfate and dermatan sulfate changes in periarticular connective tissue of control and immobilized knees of dogs, Clin. Orthop. **51:**183, 1967.
3. Akeson, W.H., Amiel D., and Woo, S.L.-Y.: Immobility effects on synovial joints: the pathomechanics of joint contracture, Biorheology **17:**95, 1980.
4. Akeson, W.H., Eichelberger, L., and Roma, M.: Biochemical studies of articular cartilage. II. Values following denervation of an extremity, J. Bone Joint Surg. **40A:**153, 1958.
5. Akeson, W.H., Miyashita, C., Taylor, T. LaViolette, D., and Amiel D.: Experimental arthroplasty of the canine hip: extracellular matrix composition in cup arthroplasty, J. Bone Joint Surg. **51A:**149, 1969.
6. Akeson, W.H. et al.: The connective tissue response to immobility: biochemical changes in periarticular connective tissue of the immobilized rabbit knee, Clin. Orthop. **93:**356, 1973.
7. Akeson, W.H., et al.: Collagen cross-linking alterations in joint contractures: changes in the reducible cross-links in periarticular connective tissue collagen after nine weeks of immobilization, Connect. Tissue Res. **5:**15, 1977.
8. Akeson, W.H., et al.: Rapid recovery from contracture in rabbit hindlimb, Clin. Orthop. **122:**359, 1977.
9. Alm, A., et al.: The anterior cruciate ligaments: a clinical and experimental study on tensile strength, morphology and replacement by patellar ligament, Acta Chir. Scand. (Suppl.) **445:**15, 1974.
10. Amiel, D., et al.: The effect of immobilization on the types of collagen synthesized in periarticular connective tissue, Connect. Tissue Res. **8:**27, 1980.
11. Amiel, D., et al.: The effect of immobilization on collagen turnover in connective tissue: a biochemical-biomechanical correlation, Acta Orthop. Scand. **53:**325, 1982.
12. Amiel, D., et al.: Tendons and ligaments: a morphological and biochemical comparison, J. Orthop. Res. **1:**257, 1984.
13. Asboe-Hansen, G., ed.: Connective tissue in health and disease, Copenhagen, 1954, Munksgaard.
14. Baer, E., et al.: Structure hierarchies in tendon collagen: an interim summary, J. Colston Papers **26:**189, 1975.
15. Bailey, A.J.: The nature of collagen. In Florkin, M., and Stotz, E., eds.: Comprehensive biochemistry, Amsterdam, 1968, Elsevier.

16. Bailey, A.J., Robins, S.P., and Balian, G.: Biological significance of the intermolecular crosslinks of collagen, Nature **251**:105, 1974.

17. Bayles, T.A.: The biology of connective tissue cells. Arthritis and Rheumatism Foundation Conference Series No. 7, New York, 1962, Arthritis and Rheumatism Foundation.

18. Bayliss, M.T., and Venn, M.: Chemistry of human articular cartilage. In Maroudas, A., and Holboro, E.J., eds.: Studies in joint disease. 1, Turnbridge Wells, England, 1980, Pitman Medical Publishing Co., Ltd., p. 2.

19. Benninghoff, A.: Form und Bau der Gelenkknorpel in ihren Beziehungen zur Funktion, Z. Anat. Entwicklungsgesch **76**:43, 1925.

20. Bloom, W., and Fawcett, D.W.: A textbook of histology, ed. 10, Philadelphia, 1975, W.B. Saunders Co.

21. Booth, F., and Tipton, C.M.: Ligamentous strength measurements in prepubescent and pubescent rats, Growth **34**:177, 1970.

22. Brooke, J.S., and Slack, H.G.B.: Metabolism of connective tissue in limb atrophy in the rabbit, Ann. Rheum. Dis. **18**:129, 1959.

23. Bullough, P., and Goodfellow, J.: The significance of the fine structure of articular cartilage, J. Bone Joint Surg. **50B**:852, 1968.

24. Burleigh, P.M.C., and Poole, A.R.: Dynamics of connective tissue macromolecules, New York, 1975, American Elsevier Publishing Co., Inc.

25. Bywaters, E.C.L.: The metabolism of joint tissues, J. Path. Bacteriol. **44**:247, 1937.

26. Cabaud, H.E., et al.: Exercise effects on the strength of the rat anterior cruciate ligament, Am. J. Sports Med. **8**:79, 1980.

27. Clark, W.E.L.: The tissues of the body, ed. 6, Oxford, 1971, Clarendon Press.

28. Convery, F.R., Akeson, W.H., and Keown, G.H.: The repair of large osteochondral defects: an experimental study in horses, Clin. Orthop. **82**:253, 1972.

29. Cooper, R.R., and Misel, S.: Tendon and ligament insertion, J. Bone Joint Surg. **52A**:1, 1970.

30. Eichelberger, L. Akeson, W.H., and Roma, M.: Biochemical studies of articular cartilage. I. Normal Values, J. Bone Joint Surg. **40A:** 142, 1958.

31. Engel, A., and Larsson, T.: Aging of connective and skeletal tissue (symposia 1-3), Solna, Sweden, 1969, Nordiska Bokhandelns.

32. Enneking, W.F., and Horowitz, M.: The intraarticular effects of immobilization on the human knee, J. Bone Joint Surg. **54A**:973, 1972.

33. Evans, E.B., et al.: Experimental immobilization and remobilization of rat knee joints, J. Bone Joint Surg. **42A**:757, 1960.

34. Franzblau, C.: Elastin. In Florkin, M., and Stotz, E.H., eds.: Comprehensive biochemistry, vol. 13, Amsterdam, 1971, Elsevier Publishing Co., p. 659.

35. Fung, Y.C.B.: Elasticity of soft tissues in simple elongation, Am. J. Physiol. **213**:1532, 1967.

36. Fung, Y.C.B.: Biorheology of soft tissues, Biorheology **10**:139, 1973.

37. Gabbiani, G., et al.: Granulation tissue as a contractile organ, J. Exp. Med. **135**:719, 1972.

38. Gallop, P.M., Blumenfeld, O.O., and Seifter, S.: Structure and metabolism of connective tissue proteins, Annu. Rev. Biochem. **41**:617, 1972.

39. Gallop, P.M., et al.: Isolation and identification of α-amino aldehydes in collagen, Biochemistry **7**:2409, 1968.

40. Gelman, R.A., and Blackwell, J.: Interaction between collagen and chondroitin-6-sulfate, Connect. Tissue Res. **2**:31, 1973.

41. Glimcher, M.J., and Krane, S.M.: The organization and structure of bone, and the mechanism of calcification. In Gould, B.S., ed.: Treatise on collagen, vol 2. Biology of Collagen, New York, 1968, Academic Press, p. 67.

42. Grant, M.E., and Prockop, D.J.: The biosynthesis of collagen. I, N. Engl. J. Med. **286**:194, 1972.

43. Gregory, J.D.: Multiple aggregation factors in cartilage proteoglycan, Biochem. J. **133**:383, 1973.

44. Hall, M.C.: Cartilage changes after experimental immobilization of the knee joint of the young rat, J. Bone Joint Surg. **45A**:36, 1963.

45. Hardingham, T.E., and Muir, H.: The specific interaction of hyaluronic acid with cartilage proteoglycans, Biochem. Biophys. Acta. **279**:401, 1972.

46. Harkness, R.D.: Biological functions of collagen, Biol. Rev. **36**:399, 1961.

47. Hascall, V.C., and Sajdera, S.W.: Protein polysaccharide complex from bovine nasal cartilage: the function of glycoprotein in the formation of aggregates, J. Biol. Chem. **244**:2384, 1969.

48. Heikkinen, E., and Vuori, I.: Effect of physical activity on the metabolism of collagen in aged mice, Acta Physiol. Scand. **84**:543, 1972.

49. Heinegaard, D., and Hascall, V.C.: Aggregation of cartilage proteoglycans. III. Characteristics of the proteins isolated from trypsin digests of aggregates, J. Biol. Chem. **249**:4250, 1974.

50. Hultkrantz, W.: Über die Spaltrichtungen der Gelenkknorpel, Verhandlungen der Anatomischen Gesellschaft **12**:248, 1898.

51. Jaffe, F.F., Mankin, H.J., Weiss, C., and Varins, A.: Water binding in the articular cartilage of rabbits, J. Bone Joint Surg. **56A**:1031, 1974.

52. Kang, A.H., and Gross, J.: Relationship between the intra- and intermolecular cross-links of collagen, Proc. Natl. Acad. Sci. USA **67**:1307, 1970.

53. Klein L., Dawson, M.H., and Heiple, K.G.: Turnover of collagen in the adult rat after denervation, J. Bone Joint Surg. **59A**:1065, 1977.

54. Klein, L., et al.: Isotropic evidence for resorption of soft tissues and bone in immobilized dogs, J. Bone Joint Surg. **64A**:225, 1982.

Because of their oblique arrangement, muscle fibers seldom extend for the entire length of the muscle belly. In most muscles the fiber length is less than half the muscle length. The fiber length is an important determinant in the amount of shortening possible in the muscle. **The force produced is proportional to the cross-sectional area and orientation of the muscle fibers.** Simply put, by geometric arrangement some lower extremity muscles are better suited for tension production and others are better suited for larger excursions and faster shortening.[64] The quadriceps group, for example, is better suited for force production than are the hamstrings, although the maximal shortening velocity of the hamstring group should be significantly faster than the quadriceps.

In addition to the skeletal muscle fibers, there is a fibrous connective tissue framework within the muscles. The tendons often are spread out on the surface or within the muscle substance, giving a wide area for attachment of muscle fibers. Connective tissue surrounds the whole muscle (epimysium), the bundles of fibers (perimysium), and the individual fibers themselves (endomysium). This connective tissue framework is continuous within the muscle and attaches into the tendon of insertion. The area of the muscle-tendon junction is a specialized region connecting the fibers into the tendon.

The location at which the motor nerve enters the muscle is called the **motor point.** The nerves then branch multiply to send a motor branch to each muscle fiber. A single motor nerve fiber innervates many muscle fibers. A motor nerve and all the muscle fibers that it innervates is called a **motor unit.** A single alpha motor neuron can innervate from 10 to 2000 muscle fibers, which act together as a functional unit.[18] The nerve fiber approaches the muscle fiber and forms a motor end-plate where the excitation from the nerve passes to the muscle. The motor end-plate has a characteristic location on the muscle fiber at approximately the midpoint of the length of the muscle fiber.

Ultrastructure

The contractile mechanism of muscle has been elucidated over the past 30 years. The orderly striation of muscle fibers seen under the light microscope is a result of the high degree of molecular order in the contractile proteins. The cytoplasm of the syncytial muscle fiber consists of many longitudinally arranged **fibrils.** The fibrils have a prominent period of repetition of several microns (Fig. 2-1). The repeating unit is the **sarcomere.** The banded arrangement is caused by the repetition of dark and light bands (Fig. 2-2). With electron microscopy the dark bands are seen to be made of **thick filaments** with small projections called **cross-bridges** covering the filament except for its center. The primary constituent protein of the thick filaments is **myosin.** Many thick filaments are bound together in a hexagonal arrangement connected along their centers at the M line.

The light band is made up of **thin filaments** and are smaller than the thick filaments. They are made up primarily of **actin,** a protein that forms the bulk of the filament. There are also regulatory proteins, **tropomyosin** and **troponin,** which regulate the process of contraction. With contraction and muscle shortening the light bands get narrower and the dark bands do not change in length.

H.E. Huxley and A.F. Huxley[31] proposed the sliding filament theory to account for muscle shortening. The thin filaments of the I band slide into the thick filament array of the A band. The cross-bridges of the thick filaments provide the force for active shortening (Fig. 2-1). The bridges can attach to the thin filaments, and their angle changes such that the thin filament array is pulled into the thick filament array. Repeated cycles of cross-bridge attachment and release create shortening. The

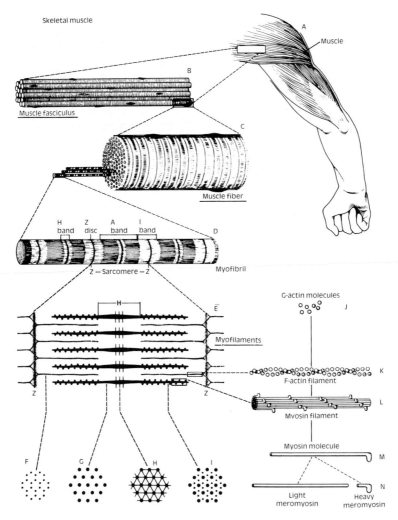

Fig. 2-1 ■ Organization of skeletal muscle shown at gross, microscopic, and molecular levels.
From Bloom, W., and Fawcett, D.W.: A textbook of histology, Philadelphia, 1975, W.B. Saunders
Co., p. 306.

myosin molecule is an enzyme that splits adenosine triphosphate (ATP) to provide the energy for contraction. The polarity of the thick filaments is opposite on either end of the thick filament; therefore, the thin filaments in either half of the A band are pulled toward the center.

The entire process is under the control of calcium, which is stored in membrane-bound areas of the cytoplasm, the sarcoplasmic reticulum. An action potential in the muscle membrane causes calcium release. The calcium binds to the regulatory proteins and allows interaction of the thick and thin filaments, producing force. The calcium is rapidly collected back into the sarcoplasmic reticulum when muscle activation by the nerve ceases and filament interaction ceases.[46]

The proteins discussed here make up the structural elements of the sarcomere. In addition, there are many enzyme systems to supply the contractile proteins with the high-energy compound ATP, which is the immediate source of energy. For the most part, these enzymes are not part of the sarcomere but soluble in the cytoplasm or contained within the mito-

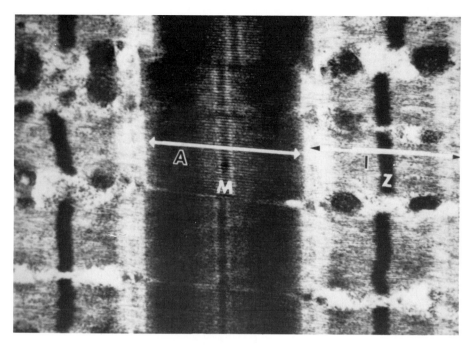

Fig. 2-2 ■ Ultrastructure of sarcomere or repeating unit of skeletal muscle.
From Garrett, W.E., Jr., Mumma, M., and Lucareche, C.L.: Orthop. Clin. North Am. **14**, 1983.

chondria. The oxidative enzyme system is mitochondrial and requires a continuous supply of oxygen for its function. The glycolytic enzymes, on the other hand, can supply ATP in the absence of oxygen, but the efficiency is lower, and metabolic end products such as lactic acid are produced in excess.

Fiber-type differences

Within a muscle the fibers are not all identical. Differences in muscle fiber structure and function have been noted since the time of Ranvier in the nineteenth century. Currently three major classes of fiber type are recognized as being structurally, physiologically, and metabolically distinct.[15] The **Type II** fiber is a physiologically faster fiber than the **Type I** fiber. In response to a motor nerve stimulus, a Type II fiber generates peak tension and falls back to baseline level more quickly than a Type I fiber.

The slower Type I fiber has the advantage of being more resistant to fatigue than the Type II fiber. The Type II fibers are subdivided further. Type II is fast-contracting and subject to fatigue, and Type IIa is intermediate between the Type I and IIb fibers. It is fast-contracting and is also relatively resistant to fatigue.

The fiber types are also distinguishable histochemically. The actomyosin ATP-ase reaction allows identification of all three major fiber types. Histochemical staining for the mitochondrial enzyme systems correlates well with fatigue resistance of the fibers being increased in Types I and IIa. Reactions to the glycolytic enzyme systems are increased in the Type II fibers.

Biochemically the structural proteins in the sarcomere are also distinct. Myosin, tropomyosin, and troponin have distinct structural isomers in the different fiber types.[11,41] The myosin in the fast fibers hydrolyzes ATP at a faster rate that is consistent with its faster speed of shortening. Recent investigations are showing more heterogeneity in the structural pro-

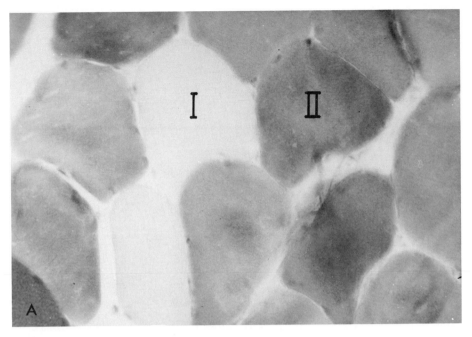

Fig. 2-3 ■ Fiber typing of human skeletal muscle using actomyosin, adenosine-triphosphatase activity.
From Garret, W.E., Jr., Mumma, M., and Lucareche, C.L.: Orthop. Clin. North. Am. **14**, 1983.

teins than had been previously expected. Rather than three distinct fiber types, there appears to be a discrete number of basic sets of structural protein isomers for the fast and slow muscles.[8,55]

Histochemical analysis of human muscles shows that there are discrete differences between muscles in regard to the fiber-type composition. Human muscles are made up of *mixtures* of the fiber types (Fig. 2-3). In general, muscles with similar functions have similar fiber types. The tonic or postural muscles are usually situated closer to the skeleton and have more Type I fibers. In contrast, the phasic, or faster-contracting, muscles lie more on the surface and have a higher proportion of Type II fibers.[34] In general, muscles with higher proportions of Type II fibers contract more rapidly than do muscles with predominantly Type I fibers. These findings have implications regarding human muscular performance. People with higher percentages of Type II muscle fibers in the quadriceps are able

to generate *more* knee extensor force than those with fewer Type II fibers.[58a] Similarly, athletes who demonstrate excellence in sprint events have a relatively high percentage of Type II fibers, while elite distance runners have predominantly Type I fibers.[37,54]

■ MUSCLE INJURIES

Muscles can be injured by several different mechanisms with separate pathologic processes. There has not been adequate basic research regarding muscle injury to elucidate the precise changes with injury, and experimental and scientific data regarding prevention and rehabilitation are often lacking. The general types of muscle injuries will be discussed first.

Muscle cramps

Ordinary muscle cramps are common following athletic exercise and are frequent even in healthy young people not involved in athletics. They occur most fre-

thors have proposed that strength imbalance or specific weakness might be a factor related to the pathogenesis of a strain.[9,10,27] Athletes who are conditioned suffer fewer strains than those who are out of condition. Specifically, **strength training** has been proposed as a means of preventing strain.

Training or muscle strengthening certainly increases the contractile power of the muscle-tendon unit. In addition, training is known to increase the strength of ligaments[59] and tendons.[61] Therefore the connective tissue elements within the muscle may also be responsive to conditioning. If the weakest point in the muscle-tendon unit is at the musculotendinous junction, this area may respond to training by becoming stronger just as with the muscle contractile substance, the ligaments, and the tendons.

Activated muscle does not necessarily shorten. Even with maximal effort, muscle may shorten, lengthen, or keep a constant length, depending on the opposing force.

TYPES OF MUSCLE CONTRACTION
- Isometric—constant length
- Isotonic—constant load with change in length
  Eccentric—lengthening
  Concentric—shortening
- Isokinetic—constant speed

Activated muscle that is neither lengthening or shortening is undergoing an **isometric** contraction. If the muscle is shortening the contraction is **concentric;** if it is lengthening because the opposing force exceeds the force of the muscle, the contraction is termed **eccentric.** Eccentric contractions are frequently implicated in muscle strains. Just as eccentric work produces more delayed muscle soreness, it also can produce a strain. Quadriceps or rectus femoris strains are often associated with a fall or forceful landing that causes the knee to bend while the muscle resists the force. Partial tears of the gastrocnemius frequently occur as the plantar-flexed foot with the activated gastrocnemius is forced into dorsiflexion. Similarly, hamstring strains may occur during intense bursts of speed when the hamstring is undergoing its function of decelerating the rapidly extending knee and therefore contracting while being forcefully lengthened. A.V. Hill[28] demonstrated that muscle force increases rapidly following the quick stretch of an activated muscle. This tension increment is soon dissipated, but there is potentially a time when the tension is the muscle-tendon unit approaches the tension necessary to disrupt its weakest link.

The ability of a muscle to generate tension may be related to its propensity to strain. Certainly, the most powerful phasic muscles of the lower extremity are most likely to be strained. Similarly, strains are more common in faster or more "explosive" athletes. The ability of a muscle to generate tension is related to its fiber type. The more phasic muscles have a higher proportion of Type II fiber. Fiber type is variable in individuals. The ability of an individual to generate maximal strength is directly related to the percentage of Type II fibers.[58] **The muscles in the lower extremity that are most subject to strain possess a higher proportion of Type II fibers to other muscles in the lower extremity or even to their protagonists.**[22]

Some consideration should be given to the relationship between muscle strains and flexibility. There is now a widespread belief in the value of flexibility in preventing injury.[17,47,62] However, there are studies showing no relation between muscle tightness and the frequency of injuries.[16,33,36] There is also uncertainty regarding the efficacy of a stretching program in altering flexibility of muscle.

Compartment syndromes

Much interest has been directed to the diagnosis, management, and scientific basis for compartment syndromes in recent years. This syndrome is a pathologic condition of skeletal muscle characterized by increased interstitial pressure within an anatomically confined muscle compartment that interferes with the circulation and function of the muscle and neurovascular components of the compartment. The pressure elevation within the muscle compartment may be caused by many different factors. Most frequently, transient ischemia is the inciting incident, as it causes muscle edema once some circulation is restored. Hemorrhage within the compartment or direct trauma to muscle can also cause pressure elevation or a compartment syndrome. Much of the current emphasis on compartment syndromes is the result of the clinical observation that if the compartment syndromes are recognized the elevated pressure may be relieved (usually by incising the investing fascia), and the circulation and function of the compartment muscle and neurovascular components can be restored.

The pathophysiology of compartment syndrome has been investigated by a number of laboratories.[26] Increased pressure in the compartment results from increased fluid. The fluid increase can come from hemorrhage, intracellular edema, or extracellular edema. The pressure within the compartment can be measured by several techniques including needle manometer,[63] wick catheter,[44] solid-state transducer,[42] and noninvasive auscultation.[65] Threshold pressures above which significant muscle damage can occur have been proposed to be 30 to 40 mm Hg[26] or to within 10 to 30 mm Hg of diastolic blood pressure.[63]

When the intracompartmental pressures reach these elevated levels it is postulated that capillary perfusion is compromised, and the skeletal muscle within the compartment is subject to ischemic injury. The level of pressure necessary to interfere with capillary circulation will not necessarily occlude major arteries running through the compartments; therefore the presence of a pulse distal to the compartment will not rule out the presence of a compartment syndrome. Clinical evaluation relies on pain, increased compartment pressure noted with palpation, and altered nervous function as noted by paresthesias in the sensory distribution of nerves within the compartment. Abnormalities in nerve function with increasing intracompartmental pressure have been demonstrated by Matsen et al.[41a] The introduction of the various objective methods of measuring tissue pressure as described previously have been extensively in clinical situations to increase the reliability of the diagnosis.

Acute compartment syndromes have been associated with a variety of injuries common in athletics.[35] Direct trauma to bone or soft tissue is most frequently noted. A review by Mubarak[44] stresses the association of compartment syndromes and fractures. Tibial shaft fractures make up a large proportion of the fractures leading to compartment syndromes. However, direct soft tissue injury and muscle trauma also can cause elevated pressure and compromise tissue perfusion. The cause of the increased pressure can be edema, hemorrhage, or a combination of the two.

In addition to direct trauma, indirect injury caused by exertion is well recognized as a cause of compartment syndromes. The indirect injuries can be acute or chronic. They have been reviewed well recently by Veith[60] and Mubarak.[44] Though the acute syndromes are not well understood, several factors deserve mention. Intense muscular activity alone causes a large rise in the interstitial pressure, which might prevent normal capillary perfusion. Intermittent pressure levels greater than 100 mm Hg are common during some exercises.[42] Therefore muscle perfusion will be possible only intermittently when the pressure falls between muscular contractions. Increasing exercise causes an increase in muscle volume as large as 20%, which is associated with increased blood content and intracompartmental fluid accumulation. The increased fluid component will likely raise tissue pressure measurements at rest. Therefore the combination of intermittent high pressures associated with muscle activity and elevated rest pressures caused by compartment fluid expansion can predispose an athlete to an acute compartment syndrome.

Acute exertional compartment syndromes are not common.[44] They are usually associated with intense muscular activity, particularly in individuals unaccustomed to such activity, such as military recruits. These syndromes are associated with muscle activity and elevated rest pressure. Compartment fluid expansion can predispose an athlete to an acute compartment syndrome, diagnosed by the same clinical principles noted earlier. Confirmation of compartment pressures

by one of the techniques listed previously is preferable. Treatment also should include decompression of the muscle and neurovascular components by fascial release.

Chronic exertional compartment syndromes are more frequently seen clinically than the acute form and have received considerable attention in the literature recently. The presenting complaint of the patient is usually pain or a deep ache over the anterior or lateral compartments. The discomfort usually occurs after a relatively long exercise period and is usually severe enough to cause the athlete either to rest or to reduce the intensity of the exercise. The symptoms are often bilateral.[52,57] Sensory changes may also be present. Muscle hernias may be present at times near the fascial opening, through which the distal branch of the superficial peroneal nerve passes to reach the subcutaneous tissue.[44]

Chronic or recurrent compartment

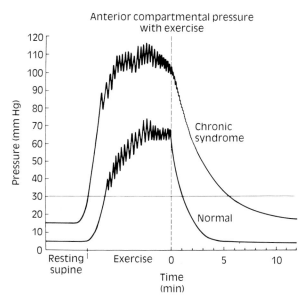

Fig. 2-9 ■ Illustrative anterior compartment pressures recorded in patient with chronic anterior compartment syndrome compared to normal. Note higher resting pressure, higher exercise peak pressure, and slower return to resting pressure in chronic compartment syndrome.
From Mubarak, S.J.: Compartment syndromes and Volkmann's contracture, Philadelphia, 1981, W.B. Saunders Co., 1981.

syndrome is difficult to diagnose clinically. Corroboration with objective pressure measurements is desirable. The resting pressure values may be slightly higher in patients who have the chronic syndrome, as measured by several techniques. However, the primary characteristic distinguishing the chronic condition is pressure elevation above normal at exercise and a slower return to resting values at the end of exercise.[60] These findings have consistently identified the chronic compartment syndromes (Fig. 2-9).

Treatment of chronic or recurrent compartment syndromes has been elective fasciotomy of a single compartment if conservative measures and activity alteration are unsuccessful.[44,60] Postoperative results in a relatively small number of cases have been gratifying subjectively, and pressure measurements have returned toward normal. One should be aware that fascial release adversely affects the strength of a muscle, and therefore this procedure should not be advocated without accurate diagnosis and counseling.[21]

Some mention should be made of the syndrome variously called "shin splints" or "medial tibial syndrome." Previously, this syndrome of exercise-related pain localized to the medial aspect of the distal third of the tibia had been ascribed to a recurrent deep posterior compartment syndrome.[51] However, objective measurement of pressure within the anterior and posterior compartments has not shown any pressure elevation.[12] The entity of "shin splints" or "medial tibial syndrome" is most likely a stress reaction of the bone or muscle origin from the bone in response to repetitive use.

REFERENCES

1. Abraham W.M.: Factors in delayed muscle soreness, Med. Sci. Sports **9**:11, 1977.
2. Almekinders, L.C., Garrett, W.E., and Seaber, A.V.: Histopathology of muscle tears in stretching injuries. Presented at the Orthopaedic Research Society, Atlanta, 1984.
3. Almekinders, L.C., Garrett, W.E., and Seaber, A.V.: Pathophysiologic response to muscle tears in stretching injuries. Presented at the Orthopaedic Research Society, Atlanta, 1984.
4. Apple, D.V., O'Toole, J., and Annis, C.: Professional basketball injuries, Phys. Sports med. **10**(11):81, 1982.
5. Asmussen, E.: Observations on experimental muscular soreness, Acta Rheum. Scand. **2**:109, 1956.
6. Berson, B.L., Rolnick, A.M., Ramos, C.G., and Thornton, J.: An epidemiologic study of squash injuries, Am. J. Sports Med. **9**:103, 1981.
7. Besson, C., Rochcongar, P., Beauverger, Y., Dassonville, J., Aubree, M., and Catheline, M.: Study of the valuations of serum muscular enzymes and myoglobin after maximal exercise test and during the next 24 hours, Eur. J. Applied Physiol. **47**:47, 1981.
7a. Brewer, B.J.: Mechanism of injury to the musculotendinous unit. In Reynolds, F.C., ed.: American Academy of Orthopaedic Surgeons Instructional course lectures, vol. 17, St. Louis, 1960, The C.V. Mosby Co., p. 354.
8. Bronson, D.D., and Schachat, F.H.: Heterogeneity of contractile proteins. J. Biol Chem **257**:3937-3944, 1982. Bryk, E., and Grantham, S.A.: Shin splints: a chronic deep posterior ischemic compartmental syndrome of the leg? Orthop. Rev. **12**(4): 29, 1983.
9. Burkett, L.N.: Causative factors in hamstring strains, Med. Sci. Sports **2**:39, 1970.
10. Christensen, C.S., and Wiseman, D.C.: Strength, the common variable in hamstring strain Athl. Training **7**(2):36, 1971.
11. Cummins, P., and Perry, S.V.: Troponin I from human skeletal and cardiac muscles, Biochem. J. **171**:251, 1978.
12. D'Ambrosia, R.D., Zelis, R.F., Chuinard, R.G. and Wilmore, J.: Interstitial pressure measurements in the anterior and posterior compartments in athletes with shin splints, Am. J. Sports Med. **5**:127, 1977.
13. Denny-Brown, D.: Seminars on neuromuscular physiology, Am. J. Med. **15**:368, 1953.
14. DeVries, H.A.: Quantitative electromyographic investigation of the spasm theory of muscle pain, Am. J. Phys. Med. **45**:119, 1966.
15. Dubowitz, V., and Brooke, M.H.: Muscle biopsy: a modern approach, ed. 2, Philadelphia, 1973, W. B. Saunders Co.
16. Ekstrand, J., and Gillquist, J.: The frequency of muscle thightness and injuries in soccer players, Am. J. Sports Med. **10**:75, 1982.
17. Ekstrand, J., Gillquist, J., and Liljedahl, S.O.: Prevention of soccer injuries: supervision by doctor and physiotherapists, Am. J. Sports Med. **11**:116, 1983.
18. Feinstein, B., Lindegard, B., Nyman, E., and Wohlfart, G.: Morphologic studies of motor units in normal human muscles, Acta Anat. (Basel) **23**:127, 1955.
19. Friden, J., Sjostrom, M., and Ekblom, B.: A morphological study of delayed muscle soreness, Experientia **37**:506, 1981.

20. Friden, J., Sjostrom, M., and Ekblom, B.: Myofibrillar damage following intense eccentric exercise in man, Int. J. Sports Med. **4**:170, 1983.

21. Garfin, S.R., Tipton, C.M., Mubarak, S.J., Woo, S.L.-Y., Hargens, A.R., and Akeson, W.H.: Role of fascia in maintenance of muscle tension and pressure, J Appl. Physiol. **51**:317, 1981.

22. Garrett, W.E., Califf, J.C., and Bassett, F.H.: Histochemical correlates of hamstring injuries, Am. J. Sports Med. **12**:98, 1984.

23. Garrett, W.E., Seaber, A.V., Boswick, J., Urbaniak, J.R., and Goldner, J.L.: The recovery of skeletal muscle following laceration and repair, J. Hand Surg. **9**:683, 1984.

24. Garrick, J.G., and Requa, R.K.: Epidemiology of women's gymnastics injuries, Am. J. Sports Med. **8**:261, 1980.

25. Grana, W.A., and Schelberg-Karnes, E.: How I manage deep muscle bruises, Phys. Sportsmed. **11**(16):123, 1983.

26. Hargens, A.R. and Akeson, W.H.: Pathophysiology of the compartment syndrome, Philadelphia, 1981, W.B. Saunders Co.

27. Heiser, T.M., Weber, J., Sullivan, G., Clare, P., and Jacobs, R.R.: Prophylaxis and management of hamstring muscle injuries in intercollegiate football players, Am. J. Sports Med. **12**:368, 1984.

28. Hill, A.V. First and last experiments in muscle mechanics, New York, 1970, Cambridge University Press.

29. Hough, T.: Ergographic studies in muscular soreness, Am. J. Physiol. **7**:76, 1902.

30. Hughston, J.C., Whatley, G.S., and Stone, M.M.: Myositis ossificans traumatica (myo-osteosis), South. Med. J. **55**:1167, 1962.

31. Huxley, H.E.: The structural basis of muscular contraction, Proc. R. Soc. Lond. [Biol.] **178**:131, 1971.

32. Jackson, D.W., and Feagin, J.A.: Quadriceps contusions in young athletes, J. Bone Joint Surg. **55A**:95, 1973.

33. Jackson, D.W., Jarrett, H., Bailey, D., Kausek, J., Swanson, J., and Powell, J.W.: Injury prediction in the young athlete: a preliminary report, Am. J. Sports Med. **6**:6, 1978.

34. Johnson, M.A., Polgar, J., Weightman D., and Appleton, D.: Data on the distribution of fibre types in thirty-six human muscles: an autopsy study, J. Neurol. Sci. **18**:111, 1973.

35. Kennedy, J.C., and Roth, J.H.: Major tibial compartment syndromes following minor athletic trauma, Am. J. Sports Med. **7**:201, 1979.

36. Kirby, R.L., Simms, F.C., Symington, V.J., and Garner, J.B.: Flexibility and musculoskeletal symptomatology in female gymnasts and age-matched controls, Am. J. Sports Med. **9**:160, 1981.

37. Komi, P.V., Rusko, H., Vos, J., et al.: Anaerobic performance capacity in athletes, Acta Physiol. Scand. **100**:107, 1977.

38. Kraus, H.: The use of surface anesthesia in the treatment of painful motion, JAMA **116**:2582, 1941.

39. Kraus, H.: Evaluation and treatment of muscle function in athletic injury, Am. J. Surg. **98**:353, 1959.

40. Krejci, V., and Koch, P.: Muscle and tendon injuries in athletes, Chicago, 1979, Year Book Medical Publishers.

41. Lowey, S., and Risby, D.: Light chains from fast and slow muscle myosins, Nature **234**:81-85, 1971.

41a. Matseu, F.A., Mayo, K.A., Krugmire, R.B., Sheridan, G.W., and Kraft, G.H.: A model compartmental syndrome in man with particular reference to the quantification of nerve function, J. Bone Joint Surg. **59**:648, 1977.

42. McDermott, A.G.P., Marble, A.E., Yabsley, R.H., and Phillips, B.: Monitoring dynamic anterior compartment pressures during exercise: a new technique using the STIC catheter, Am. J. Sports Med. **10**:83, 1982.

43. McMaster, P.E.: Tendon and muscle ruptures: clinical and experimental studies on the causes and location of subcutaneous ruptures, J. Bone Joint Surg. **15**:705, 1933.

44. Mubarak, S.J.: Etiologies of compartment syndromes. In Mubarak, S.J., and Hargens, A.R., eds.: Compartment syndromes and volkmann's contracture, Philadelphia, 1981, W.B. Saunders Co.

45. Mueller, F.O., and Blyth, C.S.: A survey of 1981 college lacrosse injuries, Phys. Sportsmed. **10**(9): 87, 1982.

46. Murray, J.M., and Weber, A.: The cooperative action of muscle proteins, Sci. Am. **230**:58, 1974.

47. Nicholas, J.A.: Injuries to knee ligaments: relationship to looseness and tightness in football players, JAMA **212**:2236, 1970.

48. Parrow, A., and Samuelsson, S.-M. Use of chloroquine phosephate: a new treatment for spontaneous leg cramps, Acta Med. Scand. **181**:237, 1967.

49. Pritchett, J.W.: High cost of high school football injuries, Am. J. Sports Med. **8**:197, 1980.

50. Prockop, D.J., and Sjoerdsma, A.: Significance of urinary hydroxyproline in man, J. Clin. Invest. **40**:843, 1961.

51. Puranen, J.: The medial tibial syndrome: exercise ischaem in the medial fascial compartment of the leg, J. Bone Joint Surg. **56B**:712, 1974.

52. Reneman, R.S.: The anterior and the lateral compartment syndrome of the leg due to intensive use of muscles, Clin. Orthop. **113**:69, 1975.

53. Ryan, A.J.: Quadriceps strain, rupture, and charlie horse, Med. Sci. Sports **1**:106, 1969.

54. Saltin, B., Henrikson, J., Nygaard, E., et al.: Fiber types and metabolic potentials of skeletal muscles in sedentary man and endurance runners, Ann. N.Y. Acad. Sci. **301**:3, 1977.

55. Schachat, F.H., Bronson, D.D., and McDonald, O.B.: Two kinds of slow skeletal muscle fibers which differ in their myosin light chain complements, FEBS Lett. **122:**80, 1980.

56. Schwane, J.A., Watrous B.G., Johnson, S.R., and Armstrong, R.B.: Is lactic acid related to delayed-onset muscle soreness? Phys. Sportsmed. **11:**124, 1983.

57. Sudmann, E.: The painful chronic anterior lower leg syndrome, Acta Orthop. Scand. **50:**573, 1979.

58. Tesch, P., and Karlsson, J.: Isometric strength performance and muscle fibre type distribution in man, Acta Physiol. Scand. **103:**47, 1978.

58a. Thortenssen, A.: Muscle strength, fibre types and enzyme activities in man, Acta Physiol. Scand., Suppl. 443, 1976.

59. Tipton, C.M., Schild, R.J., and Tomanek, R.J.: Influence of physical activity on the strength of knee ligaments in rats, Am. J. Physiol. **212:**283, 1966.

60. Veith, R.G., Recurrent compartmental syndromes due to intensive use of muscles, In Matsen, F.A., ed.: Compartmental syndromes, New York, 1980, Grune & Stratton, Inc.

61. Viidik, A.: The effect of training on the tensile strength of isolated rabbit tendons, Scand. Plast. Reconstr. Surg. **1:**141, 1967.

62. Wiktorsson-Moller, M., Oberg, B., Ekstrand, J., and Gillquist, J.: Effects of warming up, massage, and stretching on range of motion and muscle strength in the lower extremity, Am. J. Sports Med. **11:**249, 1983.

63. Whitesides, T.E., Haney, T.C., Morimoto, K., and Harada, H.: Tissue pressure measurements as a determinant for the need of fasciotomy, Clin Orthop. **113:**439, 1975.

64. Wickiewicz, T.L., Roy, R.R., Powell, P.L., and Edgerton, V.R.: Muscle architecture of the human lower limb, Clin. Orthop. **179:**275, 1983.

65. Willey, R.F., Corrall, R.J.M., and French, E.B.: Non-invasive method for the measurement of anterior tibial compartment pressure, Lancet March 13, 1982.

chapter 3

Muscle soreness and rhabdomyolysis

Paul Zabetakis

While exercise in the conditioned individual is not generally associated with discomfort, delayed muscle soreness and rhabdomyolysis frequently occur following intense muscular activity. Delayed muscle soreness can appear approximately 24 to 48 hours after strenuous exercise. Both the intensity and duration of exercise as well as the prior conditioning of the individual are factors important to the development of delayed muscle soreness. At least three theories have been proposed to explain this phenomenon. Delayed muscle soreness could be the result of structural muscle damage,[24] overstretching and injury to connective tissue,[30] or muscle spasm.[14] Support for each mechanism can be found in the literature. Under certain experimental conditions, alterations in surface electromyograms as well as elevations in both serum creatine phosphokinase and urinary hydroxyproline levels have been observed and used to support these theories, which will be reviewed here.

Rhabdomyolysis refers to a condition of skeletal muscle injury that permits the liberation of cellular contents into the circulation. Any process that interferes with the delivery, storage, or use of energy substrates to the skeletal muscle cell can result in the disruption of cellular integrity.[27] While Bywaters and Beall[11] were the first in the modern literature to describe the association of crush injuries, myoglobinuria, and renal failure, the earliest reference to the syndrome of rhabdomyolysis can be found in Old Testament Book of Numbers. The Israelites fleeing Egypt feasted on quail, "and the Lord smate the people with a very great plague" (Numbers 11: 33). Based on recent observations, sensitive individuals eating this meat develop painful muscles, paralysis, and myoglobinuria within hours.[35] Many deaths during the Exodus have been thus attributed to rhabdomyolysis following ingestion of quail.

Intense exercise can also be associated with varying degrees of muscle injury, including frank necrosis. Muscle injury in this setting is associated with a disappearance of glycogen stores and a reduction of high-energy adenosine triphosphate (ATP).[8,25] The resulting loss of cellular integrity leads to the release of intracellular

---

THEORETIC ETIOLOGIES OF DELAYED MUSCLE SORENESS

- Structural muscle damage
- Overstretching and connective tissue injury
- Muscle spasm

---

contents, including myoglobin, aldolase, creatine, creatine phosphokinase (CPK), succinic dehydrogenase, serum glutamic oxaloacetic transaminase (SGOT), lactic dehydrogenase (LDH), potassium, and phosphorus. Many such episodes of rhabdomyolysis are subclinical, associated with minor complaints of myalgias and muscle cramps. These episodes are often diagnosed serendipitously from an incidental blood chemistry or urinalysis.[26] Since these data are not routinely obtained, it is difficult to assess the true incidence of rhabdomyolysis. As will be discussed, it is suspected to be much more common than is apparent clinically.

■ DELAYED MUSCLE SORENESS

DeVries[14] in 1966 reported that sore muscles could be distinguished from normal muscles by surface electromyograms. The greater resting activity suggested to DeVries that delayed muscle soreness was caused by muscle spasms within individual muscle units. More recently, Abraham[1] studied three proposed theories on delayed muscle soreness and failed to confirm DeVries' earlier observation. The discrepancy in findings may have been related to a difference in the methods, with bipolar electrodes used by Abraham and a unipolar electrode used by DeVries. Nevertheless, Abraham did observe a delayed rise in urinary hydroxyproline excretion that appeared to correlate with the period of maximal muscle soreness (Fig. 3-1). This finding suggested to the author that injury to connective tissue or increased collagen synthesis best explained the muscle soreness occurring 24 to 48 hours after strenuous exercise.

Structural injury to the muscle has also been proposed as a mechanism for the observed muscle soreness. Abraham[1] discounted this theory based on his observation that urinary myoglobin was in fact elevated in subjects regardless of their perceived muscle soreness. In addition, the peak increase in myoglobinuria did not correlate with the maximal period of muscle soreness. In disagreement with Abraham's conclusion, Tiidus and Ianuzzo[42] observed a correlation between the magnitude of muscle soreness and the increase in muscle enzyme activity. This suggested to the authors that structural muscle damage may be responsible for the muscle soreness. As noted in Fig. 3-2, CPK rose abruptly following exercise, accompanied by a delayed rise in perceived muscle soreness, which peaked at 48 hours. The perception of muscle soreness and changes in muscle enzyme activity (CPK, LDH, and SGOT) rose in parallel as the intensity of duration of exercise was increased. Of the two, high-intensity, short-duration exercise resulted in a greater rise in enzymes and muscle soreness than low-intensity, long-duration exercise (Fig. 3-3). A plot of the change in CPK and the change in pain sensation revealed a linear correlation (Fig. 3-4), supporting the authors' conclusion that exercise-induced muscular damage results in muscle soreness. Armstrong et al.[4] have similarly observed an elevation of muscle enzyme levels following eccentric exercise in rats. Histologic studies by this group and others have in fact demonstrated myofibrillar disruption, invasion of macrophages, inflammation, edema, and myonecrosis in strenuously exercised muscles.[4,18,23] Muscle biopsies in marathon runners following a competition have likewise revealed evidence of myofibrillar lysis, dissolution of mitochondrial cristae, inflammation, and necrosis.[22,39] Recent electron microscopic and immunocytologic studies of muscle biopsies obtained 2 to 3 days after eccentric exercise have demonstrated disruption of the myofibrillar Z bands as well as the desmin filaments of the cytoskeleton.[17,18,19] Despite the immediate rise in muscle enzymes following exercise, these histologic changes were not present in biopsies taken within 1 hour of exercise and were resolved by 6 days after exercise. Hagerman et al.[22] has also observed myonecrosis and disruption of Z band architec-

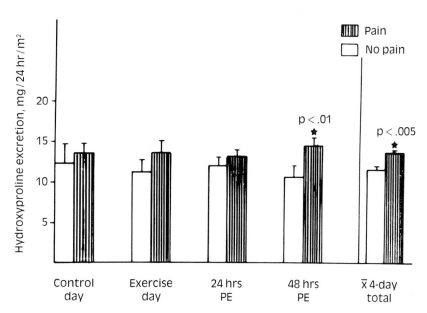

Fig. 3-1 ■ Mean hydroxyproline excretion, normalized for body size, for both soreness-inducing exercise (hatched bars) and exercise not resulting in muscle soreness (open bars). There is a significant increase in hydroxyproline excretion among subjects experiencing muscle soreness at 48 hours postexercise (*PE*).
From Abraham, W.M.: Med. Sci. Sports **9:**11, 1977.

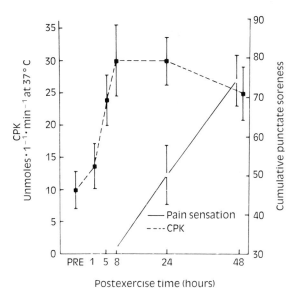

Fig. 3-2 ■ Time course for change in serum CPK activity and perceived muscle soreness following concentric-eccentric leg exercise.
From Tiidus, P.M., and Ianuzzo, C.D.: Med. Sci. Sports Exerc. **15:**461, 1983.

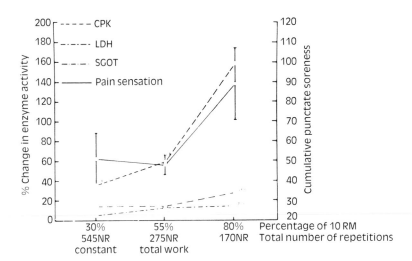

Fig. 3-3 ■ Relative effect of intensity and duration of exercise on levels of serum enzymes and perceived muscle soreness. Horizontal axis displays percentage of subject's 10 repetition maximum *(RM)* (maximum weight that could be raised 10 times) and the number of repetitions *(NR)* when total work remained relatively constant. High-intensity, short-duration exercise (80% 10 RM for 170 NR) resulted in significantly greater rise in both CPK and perceived muscle soreness than low-intensity, long-duration exercise.
From Tiidus, P.M. and Ianuzzo, C.D.: Med. Sci. Sports Exerc. **15:**461, 1983.

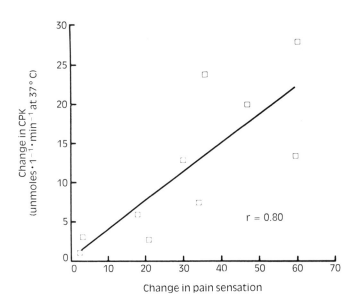

Fig. 3-4 ■ The relationship between change in CPK activity and magnitude of perceived muscle soreness following exercise of varying intensity and duration. Pearson product-moment of $r = 0.80$ was significant at $p < 0.005$.
From Tiidus, P.M. and Ianuzzo, C.D.: Med. Sci. Sports Exerc. **15:**461, 1983.

ture in biopsies obtained 1 day and 3 days after a marathon.

Taken together, these data seem to suggest that **exercise of sufficient intensity may result in muscular damage with release into the circulation of muscle enzymes.** The high mechanical stresses placed on the muscle, especially during eccentric exercise, causes disruption of Z band architecture. The delayed perception of muscle soreness appears to correlate best with the reparative process and its attendant edema formation, invasion of macrophages, inflammation, and histamine release.[4,5,21] Friden et al.[17] have proposed that the observed cytoskeletal disorganization may reflect development of sarcomeres and increased turnover of cytoskeletal and myofibillar proteins following exercise-induced muscle injury. Whether or not delayed muscle soreness is caused by muscle damage or, as discussed earlier, disruption of connective tissue, the occurrence of this syndrome is associated with a temporary reduction in an individual's ability to exercise at maximal levels.[40,42] Furthermore, overtraining may result in chronically sore muscles and, as described by Dressendorfer and Wade,[15] persistently elevated muscle enzyme levels. It would appear from these studies that muscle soreness occurring after exercise should warrant discontinuation of exercise until symptoms have resolved.

Also of note is the observation that levels of **creatine phosphokinase MB isoenzyme** (CPK-MB), generally felt to represent myocardial damage, have been found to be elevated in marathon runners.[3,39] The observed histologic changes suggest that regenerating muscle fibers, rich in CPK-MB, may account for the elevation in this isoenzyme rather than myocardial damage, as was previously thought. (Also see pp. 47-49 concerning muscle soreness.)

■ RHABDOMYOLYSIS
Etiology

A complete review of the many causes of rhabdomyolysis is beyond the scope of

this chapter. However, a list of etiologies and an overview of this subject has recently been published by Knochel[26,27] and Gabow et al.[20] Knochel has aptly classified the etiologies of rhabdomyolysis into five categories: abnormalities of energy production, hypoxia, primary muscle injury,

---

ETIOLOGIES OF RHABDOMYOLYSIS

- Abnormalities of energy production
- Hypoxia
- Primary muscle injury
- Infection
- Miscellaneous (e.g., toxins, drugs)

---

infection, and other miscellaneous causes such as toxins and drugs.[26] **Exertional rhabdomyolysis,** the subject of this chapter, is an example of muscle injury caused by abnormalities in energy production. There are also two conditions associated with enzymatic defects that result in impaired energy production in the setting of exercise. These are the absence of muscle phosphorylase (McArdle's disease) and a deficiency of the enzyme carnitine palmityl transferase (CPT-ase).

CONDITIONS IN WHICH IMPAIRED ENERGY PRODUCTION OCCURS DURING EXERCISE

- McArdle's disease (absence of muscle phosphorylase)
- CPT-ase deficiency

In McArdle's disease, absence of muscle phosphorylase prevents the use of glycogen by the muscle cell during intense exercise. This leads to a state of inadequate production of ATP, resulting in weakness, muscle cramps, and myoglobinuria. A family history of these symptoms can often be elicited. The failure of venous lactate to rise following repetitious and forceful handgrip exercise in the setting of arterial occlusion with a blood pressure cuff supports a diagnosis of McArdle's disease.[27]

CPT-ase, which facilitates mitochondrial transport of fatty acids, plays a crucial role in the normal use by muscle cells of fatty acids for energy production. Lipids, in the form of intramuscular triglycerides and circulating free fatty acids, represent a major energy substrate during prolonged low-intensity exercise, in which they are oxidized in preference to carbohydrates.[33] In the absence of CPT-ase, energy requirements of the working muscle must of necessity depend on the availability of glucose. It is not surprising then that under conditions of fasting, individuals with CPT-ase deficiency experience rhabdomyolysis and myglobinuria following exercise. A 12- to 24-hour fast will produce an increase in serum creatine phosphokinase without the expected elevation in ketones.[27]

Exertional rhabdomyolysis occurring in otherwise healthy individuals is a not infrequent consequence of intense muscular activity, especially in hot climates.[13,27,29] Of 46 skaters studied by Ono,[34] 42 had detectable levels of myoglobin in the urine. All 10 marathon runners completing a 45-kilometer race also had myoglobinuria. Since the presence of myoglobin in the urine occurs only in the setting of muscle injury, these data would suggest a relatively high incidence of rhabdomyolysis in the population studied. Smith[40] evaluated 38 naval officer candidates undergoing basic training. Subclinical rhabdomyolysis was evident in *all* candidates by minor elevations in CPK, aldolase, and SGOT levels. Four of the candidates experienced marked elevations in these enzymes associated with a reduction in the number of push-ups performed during a physical fitness test. Similar findings were reported by Demos et al.[13] when they observed myoglobinemia in two thirds of a group of Marine recruits during their training program. Thus it would appear that subclinical rhabdomyolysis may occur with greater frequency than generally appreciated.

> Subclinical rhabdomyolysis probably occurs with greater frequency than generally appreciated

Long-term studies by Knochel et al.[29] in military recruits undergoing basic training during warm weather revealed that hyperuricemia (8.2 mg%) and hyperuricosuria (1031 mg/24 hr) were prevalent findings by day 11 of the training program. The peak excretion of uric acid cor-

---

INDICATORS OF MUSCLE DAMAGE

- Myoglobinuria
- Hyperuricemia
- Hyperuricosuria
- Elevated CPK, SGOT, and aldolase

---

responded to peak levels of urine creatine and serum CPK, both indices of muscle damage (Fig. 3-5). This temporal relationship strongly suggests that increased uric acid production during training is related to nucleoprotein release from injured skeletal muscle. It is of interest in this study that with continued training, serum uric acid, urine creatine, and serum CPK levels all fell to within normal limits by day 25 of training. The uric acid excretion rate remained elevated throughout the period of observation. This study as well as others[38,43] indicates that the first 2 weeks of physical training represent the period of greatest risk for stress-induced complications, including renal failure.

Complications

Being the largest organ in the body, skeletal muscle is involved in many aspects of normal function including posture, locomotion, respiration, and metabolism. It is not unexpected then that disruption of muscle cell integrity leads to numerous and potentially life-threatening complications. Weakness, pain, and tenderness in muscles following intense ex-

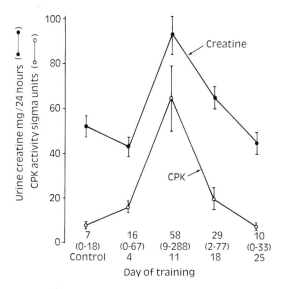

Fig. 3-5 ■ Urinary creatine excretion and serum CPK in subjects undergoing basic military training.
From Knochel, J.P., Dotin, L.N., and Hamburger, R.J.: Ann. Intern. Med. **81:**321, 1974.

CLINICAL SIGNS OF RHABDOMYOLYSIS
- Weakness
- Muscle pain
- Muscle tenderness
- Muscle swelling
- Loss of deep tendon reflexes
- Tetany
- Acute renal failure
- Compartment syndrome
- Disseminated intravascular coagulation (DIC)

ercise may be the earliest clinical signs of rhabdomyolysis. Swelling of the muscle may occur as edema fluid translocates into the damaged muscle bed. Deep tendon reflexes may also be absent in severe cases.[26] Release of potassium from damaged muscle cells can result in hyperkalemia severe enough to produce fatal arrhythmias. In addition, the liberation of phosphorus and subsequent hyperphosphatemia can bind calcium.[44] The resulting hypocalcemia places the patient at risk to develop tetany. Calcification of devitalized muscle tissue and precipitation of calcium phosphate in soft tissues and

eyes has been well described.[32] As previously mentioned, hyperuricemia and hyperuricosuria are both observed during training.[29] The elevation of serum urate in this setting is presumably the result of an overproduction of uric acid in otherwise healthy, muscular individuals.[27]

Acute renal failure following rhabdomyolysis is uncommon but does occur with enough regularity to warrant close attention by those involved in sports and athletic training. Among military recruits undergoing basic training, 10% of the cases of acute renal failure admitted to Walter Reed General Hospital from 1960 to 1966 were associated with exercise and heat stress.[37] Predisposing factors include intense exercise in a hot climate, dehydration, and the previous physical condition of the individual. The four naval candidates with the highest elevation of muscle enzymes as studied by Smith[40] were from a nonathletic subgroup. Exercise in a hot climate appears to be a rather predominant feature of many of the reported series on rhabdomyolysis-induced acute renal failure.[27-29,37,38] Several factors have been implicated as contributing to the

Part one
Basic science of
athletic injuries

**FACTORS PREDISPOSING
TO RHABDOMYOLYSIS-INDUCED ACUTE
RENAL FAILURE**

- Intense exercise in a hot climate
- Dehydration
- Unconditioned state (nonathletic)

renal failure of rhabdomyolysis. Myoglobin, while easily implicated, does not appear to be directly nephrotoxic. However, under acid conditions present during exercise, the myoglobin dissociates into ferrihemate and the globin moiety.[10] Several investigators have presented compelling evidence that ferrihemate is directly nephrotoxic through its interference with tubular function.[2,9] In all studies, dehydration and an acid urine pH appear to play a pivotal role in the development of rhabdomyolysis-induced renal failure.[27] Dehydration, if severe enough, can impair renal blood flow and result in renal injury. Likewise, during exercise, the preferential increase in blood flow to working muscles can significantly reduce renal blood flow. With intense exercise, renal plasma flow may fall by as much as 50% with a 30% to 60% fall in glomerular filtration rate.[6,12] Also of note is the observed fall in urine pH during exercise with a mean value of 4.94 reported by Barclay et al.[7] The coexistence during exercise of aciduria, dehydration, hyperuricosuria, and preferential reduction in renal blood

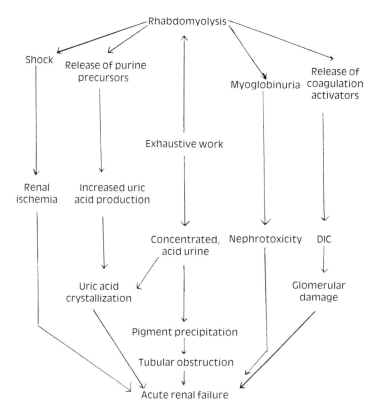

Fig. 3-6 ■ Schema demonstrating interactions of multiple factors culminating in acute renal failure following exhaustive exercise.
From Knochel, J.P. Semin. Nephrol. **1:**75-86, 1981. By permission.

would thus facilitate the development of acute renal failure, especially in the setting of rhabdomyolysis (Fig. 3-6).

Severe rhabdomyolysis can produce vascular and neurologic compromise because of muscle necrosis and edema with compartmental compression. This is particularly true of rhabdomyolysis involving muscles located in tight fascial compartments, such as the lateral thigh, soleus, anterior tibial, and gluteus.[27] Finally, evidence of disseminated intravascular coagulation (DIC) and hemorrhage can commonly be found in cases of rhabdomyolysis. The mechanism of the development of DIC is not yet well established. It is known that exercise per se is associated with an enhancement in blood coagulabil-

ity as well as a concomitant increase in fibrinolytic activity.[31] The DIC seen with rhabdomyolysis may be an extension of this process or may be related to the release of substances from damaged muscle.

Diagnosis and treatment

The diagnosis of rhabdomyolysis relies on the finding of myoglobin in the urine and elevation of serum muscle enzymes. CPK and aldolase levels are most commonly elevated following muscle injury. Levels of CPK in the range of 10,000 to 100,000 IU/L have been commonly reported.[20,26,27] Values of 500 to 2000 IU/L can be observed following uncomplicated long-distance running competitions[15,41]

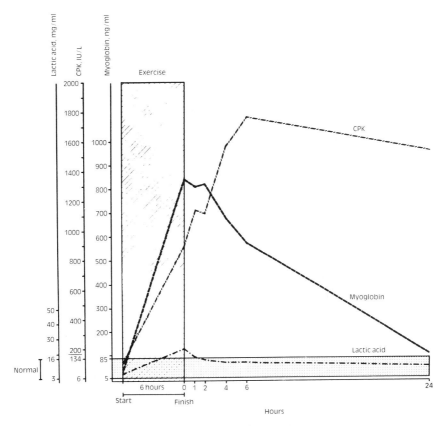

Fig. 3-7 ■ Composite values of serum myoglobin, CPK, and lactic acid from 25 athletes at the conclusion and 24 hours following a triathlon event.
From Thomas, B.D., and Motley, C.P.: Am. J. Sports Med. **12:**113, 1984. © 1984, American Orthopaedic Society for Sports Medicine

(Fig. 3-7). While the CPK is predominantly of the MM isoenzyme, the MB isoenzyme can also be elevated *without* implying myocardial damage.[3,39] This appears to be a result of regenerating muscle fibers that are rich in CPK-MB.[39] Other muscle enzymes such as SGOT and LDH can also be found elevated in this setting.

The finding of myoglobin, a red respiratory pigment, in the urine is diagnostic of rhabdomyolysis. With a molecular weight of 17,000 daltons and no specific serum binding protein, myoglobin when released from injured muscle is rapidly cleared and excreted by the kidney.[26] This is in contrast to hemoglobin, which has a larger molecular weight of 68,000 daltons and binds readily to haptoglobin. In this way free hemoglobin stains the serum red and is excreted only after all binding sites are occupied. Myoglobinemia, in contrast, does not stain the serum. Once excreted in the urine, however, both hemoglobin and myoglobin can be detected by a reaction with the orthotolidine on Hematest strips. **A positive test for "occult blood" in face of a urinalysis that fails to reveal red blood cells should alert the clinician to the possibility of either hemoglobinuria or myoglobinuria.** Other more specific tests such as radioimmunoassay, hemagglutination, immunodiffusion, or immunoelectrophoresis can also be employed to detect the presence of myoglobin. The diagnosis often relies on the constellation of findings including muscle pain and elevated muscle enzyme levels. Rapid clearance of the myoglobin may negate the importance of the urinary evaluation.

Once rhabdomyolysis has been diagnosed, appropriate therapy should be quickly instituted in the hope of avoiding major complications. Intravenous fluids sufficient to maintain normal volume status and cardiovascular stability are required. With extensive muscle damage, the associated capillary leak and interstitial edema will, in effect, translocate large volumes of fluid out of the intravascular compartment into the muscle bed. Kno-

---

TREATMENT OF RHABDOMYOLYSIS

- Intravenous fluids
- Hyperkalemia (K^+ greater than 5.5 mEq/L) → sodium polystyrene sulfonate (Kayexalate) (exchange resin)
- Hyperphosphatemia (Po_4 greater than 6.0 mg%) → aluminum hydroxide (phosphate binder)
- Avoid calcium replacement
  ? Mannitol
  ? Bicarbonate

---

chel[26,27] has reported fluid requirements of up to 10 L within 12 to 24 hours. Adequate hydration is also important for promoting a brisk diuresis to assure urinary dilution. The nephrotoxic potential of ferrihemate is enhanced in dehydration and aciduria.[2,9,10] Intravenous fluids with mannitol infusions have been shown to be beneficial in promoting diuresis and diluting the medullary interstitium in some cases of rhabdomyolysis.[16] Bicarbonate can be employed to alkalinize the urine, but it should be avoided if hypocalcemia is present.

Hyperphosphatemia, hyperkalemia, and hypocalcemia can all occur in the setting of rhabdomyolysis. Treatment of hyperphosphatemia with the phosphate binder aluminum hydroxide and treatment of hyperkalemia with the exchange resin sodium polystyrene sulfonate (Kayexalate) should be employed for phosphate levels over 6.0 mg% and potassium levels over 5.5 mEq/L, respectively. The use of calcium salts for the treatment of hypocalcemia should in general be avoided. The drop in calcium level is related to the hyperphosphotemia and soft tissue precipitation of complexes of calcium and phosphorus. In this setting, adminstration of calcium salts may result in additional tissue calcification and potentially may worsen the rhabdomyolysis.[36]

If renal failure does occur, supportive care and dialytic therapy should be employed until renal function improves. The occurrence of hypercalcemia during the

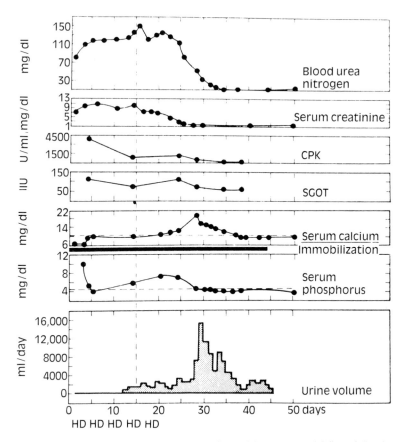

Fig. 3-8 ■ Summary of hospital course from patient with acute renal failure following rhabdomyolysis. Horizontal dotted lines represent upper limit of normal range. *HD,* hemodialysis; *CPK,* creatine phosphokinase; *SGOT,* serum glutamic oxaloacetic transaminase. From Zabetakis, P.M., et al.: N.Y. State J. Med. **79:**1887, 1979.

diuretic or recovery phase of acute tubular necrosis has been previously reported (Fig. 3-8). Several mechanisms have been proposed, including immobilization, elevated parathyroid hormone level, and resorption of calcium deposits in damaged muscle.[44] Based on the available data, limb immobilization appears to play a crucial role in the development of hypercalcemia. It is recommended that during the period of rhabdomyolysis-induced renal failure serum calcium levels be monitored closely and early mobilization attempted.

■ **SUMMARY**

Delayed muscle soreness occurs with regularity following intense muscular activity. The available data suggest that this entity is a result of structural muscle

damage with inflammation, necrosis, and disruption of myofibrillar Z bands. The delayed perception of muscle soreness appears to correlate best with the reparative process associated with edema formation, invasion of macrophages, and histamine release.

Rhabdomyolysis can be viewed as muscle injury with loss of cellular integrity that may be asymptomatic or, if severe enough, associated with muscle pain, edema, compartmental compression, hyperkalemia, hyperphosphotemia, hyperuricemia, renal failure, and DIC. The incidence of rhabdomyolysis is greatest in the setting of intense exercise in a hot climate during the first 2 weeks of exercise training, but can occur at almost any time. To avoid this complication, athletes should be warned against dehydration and intense exercise in humid climates, especially during the early stages of their conditioning program.

REFERENCES

1. Abraham, W.M.: Factors in delayed muscle soreness, Med. Sci. Sports **9**:11, 1977.
2. Anderson, W.A.D., Morrison, D.B., and Williams, E.F.: Pathologic changes following injections of ferrihemate (Hematin) in dogs, Arch. Pathol. **33**:598, 1942.
3. Apple, F.S., Rogers, M.A., Sherman, W.M., and Ivy, J.L.: Comparison of elevated serum creatinine kinase MB activities post marathon and post myocardial infarction, Med. Sci. Sports Exerc. **15**:164, 1983.
4. Armstrong, R.B., Ogilvie, R.W., and Schwane, J.A.: Eccentric exercise-induced damage to rat skeletal muscle, J. Appl. Physiol. **54**:80, 1983.
5. Asmussen, E.: Observations on experimental muscle soreness, Acta Rheum. Scand. **2**:109, 1956.
6. Barclay, J.A., Cooke, W.T., Kenney, R.A., and Nutt, M.E.: The effect of exercise on the renal blood flow in man, J. Physiol. (Lond.) **104**:148, 1946.
7. Barclay, J.A., Cooke, W.T., Kenney, R.A., and Nutt, M.E.: The effects of water diuresis and exercise on the volume and composition of urine, Am. J. Physiol. **148**:327, 1947.
8. Bergstrom, J., and Hultman, E.: A study of the glycogen metabolism during exercise in man, Scand. J. Clin. Lab. Invest. **19**:218, 1967.
9. Braun, S.R., Weiss, F.R., Keller, A.I., Ciccone, J.R., and Preuss, H.G.: Evaluation of the renal toxicity of heme proteins and their derivatives: a role in the genesis of acute tubular necrosis, J. Exp. Med. **131**:443, 1970.
10. Bunn, H.F., and Jandl, J.H.: Exchange of heme among hemoglobin molecules, Proc. Natl. Acad. Sci. USA **56**:974, 1966.
11. Bywaters, E.G.L., and Beall, D.: Crash injuries with impairment of renal function, Br. Med. J. **1**:427, 1941.
12. Castenfors, J.: Renal function during exercise, Acta. Physiol. Scand. (Suppl.) **293**:4, 1967.
13. Demos, M.A., Gitin, E.L., and Kagen, L.J.: Exercise myoblobinemia and acute exertional rhabdomyolysis, Arch. Intern. Med. **134**:669, 1974.
14. De Vries, H.A.: Quantitative electromyographic investigation of the spasm theory of muscle pain, Am. J. Phys. Med. **45**:119, 1966.
15. Dressendorfer, R.H., and Wade, C.E.: The muscular overuse syndrome in long-distance runners, Phys. Sports. Med. **11**:116, 1983.
16. Eneas, J.F., Schoenfeld, P.Y., and Humphreys, M.H.: The effect of infusion of mannitol-sodium bicarbonate on the clinical course of myoglobinuria, Arch. Intern. Med. **139**:801, 1979.
17. Friden, J., Kjorell, U., and Thornell, L.E.: Delayed muscle soreness and cytoskeletal alterations: an immunocytological study in man, Int. J. Sports. Med. **5**:15, 1984.
18. Friden, J., Sjostrom, M., and Ekblom, B.: A morphological study of delayed muscle soreness. Experientia **37**:506, 1981.
19. Friden, J., Sjostrom, M., and Ekblom, B.: Myofibrillar damage following intense eccentric exercise in man, Int. J. Sports Med. **4**:170, 1983.
20. Gabow, P.A., Kaehny, W.D., and Kelleher, S.P.: The spectrum of rhabdomyolysis, Medicine **61**:141, 1982.
21. Guyton, A.C.: Textbook of medical physiology, Philadelphia, 1981, W.B. Saunders Co., pp. 611-625.
22. Hagerman, F.C., Hikida, R.S., Staron, R.S., Sherman, W.M., and Costill, D.L.: Muscle fiber necrosis in marathon runners. Med. Sci. Sports Exerc. **15**:164, 1983.
23. Highman, B., and Altland, P.D.: Effects of exercise and training on serum enzyme and tissue changes in rats, Am. J. Physiol. **205**:162, 1963.
24. Hough, T.: Erographic studies in muscular soreness, Am. J. Physiol. **7**:76, 1902.
25. Hultman, E., Bergstrom, J., and Anderson, N.M.: Breakdown and resynthesis of phosphorylcreatine and adenosine triphosphate in connection with muscular work in man, Scand. J. Clin. Lab. Invest. **19**:56, 1967.
26. Knochel, J.P.: Rhabdomyolysis and myoglobinuria, Semin. Nephrol. **1**:75, 1981.
27. Knochel, J.P.: Rhabdomyolysis and myoglobinuria, Annu. Rev. Med. **33**:435, 1982.
28. Knochel, J.P., Beisel, W.R., Herndon, E.G., Gerard, E.S., and Barry K.G.: Renal cardiovascular, hematologic and serum electrolyte abnormalities of heat stroke. Am. J. Med. **30**:299, 1961.
29. Knochel, J.P., Dotin, L.N., and Hamburger, R.J.: Heat stress, exercise, and muscle injury: effects on urate metabolism and renal function, Ann. Intern. Med. **81**:321, 1974.
30. Komi, P.V., and Buskirk, E.R.: The effect of eccentric and concentric muscle conditioning on tension and electrical activity of human muscle, Ergonomics **15**:417, 1972.
31. Lee, G., Amsterdam, E.A., Demaria, A.N., Davis, G., La Fave, T., and Mason, D.T.: Effect of exercise on hemostatic mechanisms. In Amsterdam, E.A., Wilmore, J.H., DeMaria, A.N., editors: Exercise in cardiovascular health and disease, New York, 1977, Yorke Medical Books p. 122.
32. Meroney, W.H., Arney, G.K., Segar, W.E., and Balch, H.H.: The acute calcification of traumatized muscle, with particular reference to acute post-traumatic renal insufficiency, J. Clin. Invest. **36**:825, 1957.
33. Newsholme, E.A.: The regulation of intracellular and extracellular fuel supply during sustained exercise, Ann. NY Acad. Sci. **301**:81, 1977.

34. Ono, I.: Studies on myoglobinuria, Tohoku J. Exp. Med. **57:**273, 1953.

35. Ouzounellis, T.: Some notes on quail poisoning, JAMA **211:**1186, 1970.

36. Publicover, S.J., Ducan, C.J., and Smith, J.L.: The use of A23187 to demonstrate the role of intracellular calcium in causing ultrastructural damage in mammalian muscle, J. Neuropathol. Exp. Neurol. **37:**S544, 1978.

37. Schrier, R.W., Hano, J., Keller, H.I., Finkel, R.M., Gilliland, P.F., Cirksena, W.J., and Teschan, P.E.: Renal, metabolic, and circulatory responses to heat and exercise, Ann. Intern. Med. **73:**213, 1970.

38. Schrier, R.W., Henderson, H.S., Tischer, C.C., and Tannen, R.L.: Nephropathy associated with heat stress and exercise, Ann. Intern. Med. **67:**356, 1967.

39. Siegel, A.J., Worhol, M.J., Evans, W.J., and Silverman, L.M.: Focal myofibrillar necrosis in skeletal muscle of trained marathon runners after competition, Med. Sci. Sports Exerc. **15:**164, 1983.

40. Smith, R.F.: Exertional rhabdomyolysis in naval officer candidates, Arch. Intern. Med. **121:**313, 1968.

41. Thomas, B.D., and Motley, C.P.: Myoglobinemia and endurance exercise: a study of twenty-five participants in a triathlon competition, Am. J. Sports Med. **12:**113, 1984.

42. Tiidus, P.M., and Ianuzzo, C.D.: Effects of intensity and duration of muscular exercise on delayed soreness and serum enzyme activities, Med. Sci. Sports Exerc. **15:**461, 1983.

43. Vertel, R.M., and Knochel, J.P.: Acute renal failure due to heat injury: an analysis of ten cases associated with a high incidence of myoglobinuria, Am. J. Med. **43:**435, 1967.

44. Zabetakis, P.M., Singh, R., Michelis, M.F., and Murdaugh, H.V.: Acute renal failure: bone immobilization as cause of hypercalcemia, N.Y. State J. Med. **79:**1887, 1979.

chapter 4

Cardiovascular aspects of injury to the lower extremity

Gilbert Gleim

The cardiovascular effects of musculoskeletal injury may not be readily apparent to the orthopaedist who is not actively involved in sports medicine. On the other hand, the sports medicine physician must treat the entire athlete, and cardiovascular performance is a vital component of athletic performance. Since athletes range in age from adolescents to the elderly, cardiovascular deconditioning resulting from orthopaedic pathology takes on increasing importance as the athlete grows older.

It is important to understand that different forms of exercise do not elicit the same response from the cardiovascular system. Increasing intensities of exercise do not demonstrate a strictly linear cardiovascular stress. Peripheral training, that is, adaptation of skeletal muscle, is a factor in preventing the augmented stress response with increasing physical exertion.

Peripheral adaptations to training are extremely important when one considers injury to the lower extremity. Muscular atrophy following injury can be extremely dramatic (Fig. 4-1). Aside from the obvious decreases in strength, which are a known result of disuse atrophy, loss of muscle mass represents loss of potential declines in peripheral resistance during exercise. Additionally, we shall see that atrophy may have a greater impact on one population of muscle fibers (Type I) than on another (Type II). Cardiovascular reflexes elicited by skeletal muscle may be dependent on the relative percentages of Type I and Type II muscle, so that atrophy may alter this feedback response.

This chapter will present some basic concepts in cardiovascular physiology and skeletal muscle physiology, relating them to each other and to the other "organ systems" of the body (Fig. 4-2). Specifically, the brain acts as the seat of emotions and motor control, both of which affect autonomic nervous system function. The heart, by changing rate and stroke volume, determines cardiac output and short-term blood pressure control. Maximum oxygen consumption is primarily a

Table 4-1 ■ Simplified terminology of human skeletal muscle fiber types

Brook and Kaiser	Peter et al.*	Traditional (Padykula and Herman)
Type I	SO	Red (Dark)
Type IIa	FOG	White (Light)
Type IIb	FG	

*SO, slow oxidative; FOG, fast oxidative glycolytic; FG, fast glycolytic.

high oxidative capacity, fast glycolytic (FG) fibers a fast twitch and high glycolytic capacity, and fast oxidative glycolytic (FOG) fibers a fast-twitch and moderate oxidative and glycolytic capacity.

Finally, one also encounters the terminology of red muscle and white muscle (dark and light). Using this phraseology, the descriptions are roughly equivalent to slow and fast twitch muscle (Table 4-1).

Brook and Kaiser[10] have shown a difference in staining intensities for nicotinamide adenine dinucleotide (NADH) tetrazolium reductase and succinate dehydrogenase (SDH) between fiber types as well. For example, SDH activity is greater in Types I and IIa muscle than in Type IIb muscle.

Characteristics of types of skeletal muscle

Aside from the fact that skeletal muscle stains differently based on myofibrillar ATPase, there are significant differences between the fiber types with respect to morphology and metabolism as well.

Type I muscle is analogous to SO muscle. It is richly endowed with mitochondria, has a greater amount of myoglobin, and at least in humans has a greater capillarity.[8,33] The great number of mitochondria results in high levels of oxidative enzymes such as SDH and cytochrome C. However, this observation must be tempered by noting that enzyme profiles can be altered dramatically by training. In addition to their high oxidative capacity,

Type I muscle has a greater capacity for metabolizing free fatty acids, although this effect can also be modified with training.[35]

Type II skeletal muscle has a more extensive sarcoplasmic reticulum, a fact that may contribute to its faster twitch speed. Type II muscle usually has a larger surface area per fiber and is more richly endowed with glycolytic enzymes such as phosphofructokinase (PFK) and lactate dehydrogenase (LDH). Untrained Type II muscle does not metabolize free fatty acids well. The distinction between IIa and IIb is that IIa has more oxidative enzymes than IIb (Table 4-2).

Training-induced changes in skeletal muscle

Hermansen and Wachtlova[33] and Brodal et al.[8] demonstrated an increased capillary to fiber ratio in the muscles of trained men as opposed to untrained men. Brodal et al. showed that capillaries per square millimeter measured 305 in the untrained and 425 in the trained. Consequently, endurance training presumably increases oxygen supply to the trained muscle. Equally important may be the increased clearance of metabolites allowed by an increased perfusion potential.

In a review, Holloszy and Booth[36] demonstrated that all types of skeletal muscle increase their capacity to oxidize free fatty acids, carbohydrates, ketones, and amino acids as well as the enzyme pathways necessary for the reducing equivalents. They noted that Type I muscle shows the least change on a percentage basis, since it begins with a higher level of these oxidative enzymes. Type II muscle has the greatest potential for improvement.

Skeletal muscle training falls into two basic categories, strength and endurance. Strength training has at least two effects, and only one involves the muscle directly. Undoubtedly, initial gains in strength, which can be measured with a traditional 1 repetition maximum or with isokinetic dynamometry, are the result of more ef-

Table 4-2 ■ Characteristics of skeletal muscle

Type	Mitochondria/oxidative enzymes	Glycolytic enzymes	Capillarity	Free fatty acid metabolism
I	High	Low	High	High
IIa	Intermediate	Intermediate	Intermediate	Intermediate
IIb	Low	High	Intermediate	Low

ficient motor neuron recruitment. Hypertrophy, on the other hand, is a strength training adaptation of skeletal muscle.

Hypertrophy of skeletal muscle can be dramatically rapid. Section of the gastrocnemius muscle produced a weight gain of 40% in the synergistic soleus muscle in the rat[24] in only 6 days. No noticeable increase in muscle mass resulted if the animals were prevented from using their hind limbs. The hypertrophy of skeletal muscle is age related as well, since older muscle does not hypertrophy as rapidly as younger muscle.[50] Hypertrophy has also been induced in hypophysectomized animals, suggesting that growth hormone is not a prerequisite.[23] This treatment also indicates that a lack of thyroid hormones and adrenally derived testosterone is of no importance. Similarly, insulin does not appear to be important for hypertrophy.[23]

The hypertrophic process results from greater protein anabolism than catabolism, processes that are continuously occurring in skeletal muscle. Rapid amino acid uptake has been demonstrated in the tenotomy model noted previously.[24] The sensitive balance between uptake and breakdown will ultimately determine hypertrophy or atrophy.

The stimulus for the change in protein turnover is most likely stretch or tension.[61] Models in which a limb has been casted with the muscles in an elongated position retard the atrophic process and may induce hypertrophy. Typically, endurance exercise does not produce hypertrophy.[4,35,64] The latter study notes that, unlike endurance exercise, strength training does not increase capillary density.

Changes that occur with endurance training are likely to affect the different fiber types according to the intensity of the endurance exercise. For example, Dudley et al.[17] showed that endurance adaptation of skeletal muscle (measured as changes in cytochrome c) occurred at a lower intensity in Type IIa fibers than in IIb fibers, while Type I fibers were affected at all intensities. In this study, Type IIb changes occurred only after animals were exercising at 83% or more of maximal oxygen consumption. Similar results were obtained by Harms and Hickson,[30] who noted that exercise at 50% of maximal oxygen consumption was sufficient to induce changes in Type I mitochondrial content but much higher levels were necessary for changes in Type II mitochondria. Even high-intensity training had no effect on the myoglobin content of Type II muscle. (See Table 4-3 for summary.)

These intensity-dependent changes in endurance function of the different fiber types suggest a difference in recruitment of the muscle fibers. It should be recalled that the motor neurons innervating skeletal muscle terminate on only one fiber type. That Type I muscle is recruited first is supported by two strong lines of evidence. First, the rank order of motor neuron recruitment states that smaller motorneurons are recruited first because of their lower threshold of excitation.[32] Since Type I muscle is innervated by smaller motor neurons it is likely that these are the first fibers used for low-intensity exercise. Second, glycogen depletion studies show selective loss of glycogen from Type I muscle at low intensities, while Type II muscle is not depleted of its glycogen until high intensities are reached.[25,63] Conse-

Table 4-3 ■ Training-induced changes in skeletal muscle

	Strength training	Endurance training
Type I	Minimal or no change	Increased capillarity
	First to experience disuse atrophy	Increased myoglobin
		Some increase in oxidative enzymes occuring at all intensities
Type II	Hypertrophy	Some increase in capillarity
	Decreased capillarity	Increased myglobin in IIa, no change in IIb
	Last to experience atrophy	Increased oxidative enzymes in IIa, some increase in IIb, occurring only at high intensities

quently, it is likely that endurance changes will not occur in Type II muscle until a certain threshold intensity of exercise is accomplished.

Disuse atrophy

A well-known result of casting, surgery with immobilization, prolonged bed rest, or inactivity is atrophy of skeletal muscle. It would appear that Type I muscle is most affected by disuse. Cross-sectional areas were decreased most, on a percentage basis, in Type I muscle of guinea pig following 4 weeks of immobilization.[51] Booth[7] in a review, states that Type I muscle takes on properties of Type II skeletal muscle following immobilization, with decreases in protein synthesis occurring as early as 6 hours following immobilization. Immobilization seems to have a retrograde influence on motor neurons, an effect that can be attenuated by immobilization in a stretched position. Most recently, Templeton et al.[62] demonstrated that the normal incidence of Type I muscle in rat soleus was decreased following

4 weeks of disuse. While these studies do not provide conclusive proof that Type I muscle is affected most by disuse, they certainly provide strong support for such a hypothesis. This is not unexpected if one considers that Type I muscle is likely to be the first recruited and as a result to show the greatest changes following disuse.

■ RESPONSES TO STATIC AND DYNAMIC EXERCISE

Exercise literature abounds with the differences between the effects of isometric and dynamic exercise on the cardiovascular system. A summary of these effects follows. The intent of this review is to convince the reader that the terms "isometric" and "dynamic" may be somewhat arbitrary with respect to the cardiovascular response to exercise. From a cardiovascular focus, isometric exercise is any form of exercise that elicits intense muscular contraction to recruit Type II fibers. Dynamic exercise, on the other hand, is low-intensity exercise resulting from activation of primarily Type I muscle.

Static exercise

Lindhard[49] was the first to report the effects of isometric exercise on the cardiovascular system. He demonstrated increases in blood pressure and heart rate from bent-arm overhead hanging. The traditional test used to evoke a cardiovascular response to exercise is handgrip. Humphreys and Lind[38] demonstrated an unexpectedly large increase in blood pressure during handgrip exercise. Lind et al.[48] later demonstrated greater increases in HR and blood pressure with increasing intensity of handgrip contraction. Noticeably in these studies, SV fell with increasing intensity, although the increases in HR were sufficient to produce increases in cardiac output. In these studies there were only minor increases in oxygen consumption and no change or slight decreases in TPR.

Two theories exist to explain the in-

Part one
Basic science of
athletic injuries

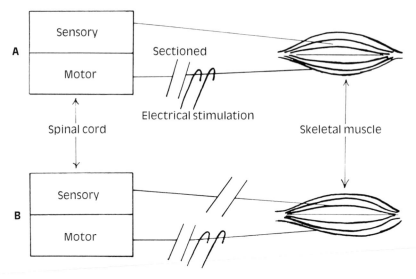

Fig. 4-5 ■ Schematic diagram of experimental procedures employed by Mitchell et al. to demonstrate reflex nature of skeletal muscle contraction on heart rate and blood pressure. **A,** Electrical stimulation of distal end of sectioned motor nerve innervating skeletal muscle caused increase in HR and blood pressure. **B,** Sensory fibers from electrically stimulated skeletal muscle were sectioned, and this prevented reflex rise in HR and blood pressure.
Data from Mitchell, J.H., Reardon, W.C., McCloskey, D.I., and Wildenthal, D.: Ann. N. Y. Acad. Sci. **301:**232, 1977.

creases in HR and blood pressure noted with exercise. The first idea, originally proposed by Krogh and Lindhard[46] is the central command hypothesis. This states that the cardiovascular centers of the brainstem receive collateral input from the motor centers whose primary role is to evoke skeletal muscle contraction. Further support for this hypothesis was provided by Asmussen.[2] Using partial curarization of the contracting skeletal muscle, it was shown that HR and blood pressure responses were increased at similar intensities of contraction following blockade. Freyschuss,[19] using a similar experimental paradigm, caused paralysis of grip through brachial artery injection of succinylcholine and noted increases in BP and HR even though no muscular contraction was taking place. The common explanation of these studies is that motor centers were issuing commands to the skeletal muscle, which could not contract. In doing so, the collaterals to the cardiovascular centers of the brainstem were also being excited, causing an increase in BP and HR.

The other explanation for the cardiovascular events during exercise is the peripheral feedback theory. Simply stated, receptors within skeletal muscle sense contraction and send afferent impulses back to the brainstem CV centers to cause reflex increases in blood pressure and HR. This theory has received ample research support.

Alam and Smirk[1] were the first to propose the peripheral feedback reflex. Most recently, work by Mitchell et al. has added the most conclusive proof of the reflex nature of this response. Mitchell et al.[52] stimulated the distal portion of severed motor nerve to hind limb muscle in anesthetized dogs and noted an increase in HR and blood pressure. When they cut the dorsal root from the area of the spinal column receiving the afferent nerves they abolished this response (Fig. 4-5). This experimentation offers irrefutable proof of the reflex.

It does not seem possible that the increases in blood pressure are the result of a localized increase in resistance of the contracted muscle. Perez-Gonzalez[54] noted

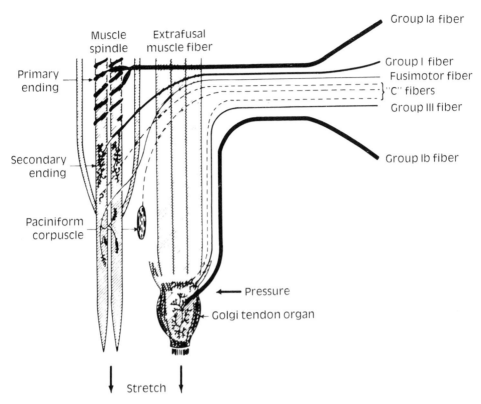

Fig. 4-6 ■ Afferent innervation of skeletal muscle, with exception of the fusimotor fibers that innervate spindle organ. Group III and "c" fibers are responsible for reflexes effecting cardiovascular system. Group I and II fibers do not evoke reflex cardiovascular responses. Nature of stimulus for Group III and "c" fibers has not been precisely defined.
From Kalia, M. Mei, S.S., and Kao, F.F.: Circ. Res. Suppl. I **48:**I25, 1981. By permission of the American Heart Association, Inc.

increases in blood pressure at 20% of maximal voluntary contraction (MVC), even though blood flow did not decrease in the contracted muscle. Further, the amount of muscle mass contracted in Mitchell's experiments is insufficient to cause a noticeable increase in TPR.

In 1973, Sato and Schmidt[58] demonstrated that Group I and II muscle afferents had no direct access to the autonomic nervous system. Since that time substantial evidence to suggest that Group III and IV afferents are responsible for the reflex has been provided. Kniffki et al.[43] showed that bradykinin, serotonin, and potassium could excite Group IV afferents, while Group III afferents were postulated to be stimulated by stretch and contraction. Kaufman et al. demonstrated

that Group IV afferents as well as some Group III afferents could be stimulated by capsaicin.[41] Therefore the precise stimuli for these receptors has not been proven, but they are collectively known as **ergoreceptors.**

Kalia et al.[40] have demonstrated that many of these fibers terminate in cardiovascular centers of the brainstem. This work provides anatomic evidence for a rather direct connection to those areas which may be responsible for increases in HR and blood pressure resulting from muscular contraction. A diagram depicting the different afferent nerves and their sources of stimulation is provided in Fig. 4-6.

Recalling that the product of HR and blood pressure, the rate pressure product, correlates highly with myocardial oxygen consumption, the implications of this reflex response are obvious. It is for this reason that **high-resistance forms of training are contraindicated in persons with coronary artery disease.** Mitchell's group has provided further evidence for a more direct effect on the myocardial circulation.[5] They demonstrated through beta-blockade and microsphere techniques that this reflex is responsible for alpha-coronary arteriole vasoconstriction. This would serve to compound the effects of a reflex increase in HR and blood pressure, since there would be increased oxygen demand with potentially decreased supply.

There is evidence that the fiber type stimulated may have an impact on the magnitude of the response of HR and blood pressure. Petrofsky et al.[56] demonstrated that if only Type I fiber is stimulated during low intensity contraction there are no significant increases in HR or blood pressure. On stimulation of Type II fibers first there were increases in these two indices of myocardial oxygen consumption. Indirect evidence in humans exists to support the notion that Type II muscle contraction is important in eliciting the increases in blood pressure. In humans, increases in blood pressure during isometric contraction were positively correlated to the percentage of Type II muscle.[20] Consequently, Type II muscle contraction may be a prerequisite for the initiation of the reflex. Recall that Type I muscle contraction occurs first and that the magnitude of the blood pressure response is related to the intensity of the contraction.

Dynamic exercise

Unlike exercise associated with intense muscular contraction (i.e., resistive strength exercise), dynamic exercise is associated with dramatic increases in whole body oxygen consumption. Further, dynamic exercise is not associated with the large increases in MAP that are found in isomet-

ric exercise. Cardiac output rises in both forms of exercise, but the fall in TPR is so great during dynamic exercise that the increased cardiac output does not cause large increases in MAP.

The range of maximal oxygen consumptions possible in various states of conditioning and sports is dramatic. It is not uncommon to find a maximal oxygen consumption of 20 ml per kg per minute (ml/kg/min) in a cardiac patient and a value of 85 ml/kg/min in an elite marathon runner. Higher values are obtained in sports in which the upper body is involved as well, such as in cross-country skiing.

There is a strong relationship between maximal oxygen consumption and cardiac output. Individuals who can attain the highest cardiac outputs during exercise will also have the highest oxygen consumptions.[3] Within an individual, the larger the exercising muscle mass, the greater the cardiac output and the higher the oxygen consumption. For this reason, oxygen consumption is usually higher for lower body exercise than upper body exercise, unless the individual has been extensively trained in the upper body.[12] Blomqvist et al.[6] have shown that the magnitude of exercising muscle determines the fall in TPR and that the slope of cardiac output vs. oxygen consumption is constant for a given individual. Obviously, if a large muscle mass has been lost as a result of disuse atrophy (i.e., thigh muscle wasting following lower extremity injury) one can expect a lower maximal oxygen consumption. There will be less exercising muscle mass and consequently less maximal work performed, and there will be less of a fall in TPR, which allows for increased venous return.

Another measure routinely assessed during the test for maximal oxygen consumption is the "anaerobic threshold" or "lactate threshold." This terminology may have been originally proposed by Wasserman et al.,[67] who noted a breakaway in bicarbonate, lactate, and minute volume at the same point during progressive exercise. They postulated that this represented a point during exercise at which the muscle tissues became hypoxic, and the hyperventilation was the body's response to the metabolic acidosis.

Since that time, much evidence corroborating their findings yet refuting their hypothesis has appeared. At this time it is currently a topic of much debate. Hagberg et al.[29] demonstrated that patients with McArdle's disease, who are incapable of producing lactate, manifest a ventilatory breakpoint during exercise as well. Also it has been shown that the lactate threshold and ventilatory threshold need not occur at the same time.[26,37] Green et al.[26] also demonstrated that lactate accumulates in skeletal muscle before the lactate threshold, and more recently it has been shown that lactate is produced in fully aerobic, working dog muscle without an increase in venous effluent lactate.[13] These findings refute the hypothesis that the lactate threshold is a result of hypoxia at the level of the exercising skeletal muscle.

In my view, the debate over whether or not the lactate threshold is caused by tissue hypoxia is missing the biologic significance of the phenomenon. The important question is, does this point represent the recruitment of Type II muscle?

It should be recalled that Type II muscle has a high glycolytic capacity because of its enzymatic characteristics. This means that the prefered fuel for metabolism is glucose and the likely end product will be lactate. Type I muscle will tend to channel any pyruvate formed into the Kreb's cycle which results in the formation of carbon dioxide and water. Increases that occur in mixed venous blood lactate are therefore likely to represent the mass recruitment of Type II muscle necessary to perform the additional work imposed.

It is well known that lactate thresholds tend to be higher in endurance athletes (i.e., represent a greater percentage of their maximum oxygen consumption) and that endurance athletes tend to have more Type I muscle. Ivy et al.[39] demonstrated strong positive correlations ($r = 0.74$ and $r = 0.70$) between percentage of Type I fibers and both the absolute and relative lactate thresholds. Komi et al.,[44] using a measure called "onset of blood lactate accumulation" (OBLA), designated as that

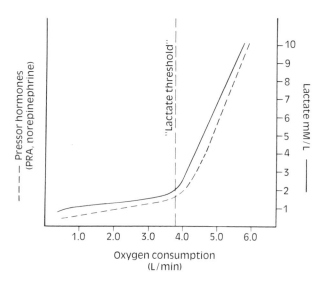

Fig. 4-7 ■ Relationship of mixed venous blood lactate to pressor hormones as oxygen consumption increases. Significance of this "lactate threshold" may be in increased amounts of these pressor hormones, representing increase in sympathetic activity.

work-rate producing a level of 4 mM per liter of lactate, showed that the power output at OBLA correlated highly with the percentage of Type I muscle (r = 0.75). It therefore seems likely that recruitment of Type II muscle is responsible for the lactate threshold.

Kotchen et al.[45] demonstrated that catecholamines and plasma renin activity (PRA) increased in parallel during exercise and that these hormones were not elevated until 70% or more of maximum oxygen consumption. Lehman et al.[47] were able to show that catecholamines paralleled mixed venous lactate during exercise. My co-workers and I recently showed that PRA and lactate also demonstrated a parallel relationship during dynamic exercise and that acute changes in plasma volume did not dictate increases in PRA.[21] The increase in mixed venous blood lactate was shown to be related to a plateau in MAP. Finally, this study also showed that following isokinetic knee extension-flexion at 50% of MVC, increases in lactate were related to increases in PRA. I feel that the biologic significance of this "lactate threshold" is that it results in the liberation of pressor hormones (Fig. 4-7) whose purpose is to maintain MAP in the face of further declines in skeletal muscle resistance to blood flow.

■ CARDIOVASCULAR EFFECTS OF ATROPHY

In the foregoing discussion I have attempted to convince the reader that it is naive to conceive of the cardiovascular and musculoskeletal systems as separate entities during exercise. Dilation within skeletal muscle is an important component in determining cardiac output, because this dilation allows for increased venous return. Atrophy results in less possible exercising muscle mass, decreasing venous return that diminishes cardiac output, and a lower maximal oxygen consumption. This means that less total work can be performed by the exercising individual.

In addition to its effects on decreasing venous return, atrophy has special effects on the skeletal muscle fiber types. The fiber type most likely to be effected by atrophy is Type I muscle. Loss of efficiency in Type I muscle will mean that it is necessary to recruit Type II muscle earlier in an attempt to accomplish additional work. This will evoke the cardiovascular reflex that increases sympathetic outflow at an earlier point during exercise (Fig. 4-8), since Type II muscle contraction appears to be the stimulus for this response.

It should be realized that only rarely in sporting activity are skeletal muscles contracting maximally. Indeed, many activities involving the lower extremity can be performed with solely Type I muscle contraction. It is useful to conceive of "dynamic" exercise as involving mainly Type I muscle contraction. "Static" or "isometric" exercise involves the additional mass recruitment of Type II muscle. Using these definitions, it can be realized that the classical definitions are inadequate in describing the effects of muscular contraction on the cardiovascular system. Indeed, low-resistance, high-repetition weight work involving mainly Type I muscle will be perceived as "dynamic" exercise by the cardiovascular system. Conversely, high-intensity dynamic exercise, such as occurs above the lactate threshold, should be perceived as "isometric" exercise from the standpoint of the cardiovascular system, since it involves the use of Type II muscle. Any time there is increased recruitment of Type II muscle there are increases in sympathetic outflow, and this will directly effect myocardial performance by causing further increases in HR and blood pressure and perhaps by promoting alpha coronary vasoconstriction.

■ ACKNOWLEDGEMENT

I am indebted to Dr. James A. Nicholas, who inspired the thinking behind this work.

Current concepts on rehabilitation in sports medicine: research and clinical interrelationships

Michael Marino

Part two
Principles of rehabilitation, reconditioning,
and athletic training

Rehabilitation is a dynamic method of preventing or reversing the deleterious effects of inactivity while returning an individual to his or her former level of activity. Rehabilitation medicine became a unique discipline after World War I, when the need to restore function to injured soldiers and polio victims became an important focus of medical care. With the

Table 7-1 ■ Neuromuscular and physical performance factors*

| | Neuromuscular and physical factors (A) | | | | | | | | | | | | | | | |
| | Performance factors | | | | | | | | | | | | | | | |
Sports	Strength	Endurance	Body type	Flexibility	Balance	Agility	Speed	Coordination	SUBTOTAL A1	Timing	Reaction time	Rhythm	Steadiness	Accuracy	SUBTOTAL A2	TOTAL A
1. Archery	1	1	0	1	2	0	0	2	7	1	0	1	3	3	8	15
2. Auto racing	2	2	1	0	1	0	0	3	9	3	3	1	3	3	13	22
3. Badminton	1	2	1	2	2	2	2	3	15	2	3	2	2	2	11	26
4. Ballet	2	3	3	3	3	3	2	3	22	3	3	3	3	3	15	37
5. Ballroom dance	1	1	1	1	2	2	1	2	11	2	1	3	1	1	8	19
6. Baseball	2	1	1	2	2	2	2	3	15	3	3	2	1	3	12	27
7. Basketball	2	3	3	2	3	3	3	3	22	3	3	2	2	3	13	35
8. Bicycling	2	2	2	1	2	1	1	1	12	1	2	3	2	2	10	22
9. Big game hunting	2	3	1	1	1	1	2	3	14	3	2	2	3	3	13	27
10. Billiards	0	0	0	0	2	1	0	2	5	2	0	3	2	3	10	15
11. Bobsledding	2	2	1	1	3	1	2	2	14	3	3	2	2	3	13	27
12. Bowling	1	1	0	1	1	0	0	1	5	2	1	3	2	3	11	16
13. Boxing	3	3	2	2	3	3	3	3	22	3	3	3	3	3	15	37
14. Bridge	0	1	0	0	0	0	0	0	1	3	1	2	2	3	11	12
15. Bull fighting	3	3	2	3	3	3	3	3	23	3	3	2	2	2	12	35
16. Calisthenics	1	1	2	2	2	1	2	2	13	2	1	3	2	1	9	22
17. Canoeing	1	2	1	1	2	1	1	2	11	3	1	2	2	2	10	21
18. Camping	1	1	0	0	2	0	0	1	5	0	0	0	0	1	1	6
19. Circus acts	2	2	1	3	3	3	2	3	19	3	2	2	2	3	12	31
20. Cricket	2	2	2	2	2	2	2	3	17	3	3	2	1	2	11	28
21. Curling	1	1	0	1	2	2	1	3	11	2	1	2	2	3	10	21
22. Diving	1	1	2	3	3	3	1	3	17	3	2	2	3	3	13	30
23. Equestrian	2	2	1	2	3	2	1	3	16	3	2	2	3	2	12	28
24. Fencing	2	3	1	2	3	3	3	3	20	3	3	3	3	3	15	35
25. Field hockey	2	2	1	1	2	2	2	2	14	2	2	2	1	1	8	22
26. Figure skating	2	2	1	3	3	3	3	3	20	3	3	3	2	3	14	34
27. Fishing (deep sea)	2	2	1	1	1	1	1	1	10	3	3	2	2	1	11	21
28. Football	3	2	3	2	3	3	3	2	21	3	3	3	3	3	15	36
29. Golf	1	1	1	2	2	0	0	3	10	3	1	3	3	3	13	23
30. Gymnastics	3	2	2	3	3	3	2	3	21	3	3	3	3	3	15	36
31. Handball	2	2	1	2	2	2	2	2	15	2	3	2	2	2	11	26

From Nicholas, J.A.: Am. J. Sports Med. **3**:243, 1976. ©1976, American Orthopaedic Society for Sports Medicine.
*0, Little or no involvement; 1, Mild involvement; 2, Moderate involvement; 3, Heavy involvement.

119

Chapter 7
Current concepts on rehabilitation in sports
medicine: research and clinical interrelationships

disappearance of polio and the heightened interest in sports and lifetime recreational activity, the focus of rehabilitation science has shifted to treat individuals suffering from the demands of sports participation.[101]

DeLorme's programs for strength through muscle overload[35] re-formed the entire concept of strength training in the 1940s, and still form the basis for some exercise programs today. O'Donoghue emphasized the importance of exercise training following surgical repair of injured knees in the 1950s.[101] In the 1960s, the concept of injury prevention through exercise evolved,[9] closely followed by the development of the isokinetic concept testing and training. In the 1970s, the

Table 7-1 ■ Neuromuscular and physical performance factors—cont'd

	Neuromuscular and physical factors (A)														
	Performance factors														
Sports	Strength	Endurance	Body type	Flexibility	Balance	Agility	Speed	Coordination	SUBTOTAL A1	Timing	Reaction time	Rhythm	Steadiness	Accuracy	SUBTOTAL A2	TOTAL A
32. Hiking	1	2	1	1	1	0	0	1	7	1	1	1	1	0	4	11
33. Hockey	3	3	2	2	3	3	3	3	22	3	3	3	3	3	15	37
34. Ice skating	2	2	2	3	3	3	3	3	21	3	2	3	2	3	13	34
35. Jai alai	3	3	2	2	3	3	3	3	22	3	3	2	2	2	12	34
36. Jockey riding	3	3	3	1	3	3	2	3	21	3	3	3	2	2	13	34
37. Judo	3	2	1	3	3	3	3	3	21	3	3	3	3	3	15	36
38. Karate	2	2	2	3	3	3	2	3	20	3	2	2	3	3	13	33
39. Lacrosse	2	2	1	1	2	2	2	3	15	2	2	2	2	2	10	25
40. Modern dance	2	2	0	2	3	2	1	2	14	1	1	3	1	0	6	20
41. Motor cycling	1	1	0	0	2	0	0	3	7	3	3	2	2	3	13	20
42. Mountain climbing	3	3	1	2	2	2	1	2	16	3	3	2	3	2	13	29
43. Paddleball	2	2	2	2	2	2	2	3	17	3	3	2	1	2	11	28
44. Polo	2	2	1	1	3	3	1	3	16	3	3	2	2	3	13	29
45. Rodeo	3	3	1	2	3	2	1	3	18	3	3	2	3	3	14	32
46. Racing	3	3	2	2	2	1	1	2	16	3	2	3	3	3	14	30
47. Rugby	2	3	1	2	3	3	3	3	23	3	3	2	1	2	11	34
48. Sailing	1	2	0	0	1	2	0	2	8	2	3	2	2	3	12	20
49. Scuba diving	1	2	0	1	2	1	0	2	9	2	3	3	2	2	12	21
50. Skiing	1	2	1	2	3	3	1	3	16	1	2	2	2	1	8	24
51. Snowmobiling	2	2	0	0	2	2	0	3	11	2	2	2	2	2	10	21
52. Soccer	2	3	1	2	3	3	3	3	20	3	3	2	2	2	12	32
53. Surfing	2	3	2	0	3	3	0	3	16	3	3	2	3	3	14	30
54. Swimming	2	2	2	2	2	1	2	2	15	2	2	3	2	3	12	27
55. Table tennis	1	1	1	1	1	2	2	2	11	3	3	2	1	3	12	23
56. Tap dance	2	2	1	1	2	2	1	3	14	3	2	3	2	3	13	27
57. Tennis	1	2	1	2	2	3	2	3	16	2	2	2	2	2	10	26
58. Tumbling	1	2	2	3	3	3	2	3	19	3	2	3	2	3	13	32
59. Volleyball	2	2	2	2	3	3	2	3	19	3	3	2	1	3	12	31
60. Water polo	2	2	2	2	1	3	2	3	17	3	3	2	1	2	11	28
61. Yachting	2	3	1	0	2	2	0	3	13	3	2	1	3	3	12	25
PERFORMANCE TOTALS	111	124	76	97	139	121	91	153		156	139	135	128	146		

Part two
Principles of rehabilitation, reconditioning,
and athletic training

practice of eccentric loading for strength development became an important part of the training program for healthy and injured athletes alike.

With the last 10 years or so, the identification and quantification of the components of athletic performance, or **profiling,** has enabled the clinician to better direct training, coaching, and rehabilitation following injury. Twenty-one performance factors have been identified[100] that address the physical, mental, and environmental demands of sports participation (Tables 7-1 and 7-2) (see Appendix I). Six fundamental categories of motion have been devised to allow the layman to comprehend how athletic skills can be altered or improved.[102] The performance de-

Table 7-2 ■ Mental, psychometric, and environmental factors*

Sports	TOTAL A	Intelligence	Creativity	Alertness	Motivation	Discipline	SUBTOTAL B	TOTAL A + B	Playing Conditions	Equipment	Practice	SUBTOTAL C	FINAL TOTAL A + B + C
1. Archery	15	1	0	2	1	3	6	21	2	2	3	7	28
2. Auto racing	22	2	3	3	3	3	14	36	3	3	3	9	45
3. Badminton	26	0	1	2	1	2	6	32	3	3	2	8	40
4. Ballet	37	1	3	3	3	3	13	50	1	1	3	5	55
5. Ballroom dance	13	1	2	2	1	1	7	26	0	0	1	1	27
6. Baseball	27	1	1	3	2	2	9	36	3	2	3	8	44
7. Basketball	35	1	1	3	3	2	10	45	1	1	3	5	50
8. Bicycling	22	1	2	2	1	2	8	30	2	2	2	6	36
9. Big game hunting	27	2	2	3	2	3	12	39	1	3	2	6	45
10. Billiards	15	0	2	1	1	1	5	20	2	2	3	7	27
11. Bobsledding	27	1	1	3	2	2	9	36	0	0	3	3	39
12. Bowling	16	0	2	2	2	2	8	24	1	2	2	5	29
13. Boxing	37	1	0	3	3	3	10	47	0	1	3	4	51
14. Bridge	12	2	2	3	2	2	11	23	0	0	3	3	26
15. Bull fighting	35	2	3	3	3	3	14	49	1	2	3	6	55
16. Calisthenics	22	1	2	2	2	2	9	31	0	0	2	2	33
17. Canoeing	21	1	2	2	2	2	9	30	3	2	2	7	37
18. Camping	6	1	2	2	2	2	9	15	3	3	2	8	23
19. Circus acts	31	1	2	2	3	3	11	42	1	2	3	6	48
20. Cricket	28	1	1	2	2	2	8	36	2	3	3	8	44
21. Curling	21	1	2	1	2	2	8	29	2	2	3	7	36
22. Diving	30	1	2	2	3	2	10	40	1	1	3	5	45
23. Equestrian	28	1	2	3	2	2	10	38	2	3	3	8	46
24. Fencing	35	1	0	3	3	3	10	45	0	2	2	4	49
25. Field hockey	22	1	1	2	2	2	8	30	2	2	2	6	36
26. Figure skating	34	1	1	3	3	3	11	45	2	1	3	6	41
27. Fishing (deep sea)	21	1	0	3	2	3	9	30	0	1	2	3	33
28. Football	36	2	1	3	3	3	12	48	2	3	3	8	56
29. Golf	23	1	2	1	2	3	9	32	2	2	3	7	39
30. Gymnastics	36	0	0	3	3	3	9	45	1	1	3	5	50
31. Handball	26	0	1	2	2	2	7	33	1	1	2	4	37

From Nicholas, J.A.: Am. J. Sports Med. **3:**243, 1976. ©1976, American Orthopaedic Society for Sports Medicine.
*0, Little or no involvement; 1, Mild involvement; 2, Moderate involvement; 3, Heavy involvement.

147

Chapter 7
Current concepts on rehabilitation in sports
medicine: research and clinical interrelationships

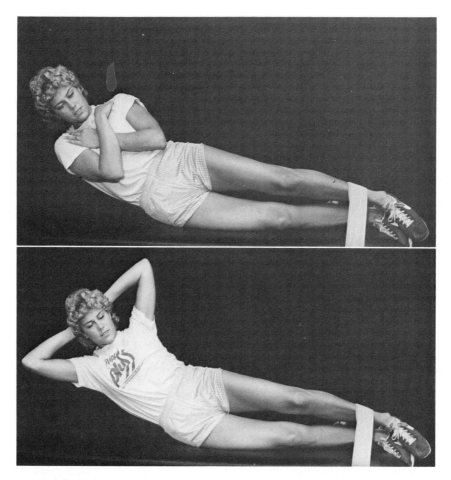

Fig. 7-22 ■ Lateral sit-up is included in all rehabilitation programs to address frequently weakened oblique muscles.

148

Part two
Principles of rehabilitation, reconditioning,
and athletic training

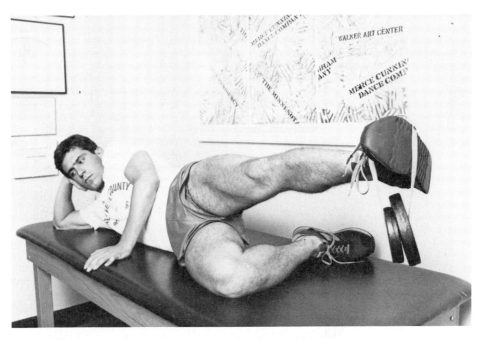

Fig. 7-23 ■ Resisted hip abduction. As with all lower extremity free weight exercises, weights are suspended from foot to strengthen all components of lower extremity link.

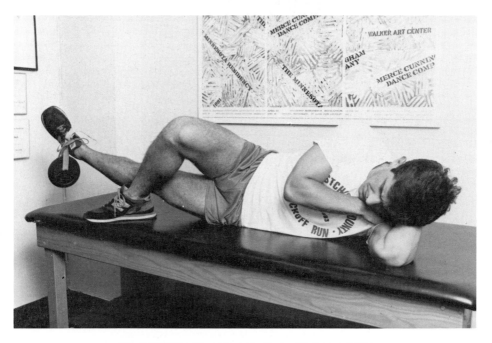

Fig. 7-24 ■ Resisted hip adduction with free weights.

149

Chapter 7
Current concepts on rehabilitation in sports
medicine: research and clinical interrelationships

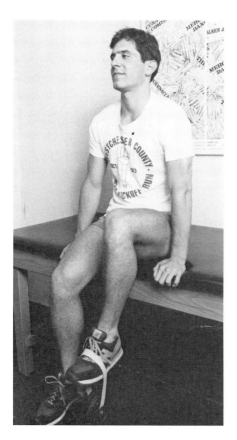

Fig. 7-25 ■ Resisted hip flexion with free weights suspended from instep of foot. Back is held erect during entire lift, which is only 8 inches off table.

hip flexors (Fig. 7-25), which anchor the quadriceps at their origin[96].

Resisted hip flexion is an important part of our rehabilitation program at IS-MAT (see Appendixes II and III [pp. 171-189]). When it is performed sitting with weight suspended from the instep, the rectus femoris is eccentrically loaded during concentric loading of the iliopsoas. There is less patellofemoral compression, as the patella remains in natural alignment in the patellofemoral groove because of the reversal of the origin and insertion of the rectus femoris. We have found this to be the most effective means of strengthening the anterior thigh without relying solely on conventional resistive knee extension and straight leg raising (Figs. 7-26 to 7-28).

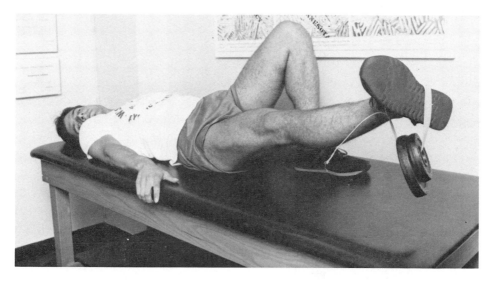

Fig. 7-26 ■ Supine straight leg raise with leg externally rotated to facilitate vastus medialis obliquus.

150

Part two
Principles of rehabilitation, reconditioning,
and athletic training

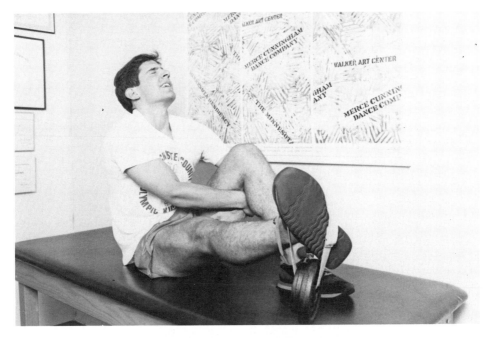

Fig. 7-27 ■ Sitting straight leg raise.

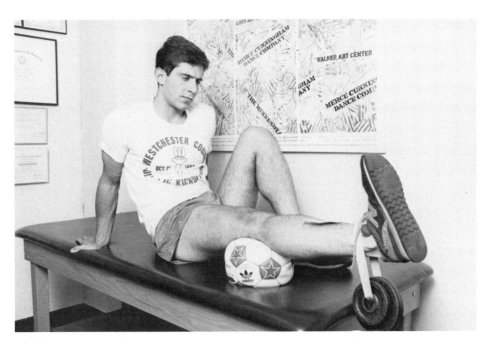

Fig. 7-28 ■ Short arc quadriceps strengthening using deflated soccer ball to control desired arc of motion.

151
Chapter 7
Current concepts on rehabilitation in sports
medicine: research and clinical interrelationships

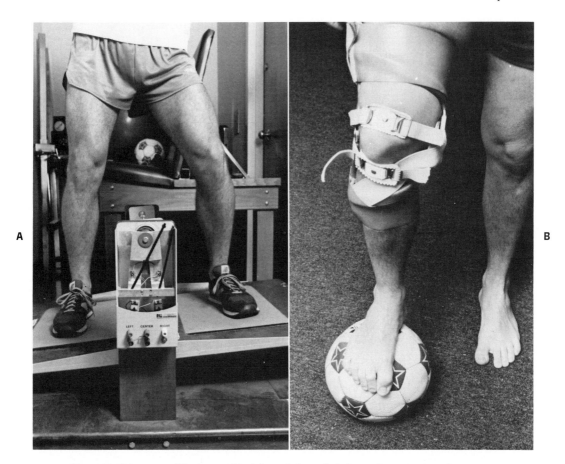

Fig. 7-29 ■ **A,** Reconditioning and training of dynamic balance, important performance demand in boxing, basketball, ballet, and football. **B,** Using soccer ball to develop weight shifting and dynamic balance in both legs following knee surgery.

We feel that muscle strengthening, like performance, should occur as a unit. Isolated strengthening exercises and machines are effective in the clinic, but their carry-over to functional activities are remote. Nowhere in normal sports activity do isolated joint motions occur. Motion results from an integrated response to the transmission and generation of forces throughout a limb, with the trunk and spine as the center. Rehabilitative exercises should integrate the muscle contractions with the performance demands that occur simultaneously during normal motion. For example, dynamic balance is an major component in downhill skiing, skateboarding, ballet, and figure skating.

Following strength exercises and as part of the actual rehabilitation program, patients practice balancing on a stabilometer to integrate reacquired motion and strength into performance-like situations (Fig. 7-29). Kinesthesis and proprioception are frequently lost following lower extremity injuries, especially following surgery. Weight-bearing exercises performed barefoot on different surfaces and with different objects stimulate sensory input (Fig. 7-29, *A*). Picking up pencils or marbles with the toes develops proprioception and dynamic balance simultaneously. Isolation of individual repetitive motions in a clinical environment is the farthest away from true athletic performance.

152

Part two
Principles of rehabilitation, reconditioning,
and athletic training

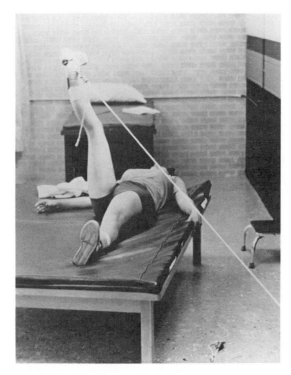

Fig. 7-30 ■ Resisted hip flexion and abduction of hip using wall pulleys.

Combining motions or patterns of motion during rehabilitation develops coordination and timing in addition to strength and motion (Fig. 7-30).

■ TRAINING PARAMETERS

At the outset of rehabilitation and following evaluation, goals must be identified with the development of the total leg as the primary target. Distinctions must be made between the development of strength and/or power, based on the performance requirements of each individual athlete. Specific rehabilitation and reconditioning exercises that mimic the athlete's on-the-field performance should be designed to redevelop each performance factor, for example, strength, balance, and anaerobic power.

Strength

Weight training is the form of exercise that has traditionally been employed to promote strength. Various forms of weight training have been documented, each reporting strength gains as a result of isometric training,[95,109,117,119] concentric training,* eccentric training,[127,135] and isokinetic training.[113,133,135,141] Ranges in strength increases have varied from 20% to over 100%, averaging 12% per week until 75% of maximal strength is obtained. Thereafter, rate of strength gain diminishes as the patient approaches his maximal strength level. These increases in strength have occurred in programs ranging from two to twelve repetition maximums and from one to six sets.† Less than maximal weight repetitions (as little as 60% of one repetition maximum) have also been demonstrated to increase strength.[5,26,30,58,113]

Increases in muscle strength develop within 6 weeks or longer.[14,28,55,58] These increments have been accompanied by al-

---

*References 10, 12, 26, 42, 113, 141, and 151.
†References 10, 11, 13, 23, 56, 112, and 138.

153

Chapter 7
Current concepts on rehabilitation in sports
medicine: research and clinical interrelationships

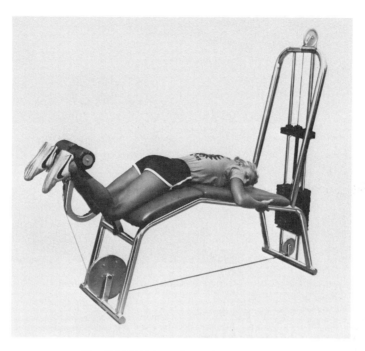

Fig. 7-31 ■ Universal exercise equipment.

terations in body composition and re-flected in an increased lean body mass, decrease in body fat, and an increase in girth measurements.[23,42,105,113,151]

Women involved in highly structured and controlled strength training programs experience similar gains in strength when compared to men on the same program, but they do not experience the same degree of hypertrophy.[151]

Isometric programs

Isometric training programs rely on contracting the muscle against fixed objects, that is, increasing tension without resultant motion. Hettinger and Muller[59] demonstrated increases of 5% of the original strength value per week as a result of one 6-second contraction per day at only 67% of maximum contraction strength.[152] Variations in contraction time (up to 45 seconds) or effort (up to 100%) did not produce significantly different gains. Although other studies have demonstrated

strength gains with isometrics, none have been able to reproduce the magnitude achieved by Hettinger and Muller.[26] Wilmore[152] reports the best results can be obtained from maximal contractions held for 6 seconds and repeated 5 to 10 times per day.

Several studies have indicated that angle-specific strength gains result from isometric training.[27] It is recommended that individuals contract the muscle at three to five angles throughout the range of motion, with 5 to 10 contractions at each joint angle.

Isotonic programs

Conventional isotonic exercise consists of raising and lowering a maximal amount of weight, whether the weight consists of large metal disks supported at the ends of a metal bar, a sophisticated system of cams and pulleys (Fig. 7-31), or a weighted towel (Fig. 7-32). All methods employ external resistance, which overloads active

Part two
Principles of rehabilitation, reconditioning,
and athletic training

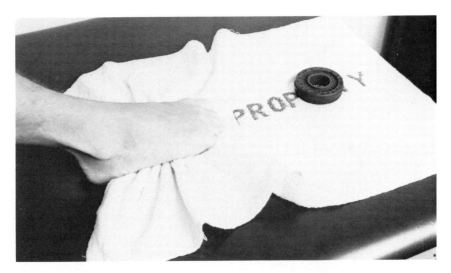

Fig. 7-32 ■ Resisted flexion of toes using weighted towel. Weak intrinsic muscles of feet are common in runners and ballet dancers.

movement. Stressing the muscles beyond the work load they are accustomed to is called the **overload principle,** and it is essential for isotonic strength gains to occur. Therefore as the muscles become stronger, they must work against proportionally greater resistance to continue gaining strength.

DeLorme[35] was the first to develop a modern strength training program that employed both the overload and progressive resistance principles. It was called the Progressive Resistive Exercise (PRE) program. Developed in 1945, this program was based on shortening the muscle against a light load for 10 repetitions and progressively increasing the resistance for each of nine additional sets of 10 contractions each. This was continued until the maximal load that could be lifted 10 times was reached, called the 10-repetition maximum,[75] the maximal amount of weight a muscle could lift through its full range of motion 10 and only 10 times. The 10-repetition maximum (10 RM) was changed weekly based on the weekly reevaluation. DeLorme was the first to use heavy resistance and low repetitions to develop strength, and light resistance and many repetitions for muscular endurance.

The shortened sequences of DeLorme and Watkins, McMorris and Elkins, and McGovern and Luscombe reported equally effective strength gains from performing three sets of 10, four sets of 10, and one set of 5 followed by one set of 10, respectively.[75] Two programs, that of Zinovieff and that of McGovern and Luscombe, reversed DeLorme's sequence and began each exercise session with 100% of 10 RM weight and decreased over 10 and three sets of 10 repetitions, respectively.[75] The rationale behind this sequence reversal was to decrease the resistance as the muscle fatigued, allowing the muscles to perform maximal work throughout the exercise period.

Current research[152] has demonstrated that three sets of five to seven maximal repetitions (5 RM to 7 RM) per session, three times per week, promote maximal strength gains.

IDEAL ISOTONIC PROGRAM

3 sets of 5 to 7 maximal repetitions, 3 times/week.

155

Chapter 7
Current concepts on rehabilitation in sports
medicine: research and clinical interrelationships

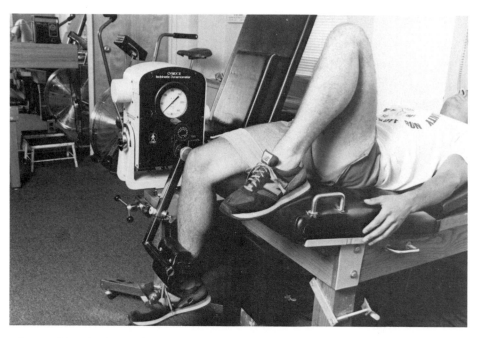

Fig. 7-33 ■ Isokinetic exercise of knee in supine position to facilitate rectus femoris-abdominal link. Note flexion of opposite hip and knee to reduce lumbar strain.

Isokinetic programs

Isokinetic exercise is a combination of the benefits of isometric and isotonic exercise, that is, the resistance is maximal throughout full range of motion at a constant velocity. Exercise is performed against a mechanism that controls limb movement at a preselected speed, thereby generating resistance in direct proportion to that applied. Unlike isotonic exercise, in which maximal loading is achieved at only the weakest point in the range of motion, isokinetic exercise permits maximal resistance at each point in the range of motion (Figs. 7-33 and 7-34).

True isokinetic devices apply maximal resistance at contractile speeds of up to 300 degrees per second for training similar to actual performance. It should be noted, however, that the specificity of isokinetic training at high speeds has not been sufficiently examined. Most athletic events, however, occur at fast velocities, and from a "specificity of training" viewpoint, it would seem reasonable to mimic those fast velocities during training.[124]

Research into the effects of strength training at different contractile speeds has yielded inconsistent results. Initial isokinetic research[94,95] showed that training at slow speeds promoted strength gains at slow contractile velocities, and training at

$$
\text{Ideal isokinetic training} \left\{ \begin{array}{l} \text{Slow} \\ \text{Medium} \\ \text{Fast} \end{array} \right\} \text{Contractile velocities}
$$

Allows strength gains at all contractile velocities.

fast speeds promoted strength gains at both fast and slow contractile velocities, suggesting that the rate of doing work was more important than the actual work done. This has since been confirmed with healthy[135] and postmeniscectomy patients.[132] Other studies have indicated that strength training is more consistent with the training velocity.[22,31,78] Although some overlap of training effects was found, the data contend that, to make strength gains at slow,

Part two
Principles of rehabilitation, reconditioning,
and athletic training

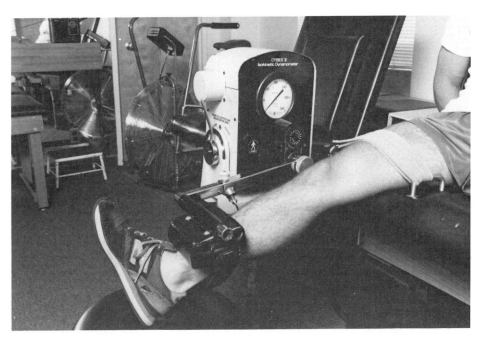

Fig. 7-34 ■ Short arc isokinetic knee extension using stool to adjust desired arc. Note external rotation of leg to strengthen screw-home mechanism of tibia on femur.

medium, and fast contractile velocities, patients must train at slow, medium, and fast speeds, respectively.[133] Clinicians should reassess muscle performance at more than one speed, since it appears that successful training at one speed may not overlap to other contractile velocities.

Variation between different methods of strength training

From the previous discussions, it can be seen that significant strength gains can be achieved from isotonic, isometric, and isokinetic training. It is up to the clinician, coach, and athlete to design a program that will promote gains necessary for the athlete's performance.

The ability to equate work loads during different forms of training (i.e., isometric vs. isotonic) is nearly impossible. One must critically assess the results obtained from different forms of weight training by examining work loads, intensities, rates, and methods of evaluation.

When comparing the differences be-
tween isometrics and isotonics, the following conclusions can be drawn:[84,152] (1) although strength gains will occur from both, isotonic exercise seems to provide greater gains; (2) muscular endurance is more effectively developed through isotonic procedures, and there is faster recovery from muscular fatigue in muscles trained isotonically; (3) isometric strength gains are angle specific; and (4) isotonically trained muscles atrophy faster than isometrically trained muscles.

Subjects trained for 5 weeks on either Nautilus or free weight equipment showed significantly equal strength gains without regard to training method or group.[127] Comparisons of the effectiveness of isokinetic over variable isotonic (Nautilus) training programs have also shown consistently equal gains in muscle strength with either training modality.[135] Yet significant gains in functional performances, that is, standing broad jump, 40-yard dash, and vertical jump, were seen in only the isokinetically trained group.

157

Chapter 7
Current concepts on rehabilitation in sports
medicine: research and clinical interrelationships

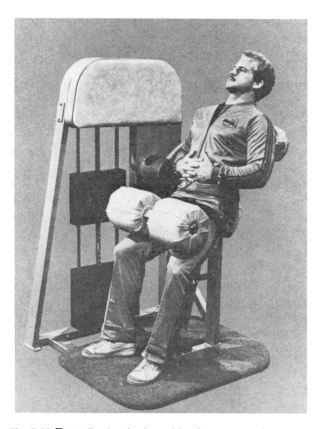

Fig. 7-35 ■ Nautilus low back machine for erector spinae group.

In athletic reconditioning, isometrics are employed during periods of immobilization or in the presence of conditions where movement is contraindicated, i.e., acute overuse tendinitis or chondromalacia. Following cast removal or a decrease in pain symptoms, isotonics or isokinetics either supplement or replace the isometric training program. Isokinetics are *not* instituted until muscle strength is well above the fair strength grade.

Much ado is being made about the necessity for eccentric weight training. Given the characteristics of an eccentric contraction, that is, increased motor unit activity and larger force generation, this concept may be valid. At ISMAT, we also emphasize the eccentric component of all our free-weight exercises. As greater loads are required for overload, eccentric exercise equipment will prove superior to free weights because they provide better mechanical efficiency and ease of lifting. Recently improved designs in Nautilus equipment now enable athletes to train the entire lower extremity link system eccentrically as well as concentrically (Figs. 7-35 to 7-43).

The greater tension developed during eccentric work may be the most effective method to stimulate adaptation in skeletal muscle.[126] The work of Komi and Buskirk[71] supports this theory, since training with maximal eccentric contractions induced more muscle growth than training with either maximal isometric or concentric contractions. Disadvantages to eccentric training include the increased risk of muscle strains because of the larger forces developed and an increased amount of muscle soreness in the initial stages of training. Eccentric weight train-

Text continued on p. 162.

158

Part two
Principles of rehabilitation, reconditioning,
and athletic training

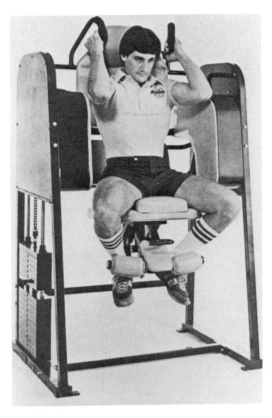

Fig. 7-36 ■ Nautilus low back machine for rectus abdominis.

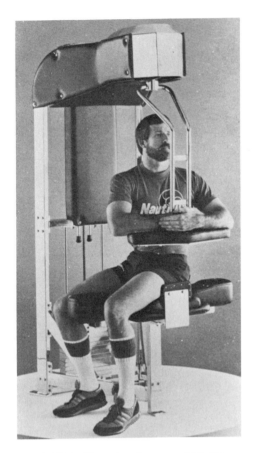

Fig. 7-37 ■ Nautilus rotary torso machine for internal and external obliques and erector spinae muscles.

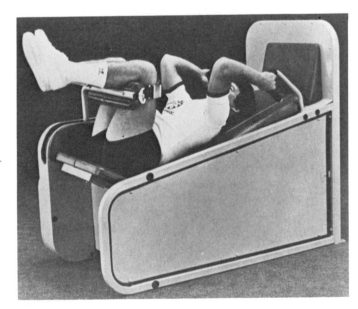

Fig. 7-38 ■ Nautilus hip flexion machine.

159

Chapter 7
Current concepts on rehabilitation in sports
medicine: research and clinical interrelationships

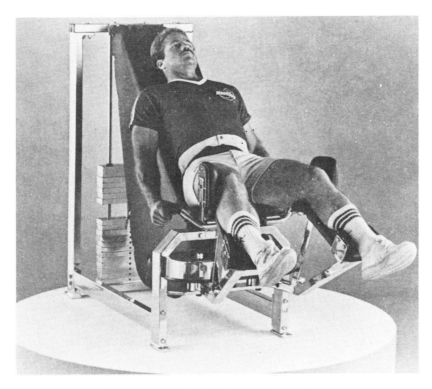

Fig. 7-39 ■ Nautilus hip abduction machine.

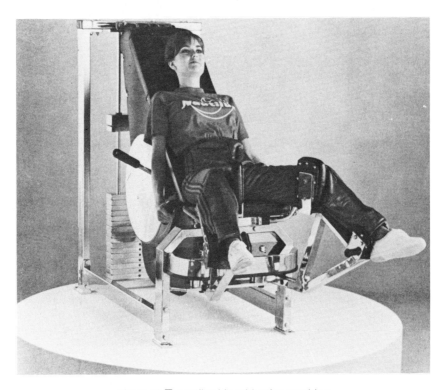

Fig. 7-40 ■ Nautilus hip adduction machine.

160

Part two
Principles of rehabilitation, reconditioning,
and athletic training

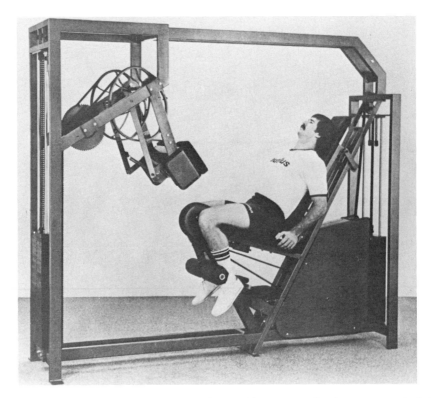

Fig. 7-41 ■ Nautilus compound leg machine for quadriceps strengthening. Leg press includes hamstrings and hip extensors strengthening.

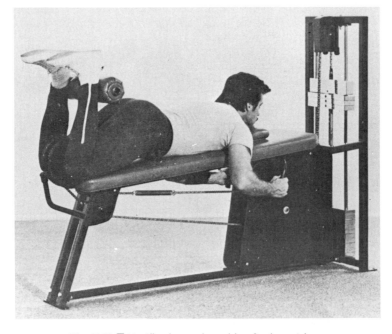

Fig. 7-42 ■ Nautilus leg curl machine for hamstrings.

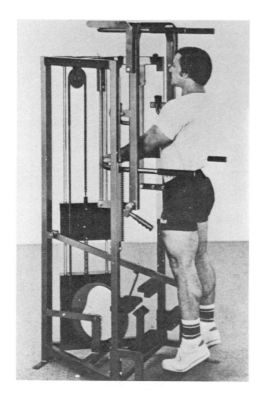

Fig. 7-43 ■ Nautilus multipurpose machine used for gastrocnemius and soleus strengthening.

Table 7-3 ■ Advantages and disadvantages of strength training equipment

	Advantages	Disadvantages
Cybex isokinetic dynamometer	Accommodating resistance at controlled velocity Permits objective assessment of muscle performance factors Reciprocal joint motions	No eccentric loading Isolated joint exercise Set-up is time-consuming Requires supervisory personnel Expensive
Orthotron	Similar to Cybex, without objective force measurement	Similar to Cybex Usable for fewer motions than Cybex
Universal Gym	Eccentric and concentric loading Circuit training Athletes can perform exercises independently	Does not accommodate resistance through range of motion Does not adequately stabilize posture No output of performance
Nautilus	Eccentric and concentric loading Circuit training Provides stabilization and support during exercise Variety of units available	Does not control velocity, although resistance accommodates to a preestablished movement arc Expensive No output of performance
Free weights	Eccentric and concentric loading Variety of motions possible Require control, stabilization, and use of entire body during exercise Inexpensive	Do not accommodate resistance through movement arc Overload muscle only at weakest point in range of motion Eccentric loading difficult and dangerous at high resistances No output

162

Part two
Principles of rehabilitation, reconditioning,
and athletic training

Table 7-4 ■ Advantages and disadvantages of cardiovascular conditioning exercises

	Advantages	Disadvantages
Endurance training	Aerobic conditioning Calorie-expending (for weight control) Associated with high ratio of high- to low-density lipoproteins Associated with low blood pressure	Overuse injury Time consuming Body-part specific No use for anaerobic power
Sprint training	Builds strength and power Builds anaerobic power	Overuse and traumatic injury No modification of "risk factors" Nonaerobic Body-part specific Decreases flexibility
Interval and Fartlek*	Some aerobic training Builds strength and power Tends to exercise larger muscle mass ? Modification of "risk factors"	Overuse and traumatic injury
Circuit	Some aerobic benefit Anaerobic power Involves many muscles No modification of "risk factors"	Traumatic injuries Decreases flexibility

*Fartlek training is similar to interval training in terms of effect. The difference is that Fartlek training uses unequal rest/exercise intervals and is usually performed on uneven terrain.

ing equipment, such as Eagle or Nautilus, minimizes the hazards of lowering large amounts of weight eccentrically. Whether working concentrically, isokinetically, or eccentrically, the focus should not be on the type of muscle contraction but on the strengthening and retraining of the entire lower extremity linkage system (Tables 7-3 and 7-4).

■ ELECTRICAL STIMULATION FOR STRENGTH GAINS

Much evidence yields to the premise that the force of maximal muscle contractions is the stimulus for strength gains. A question raised recently is whether the maximal force generation must be voluntarily elicited; can it be involuntarily generated via electrical stimulation? This idea of electrically stimulating healthy muscle tissue to promote strength gains was first reported by Dr. Yakov Kots of the Soviet Union. He reported 10% to 30% greater isometric force generation in healthy

muscle with electrical stimulation than with voluntary contraction. He also demonstrated 30% to 40% increases in muscle strength in already highly-trained athletes.[72] Unfortunately, detailed descriptions of Kots' methods are unavailable.

Therapeutic use of electrical stimulation (ES) to retard atrophy during immobilization is well known, but the effect of ES application to healthy tissue is just beginning to be studied. Although it appears logical on a theoretic basis, research has yet to duplicate the results of Kots.

The Soviet technique of ES is thought to use an interrupted medium-frequency sinusoidal current of 1600 to 2500 cycles per second, modulated by interruptions of 10 msec duration between continuous outputs of 10 msec duration.[72] The intensity is the maximal amount of current a patient can tolerate without pain. Current is most commonly applied using the bipolar technique. Only one commercially available ES unit, the Electrostim 180

163

Chapter 7
Current concepts on rehabilitation in sports
medicine: research and clinical interrelationships

(Numed, Joliet, Ill.) claims to reproduce Kots' current. A thorough description of the unit with appropriate treatment parameters was performed by Owens and Malone.[111]

A treatment session consists of 10 tetanic contractions, each lasting 10 seconds and followed by a 50-second rest period. Ten contractions simulate a maximal work load, paralleling DeLorme's 10 RM principle for strength gains. Optimal gains were reported after 20 to 25 treatment sessions administered over 4 to 5 weeks.

For ES to result in strength gains Kots states that the current must be of sufficient intensity to evoke a maximal tetanic contraction in all muscle fibers, and to recruit all muscle fibers the current must produce little or no pain.[72]

Many studies are available now that compare the effects of ES with different muscle contractions in both healthy and immobilized situations. Although initial clinical studies[86,106] did not support the effectiveness of ES for development of muscle strength, new stimulation devices and tighter research protocols have found otherwise.

The immediate effects of ES, that is, depletion of ATP, creatine phosphokinase, and glycogen stores and increased formation of lactate[41] are similar to those found following intense isometric exercise. Long-term ES, that is 4 to 5 weeks, did not cause any significant changes in enzyme activities, muscle fiber characteristics, or mitochondrial properties in human quadriceps.[41] However, significantly increased tissue contractile proteins, decreased collagen content, and elevated levels of muscular fuels, mitochondral contact, and oxidative metabolism, which produced a delayed onset of fatigue, were found following in vivo electrical stimulation of the gastrocnemius muscles of intact frogs.[45]

Two weeks of either superimposing ES on a maximal voluntary contraction or training with maximal voluntary contractions alone produced similar gains in muscle strength.[32] Five weeks of ES alone or isometric quadriceps exercise alone both produced statistically significant increases in muscle torque.[77] Isometric abdominal strength and endurance were increased after a 5-week program of ES.[58] Ankle evertor muscle strength was also increased, consistent with isometric strength gains after 3 weeks of ES.[115]

The effect of ES on dynamically measured muscle strength has been less dramatic. In a study by Halback and Straus,[53] two groups were trained for 3 weeks each with either isokinetics or electrical stimulation. The isokinetic group demonstrated twice as much gain in isokinetic torque as did the group that performed ES alone. This appears consistent with the findings of Eriksson and Haggmark et al. that the effects of ES appeared more "position-specific" and less "speed-specific" than those of voluntary training with slow isokinetic contractions.[40] Romero et al. also felt that ES had little carry-over to affect dynamic or high-speed muscle strength.[123]

Electrical stimulation for immobilized muscle

ES during immobilization has become a popular means of retarding atrophy and minimizing the effects of inactivity on injured or immobilized muscle tissue. Studies comparing conventional isometric exercise and ES in conjunction with isometric exercises have come out clearly in favor of the ES group.[40,140,150]

A group of patients[40] undergoing rehabilitation following anterior cruciate reconstruction received standard isometric quadriceps-setting exercises during plaster immobilization. A similar group received the same, but underwent ES through a hole in the cast for 1 hour a day, 5 days a week, for 4 weeks. The stimulated group showed better clinical muscle function and significantly higher succinate dehydrogenase (SDH) activity as determined by muscle biopsy. (SDH activity is a measure of the mitochondral oxidative capacity.)

Part two
Principles of rehabilitation, reconditioning,
and athletic training

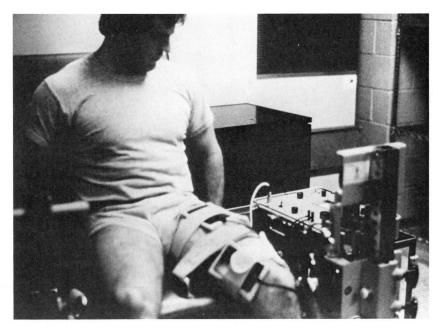

Fig. 7-44 ■ Using Electro-Stim 180 to facilitate maximal quadriceps contraction during isokinetic rehabilitation exercises.

Twenty treatments of ES to the quadriceps femoris of 50 patients with chondromalacia patellae demonstrated an increase in quadriceps strength ranging from 25.3% to 200%. Quadriceps girth increased 5.1%. The authors also found the results were directly proportional to the frequency and intensity of the treatment.[66]

At ISMAT, especially with the professional and competitive athletes, we have found the EMS 180 to be an effective adjunct to either isokinetic or isotonic weight training. Units can be used during immobilization, before exercise (Fig. 7-44), or simultaneously with isokinetic equipment to facilitate the intensity of a weak muscle contraction. Subjectively, patients report improved muscle tone at a more rapid rate when ES accompanies rehabilitation exercises.

■ FLEXIBILITY

Flexibility is the ability to move unresisted through full range of motion and is as important to an athlete as strength,

cardiovascular conditioning, or timing. Flexibility is an important trait because the fullest muscle-tendon length gives a more efficient contraction.[101]

Flexibility is only one by-product of stretching, and is best achieved through a series of slow, steady, sustained stretches of the muscle-tendon unit (Fig. 7-45). As muscle fibers become more flexible, extensible, and elastic, greater range of movement is permitted, thus decreasing the excessive stress applied to muscles and muscle fibers during activity.[131] Flexible muscles reduce the chance of injury.[69,131]

Stretching exercises are an important aspect of rehabilitation, where early mobilization may limit the loss of motion, retard atrophy, prevent permanent tissue scarring, preserve joint range, disperse edema, reduce pain, and stimulate reciprocal muscle function.[125]

Assessment of joint motion

Both active and passive range of individual joint motions are most accurately

165

Chapter 7
Current concepts on rehabilitation in sports
medicine: research and clinical interrelationships

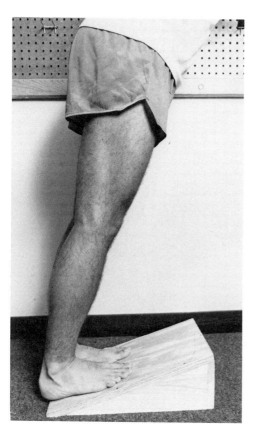

Fig. 7-45 ■ Passive stretching of gastrocsoleus group.

measured with a goniometer.[88] During rehabilitation or reconditioning, this is the most objective means of measuring progress. Goniometric measurements are time consuming, however, and do not readily lend themselves to rapid measurement of many motions or to many individuals, as in screening programs. It is also difficult for the individual to measure his or her own progress without the help of an experienced trainer, therapist, or physician.

In these situations, functional tests of flexibility are used. Perhaps the most well-known and most frequently documented are the Nicholas tests of flexibility,[99] which are used more as a guide to an individual's joint characteristics rather than as a demonstration of progress during a rehabilitation program. Nevertheless, baseline flexibility data of the uninvolved limb are

essential when assessing an athlete's ability to return to play.

For more practical purposes, we use the sit-and-reach test to assess low back and lower extremity flexibility, the back hyperextension test to assess trunk flexibility, and the shoulder mobility test to assess upper body flexibility.

Sit-and-reach test (Fig. 7-46)

To measure the sit-and-reach, the individual sits on the floor with the legs extended directly in front and the knees in extension. The dorsiflexed feet are placed against a box or stool to which a yardstick is attached, with the 14-inch mark placed at the point where the feet contact the box. Placing the middle fingers of both hands one on top of the other, the individual reaches forward slowly as far as possible along the yardstick for three consecutive tries. On the third attempt, the reach is held for 1 second while the distance reached is recorded. The examiner is careful to monitor that the knees are kept extended and that the subject does not bounce into position. Standards for an athletic population are presented according to Wilmore[141] (Table 7-5).

Back hyperextension

The back hyperextension test is a measure of lower back flexibility and is performed with the subject prone, lying on the floor. With the feet stabilized, the subject arches the back and, keeping the arms at the sides, attempts to lift the chin as far off the floor as possible. An examiner measures the distance between the floor and the sternal notch. Then the subject sits upright on the floor with the back and buttocks against a wall, and the perpendicular distance between the sternal notch and floor is measured again. The flexibility score is computed by dividing the hyperextension height by the seated height and multiplying by 100. Dividing the hyperextension height by the seated height provides an estimate of the angle of flexibility, and partially negates the advan-

Part two
Principles of rehabilitation, reconditioning,
and athletic training

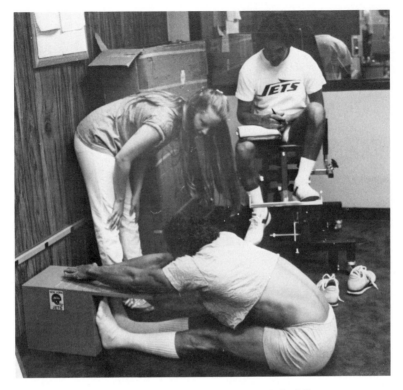

Fig. 7-46 ■ Assessment of sit-and-reach flexibility.

Table 7-5 ■ Standards for the sit-and-reach and back hyperextension flexibility tests

	Sit and reach	Back hyperextension
Excellent	22 inches or greater	56 or greater
Good	20 to 21 inches	46 to 55
Average	14 to 18 inches	36 to 45
Fair	12 to 13 inches	26 to 35
Poor	11 inches or less	25 or less

From Wilmore, J.H.: Training for sport and activity: the physiological basis of the conditioning process, ed. 2, Boston, 1982, Allyn & Bacon, Inc.

tage of having a long trunk.[141] Standards are presented in Table 7-5.

Shoulder mobility

A simple test of shoulder mobility is performed by having the subject touch his hands behind his back, once with the right arm going behind the head and the left hand from behind the back, then vice versa. These two tests give adequate indication of the internal and external rotation of the shoulder joints. Measurement can be made in either of two ways: (1) the vertebra that each middle finger can reach is recorded, or (2) the distance the hands overlap is recorded. If the hands do not touch, this is recorded in negative numbers.

Clinical limitations of range of motion
Muscle

The principal sources of passive resistance at the extremes of joint motion are primarily connective tissue structures, i.e., ligaments, joint capsules, tendons, and the connective tissue framework and sheath within and around the myofibrillar elements of muscle.[128] In an injured state, scar tissue, adhesions, and fibrative con-

167

Chapter 7
Current concepts on rehabilitation in sports
medicine: research and clinical interrelationships

tractures, all forms of connective tissue, may limit range of motion as well.

Connective tissue, which is viscoelastic in nature, by definition exhibits both elastic and plastic qualities. (Elastic tissues return to their original state after deformation. Plastic tissues do not return to their original state and exhibit some degree of deformation after loading.) Range of motion exercises therefore should be designed to promote plastic deformation of connective tissue elements.[128] Exercises should take into account such external factors as applied tensile force intensity and duration of loading.

Muscle spasm vs. contracture. It is important to differentiate between a muscle spasm and a muscle contracture. A muscle spasm is a prolonged, continuous contraction of muscle and is usually the most common manifestation of musculoskeletal pathology. Spasms are frequently associated with contusions and strains. For the most part, muscle spasm is a secondary reaction of guarding or splinting phenomenon to protect a pathologic condition or prevent painful movement, as in an unreduced dislocation or untreated fracture. Muscle spasm may also be a primary manifestation of a viral infection.[157]

A contracture, on the other hand, is a physical shortening of the connective tissue of muscle that is not alleviated by conventional stretching techniques. Some authors feel a contracture can be reduced through physical therapy.[157]

Synovium

The synovium can limit range of motion. The following five signs, outlined by Zohn and Mennell[157] will help in the differentiation:

1. Redness. An increase in circulation around joints, or erythema, is a common sign of synovitis.
2. Heat. Intracapsular inflammation is also a sign of synovitis.
3. Stiffness, or increased resistance to movement through the available

range of motion, is usually caused by inflammation of the synovium and capsule.

4. Discomfort. The synovium is insensitive to pain, and accompanying pain is caused by involvement of adjacent well-innervated capsule and ligaments. Pain from synovitis is usually diffuse, poorly localized, and present usually at the extremes of motion.
5. Swelling, either caused by the presence of fluid or swelling of the soft tissues themselves.

Treatment of limitations of range of motion

High-force, short-duration stretching attacks the elastic tissue components, whereas low-force, long-duration stretching facilitates plastic deformation.[128] Elevated tissue temperatures have also been shown to reduce stiffness, thereby increasing the extensibility of connective tissue.[128] Combining low-force, long-duration stretching with moist hot packs has been shown to be an effective means of promoting permanent elongation of connective tissue in the injured muscle.[128] Prentice,[114] on the other hand, found cold to be more effective than heat in stretching muscle tissue for relaxation. Whether heat or cold is used, prolonged stretching still appears to be the most consistently effective means of reducing a muscle contracture.

Some therapists feel that passive stretching is harmful to muscle tissue. Not only is it painful, but it may elicit a stretch reflex contraction in the agonist muscle if the spinal cord is intact.[25]

Like any component of training, there are various methods of achieving increased range of motion through stretching. Stretching consists of applying a force to lengthen the muscle against its own resistance. It can be applied actively, through contraction of antagonist muscle groups, or passively, through external application of resistance. Some authors[70,125,131] feel that active or active-assisted stretching is far more effective to promote movement and less damaging to sensitive joint tissues.

Dynamic stretching is most frequently performed two ways, ballistically, or using the neurophysiologic mechanisms of inhibition developed by Knott and Voss.[70] **Static stretching**, the most common technique, consists of simply holding the lengthened position for a period of time, followed by relaxation. Ballistic stretching uses body momentum to force muscle tissues to elongate, usually against their own resistance. This bouncing stretch is thought to elicit muscle spindle activity and the quick stretch reflex, which only facilitates contraction of the muscle. Ballistic stretching may induce minute muscle tears as a result of misjudging stretch tolerance,[131] and is to be *avoided*.

Proprioceptive neuromuscular facilitation

Proprioceptive neuromuscular facilitation (PNF) has been shown to be the most effective means of increasing range of motion while increasing strength, especially in athletes.[61,70,114,131] PNF is the clinical application of basic neurophysiologic principles to promote strength, increase range of motion, facilitate the normal developmental sequence, and promote stability. The theory behind PNF states that functional movement does not occur in cardinal planes, such as pure flexion or extension, but occurs in three-dimensional spiral, or diagonal, patterns that incorporate all motions of a joint, such as flexion, adduction, and external rotation of the shoulder, or flexion, abduction, and internal rotation of the hip. Normal movement is facilitated through stimulation of proprioceptors and reflex responses by maximal resistance, stretch, touch, pressure, traction, and verbal commands.

For athletic applications, the four PNF neurophysiologic principles described here are easily applied.

Autogenic inhibition (AI). When a muscle contracts, it is inhibited by its own Golgi tendon organs. AI is used when relaxation is desired and an increase of range of motion is needed. The therapist calls for a hold or isotonic contraction of the agonist in the fully elongated position, followed by a command to relax. The therapist then attempts to elongate the muscle further in combination with a contraction of the antagonist muscle.

Reciprocal inhibition (RI). RI is based on the principle that when a muscle contracts its antagonist is inhibited. It is used when smooth, reciprocal movements are desired at a slower or faster rate, or when the goal is relaxation of the antagonist.

Successive induction (SI). When a muscle contracts its antagonist is prepared for contraction. SI is used when muscle imbalance exists between two antagonists. The therapist calls for a contraction in the stronger musculature, followed by a contraction in the weaker. This can be done with active motion, reciprocal isotonic or isokinetic equipment, or isometrics.

Irradiation. Irradiation is the overflow of neural stimulation between adjacent anterior horn cells to elicit a better motor response. Irradiation can be used to facilitate the weaker muscle in a pattern where the rest of the muscles are strong.

■ ■ ■

As seen from the techniques just described, PNF is not only facilitory. Inhibitory techniques such as contract relax (CR), and hold relax (HR) are used to promote flexibility by decreasing resistive antagonistic tone in opposing muscles.

CR is the isotonic contraction of the antagonist, allowing range of motion in rotation against maximal resistance but no movement in the other components, followed by a period of relaxation. The therapist moves the limb passively into the agonist pattern to the point where limitation is felt, elicits a maximal antagonist contraction, then instructs the patient to relax. Having felt the patient "let go," the therapist again moves the part passively

179

Chapter 7
Current concepts on rehabilitation in sports
medicine: research and clinical interrelationships

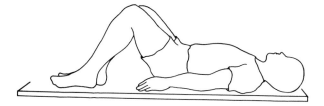

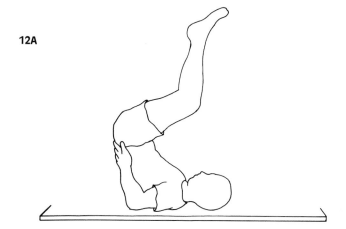

12A

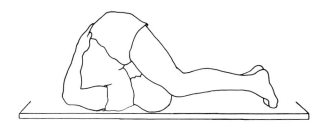

12B

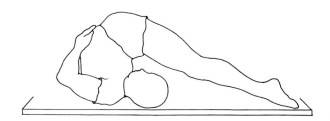

Part two
Principles of rehabilitation, reconditioning,
and athletic training

Exercise 3. Posterior hip, lower back, and iliotibial band stretch (Fig. 13)

Starting position: Lie on your back with your arms out to the sides.

Action: Lift your right leg over your left leg, placing your left hand on the back of your right thigh. Keep your right arm extended out to the side and both shoulders flat on the table. If possible, try to extend your right knee out to accentuate the stretch. Repeat on the opposite side.

Exercise 4. Posterior thigh, back, and iliotibial band stretch (Fig. 14)

Starting position: Sit comfortably on the floor or mat with your legs out in front of you.

Action: With your left leg straight, put your right foot flat on the ground on the opposite side of your left knee. Reach over your right leg with your left arm so that your elbow is on the outside of your right leg. Slowly turn your head and look over your right shoulder and, at the same time, turn your upper body toward your right arm. Keep your hips flat on the floor at all times. Repeat this exercise on the opposite side.

NOTE: If you do not feel a stretch at all while doing this exercise, then begin the exercise with your left knee bent and rotated next to the right hip.

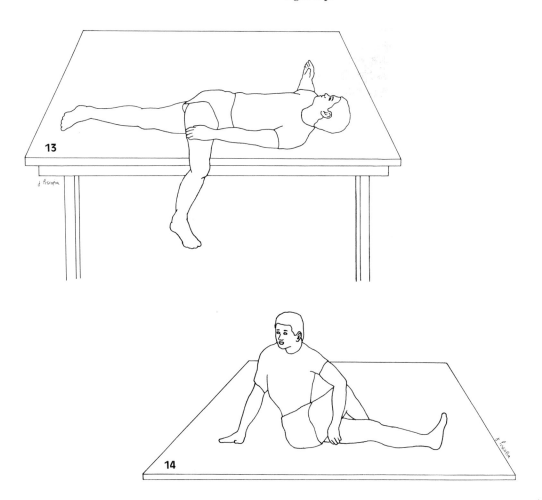

181

Chapter 7
Current concepts on rehabilitation in sports
medicine: research and clinical interrelationships

Exercise 5. Anterior thigh stretch (Fig. 15)

Starting position: Stand on a level surface with one arm holding onto a chair or wall for support.

Action: With the free hand, grasp the instep of the foot and bring the heel of the foot back toward your buttocks. When you experience a stretching sensation in the front portion of the thigh, hold the leg at that position.

NOTE: You should be standing straight up throughout the entire exercise. Do not bend forward.

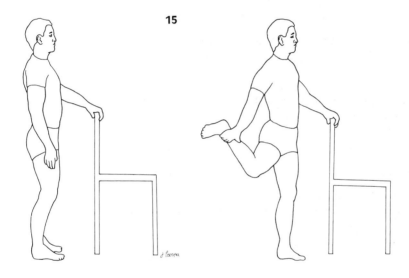

15

Part two
Principles of rehabilitation, reconditioning,
and athletic training

Exercise 6. Anterior thigh stretch (Fig. 16)

Starting position: Lie on your back on a table with the leg that has to be stretched hanging over the side of the table. Pull your right knee toward your chest and use your right arm to hold it.

Action: Grasp the instep of the foot and bring the heel back in the direction of the buttocks. Avoid arching your back.

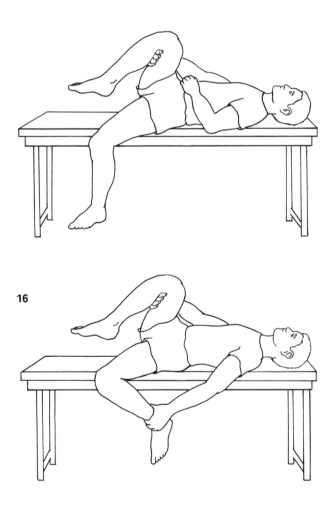

16

183

Chapter 7
Current concepts on rehabilitation in sports
medicine: research and clinical interrelationships

Exercise 7. Anterior thigh stretch (Fig. 17)

Starting position: Kneel on your hands and knees on a floor or mat.

Action: Bring your right foot up next to your right hand. Rock forward, keeping your left leg relaxed. Reach back with your right hand and grab the left foot. Pull the left foot up toward your buttocks, keeping your hips forward. Hold this stretch for 5 seconds. Let go of your left foot and return to the original supporting position. Support your body weight on your left foot, lifting your left knee up off the mat. Bending your elbows, drop your trunk forward, keeping your left knee straight, until you feel a stretch in the front of the left thigh. Hold this position for 5 seconds. Relax and repeat on the opposite leg.

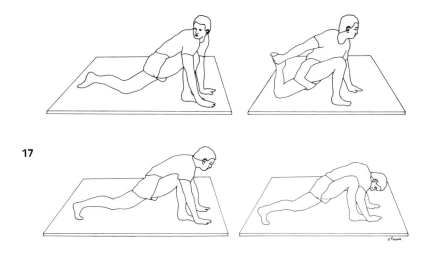

17

Part two
Principles of rehabilitation, reconditioning,
and athletic training

Exercise 8. Posterior thigh stretch (Fig. 18)

Starting position: Sit with your legs straight out in front of you and your knees flat on the mat (Fig. 18A).

Action: Slowly reach your hands out towards your toes, grasping onto your legs. Continue reaching until you experience a stretching sensation in the posterior portion of your legs. Hold that position by grasping the legs. As the stretching sensation diminishes, reach further down your legs (Fig. 18B).

NOTE: Make sure both knees remain straight throughout the exercise. If you are unable to stretch comfortably, hold onto your legs to obtain the stretch and use a towel hooked around your feet to support the stretch (Fig. 18C).

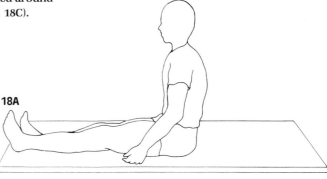

18A

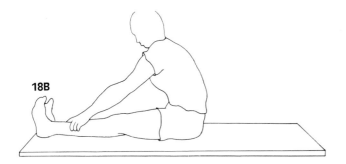

18B

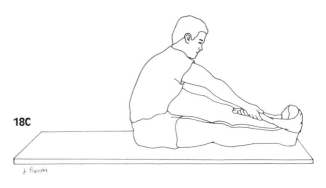

18C

J. Piscopia

205

Chapter 8
Principles of therapeutic modalities:
implications for sports injuries

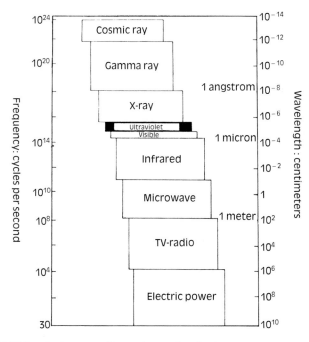

Fig. 8-5 ■ The electromagnetic spectrum of radiant energy.

From Anderson, W.T.: Instrumentation for ultraviolet therapy. In Licht, S., ed.: Therapeutic
electricity and ultraviolet radiation, ed. 2, New Haven, 1967, Elizabeth Licht, Publisher.

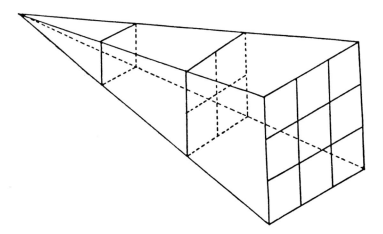

Fig. 8-6 ■ Schematic illustration of the inverse square law, showing that when
radiation is from a point source, as in microwave diathermy or infrared lamps, the
intensity of radiation falling on a surface is inversely proportional to the square of
the distance of the surface from the source.

From Stoner, E.K.: Luminous and infrared heating. In Licht, S., ed.: Therapeutic heat and cold, New
Haven, 1965, Elizabeth Licht, Publisher.

206

Part two
Principles of rehabilitation
reconditioning, and athletic training

one surface separating the two media. This is called *refraction*. Penetration occurs when beams of radiant energy pass through a medium without becoming incorporated into the medium or affecting the medium; it is also called *transmission*. *Absorption* is the incorporation of energy from one medium to another, resulting in a physiologic or chemical change (e.g., phosphorescence).

When radiant energy is administered from any source, the intensity of the radiation varies inversely with the square of the distance from the source (Fig. 8-6). This is called the inverse square law.

RADIANT ENERGY

Inverse square law

Intensity is inversely related to the square of the distance from the source

Cosine law

Radiation is maximum when the angle of application is perpendicular to the surface

---

The cosine law states that patients receive maximum radiation if the source of radiation is positioned at right angles to the irradiated surface. As the angle of application deviates from 90 degrees, treatment effectiveness decreases.

■ ELECTROTHERAPY

Electricity is the flow of electrons between two charged points or bodies. Charged atoms, either positive or negative, are classified by the relative amount of electrons (negative) to protons (positive) located in the nucleus of an atom. An atom with more electrons than protons is negatively charged, while an atom with more protons than electrons is positively charged. Electrons will flow from an area of high concentration to an area of low concentration (i.e., from a negatively charged point to a positively charged point). This difference in electrical charge or potential of two points is called the electromotive force

(EMF). EMF is the driving force behind electron flow.

The electrical potential of a point or body (EMF) is determined by the direction and amount of electron movement. The higher the concentration gradient, the more electrons will flow and the higher the electron potential will be. Electrical potential is expressed in volts (V). The amount of volts, or voltage, depends on the relative number of electrons that flow across the concentration gradient. If the charge of the two points is the same, there will be no concentration gradient and no flow of electricity. The poles or terminals of a battery or electrical stimulator are charged points, and when they are connected, this causes the flow of electricity from the negative to the positive pole.

Electricity flows between two points of different electrical potential only if they are connected by a conductor. A conductor is any material that will carry the flow of electrons. A good conductor is composed of atoms that have more electrons than protons, called free electrons. Metals such as copper, aluminum, and silver have many free electrons and good conductors. The more free electrons, the better the conductor, and the more easily current will flow. Compounds composed of atoms in which the number of protons equals the number of electrons are nonconductors. Glass, air, and rubber are examples of nonconductors; these have no free electrons. Nonconductors can be used to insulate conductors and prevent the flow of electricity.

Since there are no pure conductors of electrical energy, there is always some resistance to current flow. This resistance is measured in ohms. The better the conductor, the lower the resistance. Given a choice, electricity will always take the path of least resistance through the best conductor. Resistance not only varies with the material of the conductor but also with the length and diameter of the conductor. The longer the conductor and the

213

Chapter 8
Principles of therapeutic modalities:
implications for sports injuries

overuse and misuse syndromes in athletes.[9] Hydrocortisone, another antiinflammatory medication, is applied under the positive pole. It has been shown effective for myositis, arthritis,[47] and shinsplints.[28] Iodine, a sclerolytic agent, applied under the negative pole has been used to treat scar tissue[104] and adhesions. Salicylate, derived from acetylsalicylic acid (ASA; aspirin) dissolved in water, is applied under the negative pole for its analgesic effect.[34]

Transcutaneous electrical nerve stimulation

Pain is a sensory experience resulting from a complex pattern of stimuli, which can be generated either at the pain site[80] or displaced from the location of the stimulus (referred pain).[107] Unimodal nociceptors respond specifically to noxious stimuli.[11] Other receptors that respond to temperature changes (thermoreceptors), chemical fluctuations (chemoreceptors), or position sense and movement (proprioceptors) may all become nociceptors if the specific stimuli that excite them have a sufficiently high threshold.[80] These receptors are polymodal nociceptors. For example, when a tight joint is stretched, proprioceptors will not only respond to the changes in joint angle but also, when the available range of motion is stressed, a higher discharge frequency stimulates the perception of pain.

History

Using electrical stimulation to treat acute and chronic pain conditions is not new: the early Greeks and Romans used live torpedo fish to generate afferent electrical impulses.[106] Man-made electrical stimulators replaced fish in the eighteenth and nineteenth centuries, when medical galvanism (DC) was a common form of medical treatment. Traditionally electrical stimulation was used for its potential to evoke involuntary muscle contractions through motor nerve fiber or direct muscle stimulation.

Modern concepts

Not until 1965, with the publication of Melzack and Wall's theories on gate control of pain perception, did electrical currents become popular again for the treatment of painful conditions[69] (i.e., for its sensory as opposed to motor effects). The **gate-control theory** of pain perception states generally that a painful sensation (nociception) is transmitted to the central nervous system via small-diameter peripheral nerves, namely, the A-delta and C fibers. Melzack and Wall's theory suggests that pain-activated cells in the cord can either be facilitated or, more commonly, inhibited by input from other sensory fibers. According to Bishop,[11] the theory states that transmission of sensation is controlled by the balance of activity in small-diameter, slow-conducting fibers (A-delta and C) and large-diameter, fast-conducting fibers entering the spinal cord. According to the gate-control theory, low-level activity in the small fibers that carry impulses from the nociceptors is normally blocked at the first synapse by activity in large primary fibers and by activity in fibers descending from higher brain regions. The "gate" at the first synapse is opened by intense activity in small fibers, as would occur with intense, painful stimulation during tissue damage. A predominance of activity in large fibers closes the gate; a predominance of activity in small fibers opens the gate. Hence the gate through which pain signals are transmitted to the transmitter cells is variable.

Studies have tested[108] and confirmed[72] the gate-control theory. Patients reported temporary relief of pain that occasionally outlasted the period of stimulation. Studies that directly recorded spinal cord neurons later confirmed that those cells activated by A-delta and C fibers were inhibited by stimulation of low-threshold sensory afferents.[94]

The effectiveness of transcutaneous electrical nerve stimulation (TENS) has also been explained by stimulating increased levels of endorphins. Endorphins

Part two
Principles of rehabilitation
reconditioning, and athletic training

are endogenous opiate peptides that act as agonists at opiate receptor sites. They are released from various regions of the brainstem as well as from the pituitary gland. Enkephalins refer to the specific pentapeptides—methionine- and leucine-enkephalin—that were identified by Hughes et al. in 1975.[44] Enkephalins are composed only of a small segment of the polypeptide chain of which endorphins are composed, yet they also act as agonists at opiate receptor sites.[100] In general the actions of endogenous opiate substances are similar to those of morphine.[41]

Endogenous opioids may induce analgesia by specifically interfering with the processing of pain and preventing pain information from involving the limbic structures,[83] which mediate the affective and motivational components of the pain experience[100] by activating an efferent brainstem pain-suppression system[8] or by activating serotonergic mechanisms.[100]

Electroanalgesia, the term used to describe a decrease in pain sensation resulting from TENS, is activated by three

> **MECHANISMS OF TENS EFFECTS**
>
> Inhibition of spinal cord neurons
> Direct peripheral blockade of nerve fibers
> Indirect activation of central mechanisms of pain suppression

known mechanisms: (1) inhibition of spinal cord neurons involved in the nociceptive transmission process through activation of large-diameter, low-threshold sensory fibers; (2) direct peripheral blockade of nerve fibers or endings by electrical stimulation; and (3) in special conditions, indirect activation of brain mechanisms involved in pain suppression that lead to neurochemical inhibition of lower centers.

Not all patients experience electroanalgesia or relief of symptoms nor do all conditions respond to this therapy. Results obtained from electrical stimulation

Table 8-1 ■ Treatment mode selection chart

Mode and description	Analogous characteristics of pulse	Typical parameters	Sensation	Strength
1. Conventional (C) First choice Most frequently used mode Wide range of effectiveness in acute, chronic, and post-op pain	Similar to the rapid beat of small drums, gentle and constant, masking the pain messages just below the skin	A medium number of pulses (85 pps) of low energy (75 μsec) and low amplitude (10 mA)	Tingling (paresthesia) without muscle contraction	Comfortable

239

Chapter 8
Principles of therapeutic modalities:
implications for sports injuries

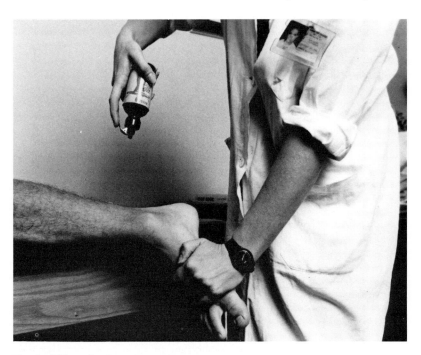

Fig. 8-18 ■ Application of ethyl chloride spray to the posterior tibial tendon using the spray and stretch technique of Travell and Simon.

ful for treating deep muscle strains and as an effective aid to reduce soreness after exercise.

Chemical sprays

Ethyl chloride and fluoromethane spray coolants have been used in sports for many years to reduce local spasm and hemorrhage caused by acute injury.[48] In rehabilitation they are used to anesthetize the skin, allowing passive lengthening of contracted muscle tissue[107,115] (Fig. 8-18). Extreme caution must be taken when applying chemical sprays, since skin temperature can be lowered to 39.2° F (4° C) and can produce second- and third-degree damage.[67] Only a few brief strokes are sufficient to decrease skin sensation. Continued spraying, which may cool the muscle, will prove counterproductive when attempting to passively elongate the muscle spasm.[107,115]

The application of ethyl chloride spray through a protective dressing, sock, or fabric sleeve lessens the danger of skin burn.[55]

Indications

Cold therapy is indicated in the treatment of most sports injuries. Inflammatory conditions can be cooled initially to decrease swelling, pain, and associated muscle spasm. Acute and chronic muscle strains and contusions, sprains, spasms, and overuse syndromes will benefit from cryotherapy. The application of cold after vigorous exercise has been shown to decrease soreness after exercise, especially in patients with chondromalacia.[45]

Ice is a frequent adjunct to intense rehabilitation exercises, where it is used to limit any overuse tendinitis or swelling that will occur from focusing on a specific joint or body.

Application of superficial cold packs under rapid pulsed pneumatic compression for ankle sprains has been effective

240

Part two
Principles of rehabilitation
reconditioning, and athletic training

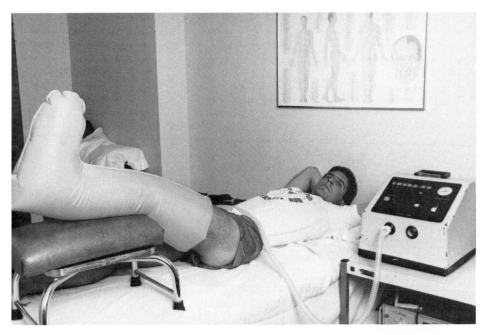

Fig. 8-19 ■ Rapid pulsed pneumatic compression to the lower leg and ankle over cold packs for reduction of edema and pain.

for reducing rehabilitation time and promoting early mobilization[86] (Fig. 8-19).

Contraindications

Application of cold is not indicated for the following conditions: inflamed kidneys, blisters, open wounds,[55] collagen diseases such as lupus erythematosus and rheumatoid arthritis, Raynaud's phenomenon, cold allergy, cryoglobulinemia, and pheochromocytoma.[67]

Precautions

Because all applications of cold are transmitted to or through the skin, frostbite can occur. Despite local, superficial regulatory changes (i.e., hunting reaction), prolonged application can cause local damage. Because of the decreases in sen-

> Avoid prolonged ice application. Frostbite can occur!

sation and collagen elasticity, vigorous physical activity should be avoided immediately after ice applications.

Treatment applications

Application of ice immediately after an injury is only part of the treatment regimen of rest, compression, elevation, and protection. Although evidence leans to

---

ICE APPLICATION SCHEDULE

12 to 20 min application per hour
Total application time 2 hours
Example:
20 min out of each hour × 6 = 120 min (2 hours)

---

less-cool temperatures, the early application of ice to lessen edema and retard the development of hematomas is a common clinical practice. Ice application should consist of repeated 12 to 20 min intervals of application for a total of 2 hours, while

chapter 9

Athletic training techniques and protective equipment

Robert C. Reese, Jr.

T. Pepper Burruss

Part two
Principles of rehabilitation, reconditioning,
and athletic training

Part II—Protective equipment

Athletic training techniques*

by Robert C. Reese, Jr.

When an athlete is injured, whether during practice or a game, the athletic trainer is often the first individual to evaluate the injury. The initial on-the-field, sideline, or training-room evaluation is an extremely important step in the overall management of athletic injury. During this early examination, the location and severity of the injury are assessed, as is the ability of the athlete to return immediately to participation. For minor injuries, additional taping or a piece of protective equipment may be all that is necessary to permit continued play. However, in more severe injuries, the initial evaluation is only the first step in the sequence of events in which the athletic trainer may be the primary individual responsible for determining the athlete's ability to return to participation. This process includes definitive diagnosis, treatment of an acute condition, rehabilitation, taping, and fabrication and application of protective devices. Optimal treatment may also include participation by several sports medicine professionals, including physicians and physical therapists. It must always be borne in mind that the ultimate goal of injury management is to return the injured player to action as soon and as safely as possible. This cannot be accomplished without definitive recognition and diagnosis of the injury.

At the time the player is first seen—on the field or the sidelines or in the training room, clinic, or office—obtaining an adequate history is imperative. What, how, when, and why should all be asked of the injured athlete. Often the history can lead to an immediate presumptive diagnosis. After a brief but thorough history is obtained, examination of the injured body part may begin. The immediate postinjury period is a "golden period" for examination. In this period no spasm has occurred that would limit stress testing. In addition, intraarticular effusion, which may limit motion, is not present as yet. It is important when examining a player on the field to control the number of people surrounding the player. The trainer or physician in charge must limit access to the player to appropriate health care individuals to allow expeditious diagnosis and first aid.

---

*Editors' note: The athletic trainer is a most valuable paramedical aide. We do not have enough of them. Their work should be recognized by state professional licensing organizations so as to encourage their employment by high schools, clubs, colleges, and other amateur athletic organizations. In general, the public does not appreciate athletic trainers as much as team physicians and athletes do. With the current fitness boom, athletic trainers are more necessary than ever.

As with diagnosis, the optimal time for intervention and acute care is immediately after the injury. Protection of the injured area is paramount, particularly in major injuries. This may take the form of a splint applied to a leg on the playing field or simply supporting the player coming off the field. Ice can easily be applied to the injured area at the sidelines. Occasionally this may precede a final diagnosis, particularly when x-ray evaluation is required.

Rehabilitation becomes the cornerstone of the natural progression of the athlete's return to sports. Often the trainer is the individual responsible for the day-to-day monitoring and adjustment of the rehabilitative process. The trainer also offers encouragement to the athlete, providing much of the impetus for faithfully continuing the outlined program. When contemplating initiation of functional rehabilitation techniques, the trainer is responsible for devising and implementing a graded, sport-specific functional program. The trainer monitors daily progress, whereas the team physician evaluates the overall appropriateness and success of the program. Finally, taping or protective devices

are fashioned to allow the athlete to return to competition or full training with minimal risks. The trainer works closely with the athlete to ensure the appropriate use, fit, and stabilization of the device.

Throughout the process, the trainer's close association with an athlete is important. This relationship is built on preinjury encounters between trainer and athlete. Thus the trainer is able to judge the athlete's psychological response to injury and help an athlete through a period of infirmity. Trainers who understand their athletes' personalities will best be able to help them deal with the disappointment or depression that may develop. In addition, the trainer will be able to judge when additional outside help may be necessary.*

■ ANKLE

In sports the ankle is one of the most vulnerable and often injured parts of the

---

*Editors' note: An equally important duty is close association with the physician. The physician and trainer must "speak the same language" and be able to make decisions based on accurate reporting and justifiable criteria.

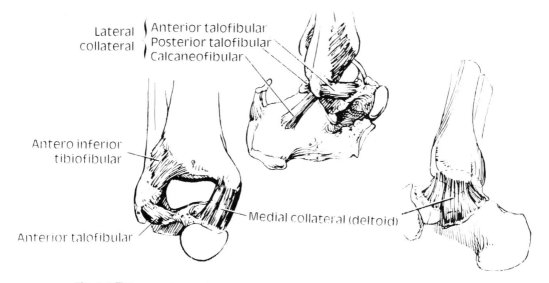

Fig. 9-1 ■ Bony anatomy of ankle.
From Baxter, D.E.: Ligamentous injuries. In Mann, R.A., ed.: Surgery of the foot, ed. 5, St. Louis, 1986, The C.V. Mosby Co.

248

Part two
Principles of rehabilitation, reconditioning,
and athletic training

body. This joint is formed by the articulation of the tibia and fibula with the talus. The ankle's bony structure and its ligamentous arrangement render it extremely stable (Fig. 9-1).

The tibia and fibula rest on the talus, an eccentric ball bearing–like bone with seven articular facets. None of these facets is parallel, and none is at a right angle to any other. Nevertheless, no matter what the position of the foot or its relation to the leg, all surfaces are constantly in contact with the adjacent bones of the foot and leg. The anatomy of the talus is well suited for ambulation on irregular surfaces. It allows maintenance of an upright position regardless of the foot position. Few parts of the body, from a purely anatomic viewpoint, are as mechanically efficient or as architecturally sound as the ankle.

Injuries
On-the-field evaluation

Injuries to the ankle, foot, and lower leg, although often serious, are rarely life-threatening. The neurovascular status of the limb following injury, however, should always be a primary consideration. After a history has been obtained and the mechanism of injury is known, one may begin palpation.

The foot is palpated laterally by holding one hand under the bottom of the foot. The thumb is used to palpate anteriorly, posteriorly, and distal to the lateral malleolus. The pressure should be firm and the anatomic location of tenderness specifically noted. The medial, anterior, and posterior soft tissue areas are likewise palpated. By moving around the malleoli, pressing at different points along the capsule and ligaments, one can quickly discover the most tender areas and the site of injury.

The bones are palpated in a "walking up" fashion, with the distal fibula and medial malleolus being located. Finally, the malleoli are squeezed together if there is no deformity or bony tenderness. If there is *no* suspicion of fracture or dislocation,

then movements through the broadest range of motion are called for to evaluate which motions produce pain. Inversion, eversion, dorsiflexion, plantar flexion, and various combinations are all performed. While the player is attempting motion at the ankle joint, the trainer or team physician should be constantly talking to and watching the player to help isolate the anatomic location of injury. One should also quickly check integrity of the tendons by applying resistance to the appropriate movements. The site of injury can easily be determined with a quick on-the-field examination; however, the degree of injury, particularly to soft tissues, can only be judged with stress testing. The overall prognosis will be rendered at a later time, usually within the next 48 hours, depending on the amount of swelling and tenderness present as the injury becomes apparent. Within 24 to 48 hours, the entire ankle may be swollen and the specific location of tenderness may become diffuse and difficult to isolate.

After a brief, general examination on the playing field, the athlete should be assisted to the sideline. Depending on the findings of the examination, the player may or may not be permitted to bear weight on the ankle. Tolerance to compression through the heel and control of the foot are valuable indicators of the degree of injury. If there is significant pain, the player should be assisted to the sidelines by the trainers, with support from other players if necessary, allowing the player to swing the leg free or lightly bear weight (Fig. 9-2). If only one trainer is available, then the athlete may lean on the trainer as a single support, placing the affected side closest to the trainer (Fig. 9-3). The injured athlete then drapes his arm behind the trainer's neck and over the trainer's shoulder. The trainer can then grasp this arm at the wrist to provide stability while the athlete is depending on the trainer for support. At the same time, the trainer's other hand is free to support the injured limb, as seen in Fig. 9-3.

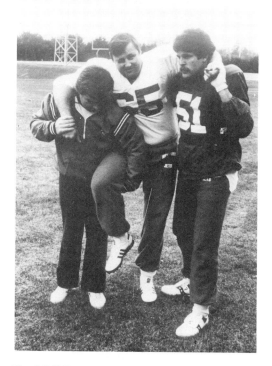

Fig. 9-2 ■ Two people assisting injured player from field. Note trainer and player holding injured player's hand, which is draped over shoulder.

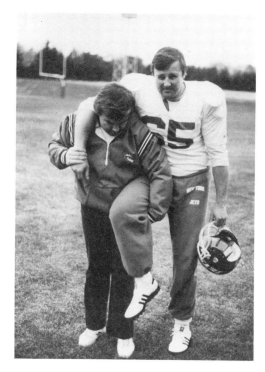

Fig. 9-3 ■ Single person assisting injured player from field.

Sideline evaluation

Once the athlete is off the field, a more detailed examination should be performed. If the athlete's ankle has protective taping, initially leave the tape in place. At this point the severity of the injury should be ascertained and a determination made as to whether or not participation can be safely continued. In many cases the pain disappears when the player is brought to the sideline. If this occurs, more tape may be added and the player asked to gingerly use the ankle. Such instances require that the trainer or team physician know the athlete well in performance and daily contact. Always give the athlete the benefit of the doubt. In a practice situation, it is preferable to keep the athlete from returning to play to reduce the risk of further injury.

Intensive treatment of mild to moderate ankle sprains*

Immediate postinjury regimen. After the athlete has been assisted to the locker room or athletic training area, and with the tape still intact, the ankle and foot are placed in a slush bucket of ice and water (Fig. 9-4). Compression is already present because of the taping. If the foot or ankle

---

*Editors' note: This program of treatment provides relatively quick and safe return to sports following a mild to moderate ankle sprain. It requires close supervision of the athlete by the trainer and physician. It is appropriate for highly organized team situations in which a full complement of athletic trainers, team physicians, or other medical personnel are available and reliable. This is most often found at the college and professional levels, although with the current interest in sports medicine, some high school and club athletes may fall into this group.

250

Part two
Principles of rehabilitation, reconditioning,
and athletic training

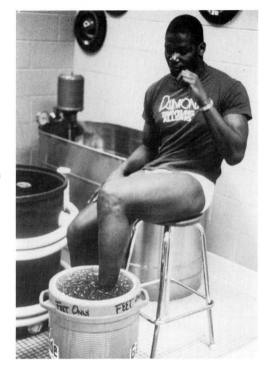

Fig. 9-4 ■ Injured foot placed in slush bucket of ice and water.

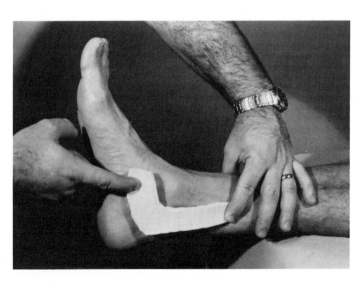

Fig. 9-5 ■ Horseshoe or L-shaped pressure placed around distal posterior and/or anterior aspect of malleolus. It is used to fill the natural gaps and provide even compression.

is not taped, a light tape cast is often applied. A small horseshoe-shaped pad is placed around the distal posterior and anterior aspect of the involved malleolus to fill the natural gap present (Fig. 9-5). Swelling will occur in these areas if compression is not placed evenly around the malleoli, hence the use of the horseshoe pad. If the ankle is well taped, however, this is not necessary.

**TREATMENT PLAN IMMEDIATELY AFTER
ANKLE SPRAIN**

- Cryotherapy, with slush bucket immersion for 15 minutes with tape in place
- Athlete takes quick shower allowing foot and ankle to "thaw out"
- Remove tape and perform examination
- Apply tape cast with pads around malleoli
- Crutches
- Elevation

The taped foot and ankle should be immersed in the ice water for 15 to 20 minutes. The level of the ice water should reach the base of the calf. Observe the athlete to make sure he or she does not remove the foot from the ice bath, since removal would mean the icing process would have to be restarted. The trainer should remain with the athlete to provide encouragment during the first 5 to 7 minutes of immersion. The foot will then become less sensitive and the ice water tolerable. In some instances a sock over the toes will be of value. When using this treatment on a regular basis or for rehabilitation purposes, small toe covers made of neoprene rubber (Fig. 9-6) are appropriate to make the ice bath more tolerable.

After the ice bath the athlete is either placed on crutches or allowed to walk with minimal weight bearing to take a quick shower, leaving the tape in place. Following the shower, the athlete returns to the training room. By this time the foot will have "thawed out." The tape is then removed. After the tape is removed and

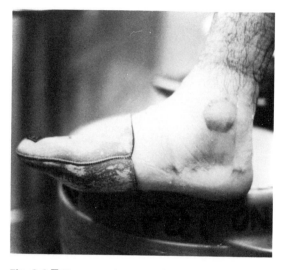

Fig. 9-6 ■ Neoprene toe cover for warmth while in ice water.

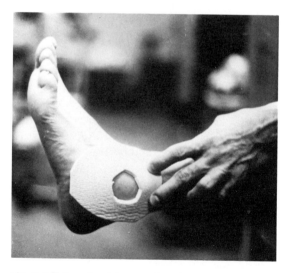

Fig. 9-7 ■ Doughnut-type pad as alternative to horseshoe or L-shaped pressure pad.

the foot is dried, another modified examination and gentle stress test is performed. At this time it should be determined whether roentgenograms will be necessary. Of course, in cases in which fracture is probable, roentgenograms are obtained as soon as possible after the injury.

An L-shaped, horseshoe, or doughnut pad (Fig. 9-7) is placed around the malleo-

Part two
Principles of rehabilitation, reconditioning,
and athletic training

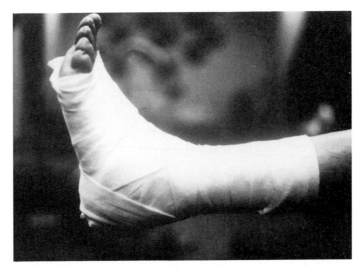

Fig. 9-8 ■ Webril cast wadding used as prewrap for tape cast application.

lus and a tape cast is applied.* The importance of the horseshoe pressure pad around the malleolus and covering the ankle ligament complex to limit swelling cannot be overemphasized.

The athlete is now allowed to leave the training area with instructions to elevate the ankle continuously. The new tape cast should have been lightly applied with multiple layers of tape over a Webril wrap (Fig. 9-8) to provide snug stability as a light but firm compression bandage. If possible the athlete should be provided with crutches to ensure adequate rest of the injured structures. It is imperative during the first 24 hours that compression, ice, elevation, and rest be strictly enforced. Telephone books may be placed beneath the foot of the bed to maintain constant elevation of the ankle and foot, whether the athlete sleeps on the side, prone, or supine.

Postinjury day 1. Active treatment of the ankle sprain begins the day after the injury. The treatment plan we prefer is commonly referred to as the Air Force treatment. The entire treatment sequence should be performed three or four times

during the day, depending on the availability of the athlete to the training room. The ideal frequency is a minimum of three times during the day.

POSTINJURY DAY 1 (NON-WEIGHT-BEARING STAGE)

Perform sequence three or four times throughout the day	Slush bucket 7 to 10 minutes with tape in place
	Remove tape
	Reimmerse 10 to 12 minutes
	Intermittent air compression for 20 minutes
	Brief examination
	Tape cast
	Maintain elevation

The tape cast, applied the previous day, should still be on the injured limb. The athlete places the foot, still enclosed in the tape cast, into the slush water ice bath for 7 to 10 minutes. The tape cast is removed and the ankle is then reimmersed for 10 to 12 minutes. After the immersion treatment is completed, and an intermittent air compression device is applied for 20 minutes (Fig. 9-9). While the foot and ankle are in the compression boot, the in-

*See p. 266 for tape cast technique.

Ferguson, however, cited a number of factors that he felt argued against the use of ankle taping.[2] The problems, he stated, included the mobile nature of the skin, loosened skin adhesive from moisture, disuse atrophy of the muscles supporting the ankle, deemphasis of conditioning programs that strengthen the muscles around the ankle, and possible increased risk of proximal injury, particularly to the knee, by loss of the "safety valve" subtalar motion. Glick, however, did not find an increased incidence of knee injuries among athletes with taped ankles.[6] Taping should never be used without an extensive rehabilitation program following injury.

A controlled clinical study by Ekstrand et al. documented a statistically significant decrease in ankle sprains among soccer players whose ankles were taped.[1] The researchers felt that ankle taping was therefore an effective and realistic means of limiting the number of ankle sprains among soccer players.

We feel that mandatory taping of all athletes is unnecessary. However, any athlete with a previous ankle injury should be taped for practice and competition. This is based on the concept that once an ankle joint is sprained and the ligaments disrupted, the ankle will always remain structurally weaker. Injury strapping clearly provides additional support. Of course, any athlete with an ankle injury or a history of ankle problems should be on an intensive rehabilitation program, developing strength in the motor units spanning the ankle. For inversion injury, particular emphasis is placed on the peroneal muscles.

Elastic vs. adhesive tape

Another controversy in ankle strapping involves the use of elastic or adhesive tape. It has long been felt that standard cotton-backed adhesive tape offers the most support, while elastic tape offers the long-lasting effect desired in ankle strapping. Some elastic tapes may have greater tensile strength, but the elastic nature allows more freedom of movement. The range of motion allowed by elastic tape, particularly at the ankle, will not preclude undesirable motion and its effectiveness is therefore questionable. The positive feature of elastic tape is its tendency to not loosen as readily as cloth-backed adhesive tape. The length of time that regular adhesive strapping will last has been debated and tested. The factors that play a role in this regard include the amount of tape applied, the technique of application, and the level and duration of activity. Rarick et al. demonstrated that as much as 40% of the net supporting strength of the strappings was lost after 10 minutes of vigorous exercise.[12] Despite this, clinical studies have clearly demonstrated the effectiveness of ankle taping in reducing ankle injury.[1,5] It therefore seems that although the initial strength is diminished, the residual strength may suffice to assist in preventing injury.

The quality and strength of adhesive tape depends on the number of cotton fibers that cross in a square inch. Tapes with a lower count of cotton fibers per square inch are easier to tear. However, they offer less support and rigidity.

Principles of taping

A number of factors in ankle taping should be considered, as follows.

1. Tight is not necessarily right in a tape job. If more strength is needed, add more tape, building up several layers rather than tightening the application.

2. To remove the tape, remember to peel the skin away from the tape and not jerk or tear the tape away from the skin. A massaging action is recommended when tape is applied directly to the skin. Remind athletes of this, particularly if they are new or if you are applying a new type of strapping that they have not had in the past.

3. When taping an ankle, flatten the foot with your stomach by pressing up against the foot as you go around it to help keep from pinching the fifth metatarsal (Fig. 9-11).

Part two
Principles of rehabilitation, reconditioning,
and athletic training

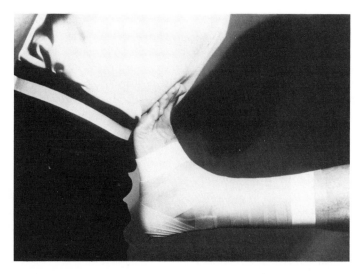

Fig. 9-11 ■ Athlete's foot flattened by pressing the trainer's stomach against foot to prevent pinching of fifth metatarsal.

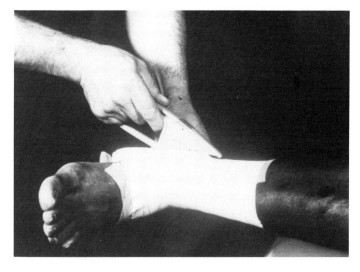

Fig. 9-12 ■ Cut tape by following natural contours of body.

4. Find a comfortable height for the training table to prevent trainer back problems that may result from improper posture and paravertebral fatigue.

5. Tape should be applied so that the tape goes where it wants to go. Tape cannot be steered. The tape must be laid down on the skin at the appropriate angle to control its direction and achieve the desired goal of the tape job. If you find that you have started with an incorrect angle and a wrinkle is going to appear in the tape, either tear or cut the tape and leave it in place. Proceed with another strip at the correct angle.

6. Tape for any joint should not be kept on for more than one practice session or contest.

7. When cutting tape from the body part, find the natural valleys and contours of the body to guide the tape-removing instrument (Fig. 9-12). Always use the blunt edge of a scissors or a tape cutter and when possible let the athlete cut and re-

move the tape. You should have the athlete cut down the unaffected side of the
joint.

8. The closer the tape is to the skin, the
more support it offers, but more care to
prevent skin problems is then necessary.
Judgments by daily observation and questioning for symptoms such as burning are
good aids to management.

Taping techniques
Gibney open basket weave

Gibney open basket weave taping is the
original ankle strapping method. Although
this technique forms the basis of many
tape jobs used today, many modifications
have improved its usefulness. Thus, the
traditional open basket weave technique is
rarely used today. The original basket
weave was left open anteriorly because of
concern about impaired blood circulation
in the foot with circumferential tape application. This concern is not necessary
unless an individual has a particular problem with circulation, since with proper
taping methods, as just described, there
should be no problems with circulation.

The tape is applied so that after the anchors are in place, a stirrup is applied
(Fig. 9-13, *A*), then a shingle, then a stirrup
(Fig. 9-13, *B*), then a shingle (Fig. 9-13, *C*),
then a stirrup, and so on (Fig. 9-13, *D*).
The important thing to learn from Gibney
strapping is the principle that tape can
work against itself. This overlapping inter-
locking technique is the basis for all athletic strapping. A law of physics is that
every action has an equal and opposite reaction. This is why it is important to have
the tape working against itself. For example, if the tape is stretched medially, it will
pull against itself on the lateral side. This
gives the athletic strappings its integrity.
This principle is true of all tape jobs.

Basic preventive taping of the ankle

It has been said that every art has a
basic form, and the basic form for ankle
strapping is the preventive tape job with
cotton-backed tape. To begin, prepare the
ankle.

BASICS OF INJURY TAPING

Athletic taping or strapping has a number
of useful attributes. First, taping supports
an injured or recovering joint very well. Second, it can limit or accent certain motions
that are essential for any joint. There are
three basic components for any taping
technique, whether applied to the ankle,
hand, wrist, knee, foot, toe, or other area.
These are the:

Anchor strips
Checkreins
Figure-8s

Anchor strips are exactly what they sound
like. These strips of tape are applied around
a section of the body, either directly or partially to the skin, to provide a firm point of
attachment for other strips of tape. Generally
they are applied twice to provide a wide area
for attachment. Anchor strips are applied
snugly but not tightly, since they are generally circumferential.

Checkreins are strips of tape placed on the
body between anchor strips to prevent or
accent certain motions. They may take any
number of forms or any shape, depending
on the goal of the taping technique. Checkreins are applied to support the joint but allow freedom of the range of motion that is
necessary to perform the athletic task required.

Figure-8s are applied in a circular motion
to create a crisscross pattern. They help
maintain the integrity of the joint while providing strength. These strips go around the
extremity in the natural contours.

Using these three basic techniques of taping, most joints and their injuries can be supported and protected by the use of tape. The
goals of any tape job or injury strapping are
to provide light, strong support, allow appropriate range of motion, provide comfort, and
cause minimal skin irritation. An adequate
tape application should be durable and long
lasting as well as relatively easy to apply.

Preparation. In the past, the ankle was
totally shaved. Tape preparation spray
(Fig. 9-14) was applied so that on removal
of the tape, the tape spray would come off
with the adhesive of the tape, as opposed
to the skin coming off with the adhesive
tape. In recent years the invention and acceptance of the thin, highly porous, poly-
urethane foam underwrap has taken the

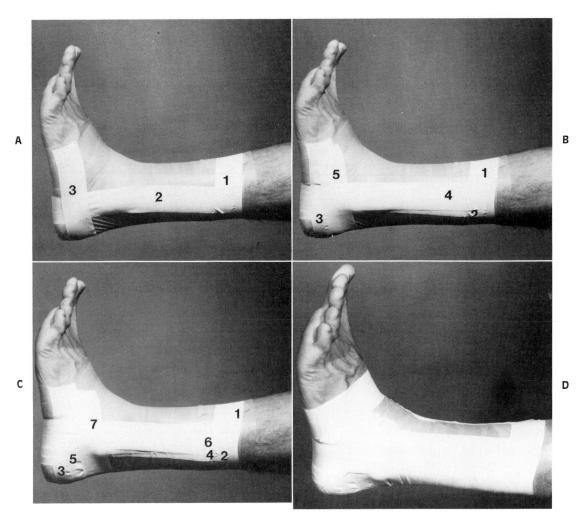

Fig. 9-13 ■ **A,** Anchor with first stirrup and shingle. **B,** Second stirrup and second shingle (overlap at least half). **C,** Third stirrup and third shingle. **D,** Completed Gibney with open front. *1,* Anchor; *2,* first stirrup; *3,* shingle; *4,* second stirrup; *5,* second shingle; *6,* third stirrup; *7,* third shingle.

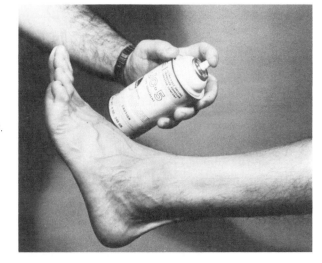

Fig. 9-14 ■ Tape preparation spray.

this can become a continuation of the figure-8 so that a figure-8 and double heel lock is created without tearing the tape (Fig. 9-34). (Note: To practice continuous application of figure-8s and heel locks, use a 2-inch Ace bandage.) An anchor strip should be placed once again at the top and the bottom after these steps have been completed.

Many athletic trainers feel that the figure-8s and the heel locks should be applied immediately after the stirrups. We feel that either is correct, but by placing the figure-8s and heel locks on top of the shingles and stirrups, the integrity of the ankle strapping is increased by tying the strapping together (Fig. 9-35).

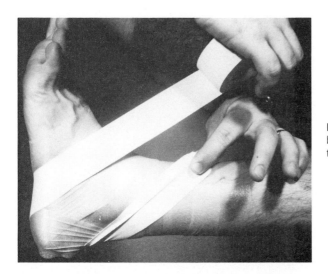

Fig. 9-32 ■ Loop heel lock. Measure length by placing nonadherent side of tape next to ankle.

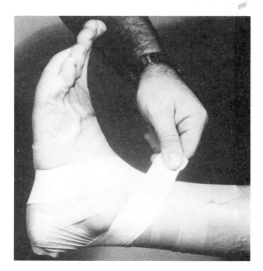

Fig. 9-33 ■ Loop heel lock application. Cross instep and encircle heel.

270

Part two
Principles of rehabilitation, reconditioning,
and athletic training

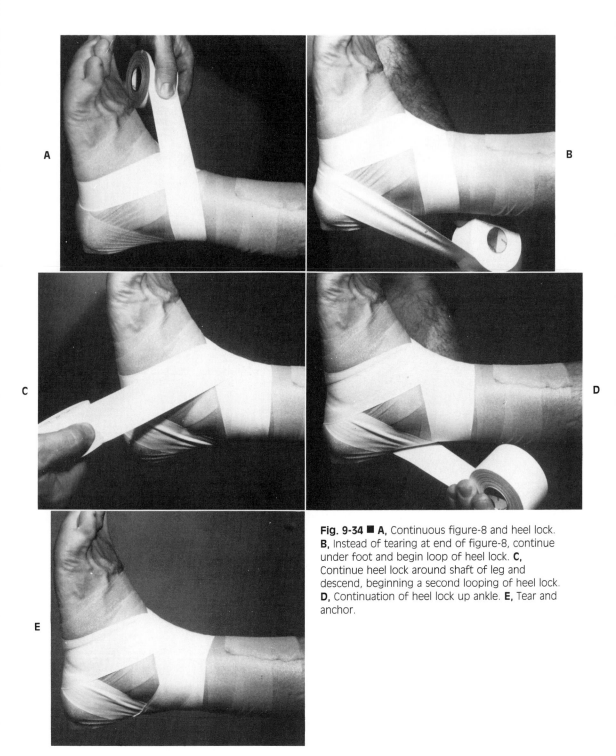

Fig. 9-34 ■ **A,** Continuous figure-8 and heel lock.
B, Instead of tearing at end of figure-8, continue
under foot and begin loop of heel lock. **C,**
Continue heel lock around shaft of leg and
descend, beginning a second looping of heel lock.
D, Continuation of heel lock up ankle. **E,** Tear and
anchor.

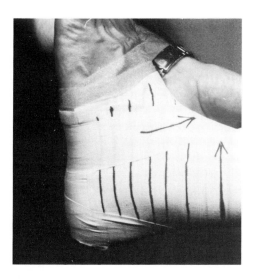

Fig. 9-35 ■ Figure-8 and heel lock applied over shingles. Follow same steps as in Fig. 9-34, *A-D*.

Ankle injury taping technique

Ankle injury strapping is also done with adhesive tape. Once again, prepare the ankle as for preventive taping. For this technique, the anchor strip should be attached to the skin at the top of the ankle. The skin should be sprayed with pretape spray to prevent skin problems. The most common ankle injury is an inversion sprain. A useful tape technique following this injury accents eversion and limits inversion. In preparing the ankle, shave a circular strip of skin from below the base of the calf muscle distally 2 to 3 inches. If this tape technique needs daily application, alternate the area of the anchor strip up and down the shaft of the lower leg with each succeeding strapping. Spread the foot when applying the bottom anchor strip around the arch or toward the forefoot. Three stirrups are applied (Fig. 9-36). However, this time they should start from the medial side, descend, cross the medial malleolus, go under the heel, and, as they cross under the heel, be given a slight lift to the outside. It is not necessary to crank or pull with great force all the way from the medial anchor strip to the outside. Use the downward portion of the stirrup as a large longitudinal anchor, and when crossing under the heel, apply

slight tension to the tape to help accent eversion and prevent inversion. Do this with all three stirrups, fanning the strips at the top to obtain a large base of support.

Next, to provide additional support to the lateral ankle complex, apply tape by starting laterally above the malleolus, proceeding distally (Fig. 9-37) and traversing the instep, the tape "splitting" the heel, and finally applying a lift (Fig. 9-38) to the outside as the tape comes up and across the lateral malleolus and instep. The next strip should start at a slightly different angle below the first strip (Fig. 9-39). Again, starting laterally but coming across the foot (Fig. 9-40) and under the arch, remember to press against the foot to spread it, give a lift to the outside as the tape passes over the fifth metatarsal and go back across the instep and tear. Following this, three or four checkreins are applied on the lateral side, keeping the foot at a minimum of 90 degrees or with as much dorsiflexion as possible (Fig. 9-41).

The checkreins are placed on the lateral side. They can be cut or torn first and then applied with the foot at 90 degrees or less. Start low and cross to the Achilles tendon, anchoring under the base of the

Part two
Principles of rehabilitation, reconditioning,
and athletic training

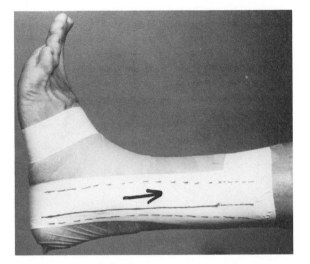

Fig. 9-36 ■ Three stirrups applied medially to laterally with lift laterally.

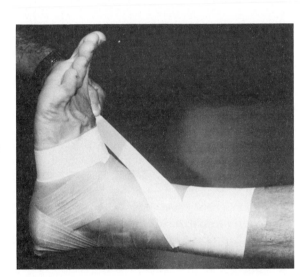

Fig. 9-37 ■ Additional lateral support: start laterally above malleolus, proceed across instep toward heel.

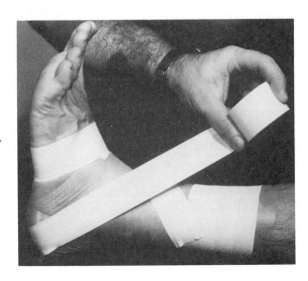

Fig. 9-38 ■ Lateral support. Split heel, apply lift, and tear, anchoring on medial side.

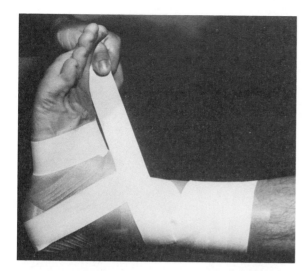

Fig. 9-39 ■ Lateral support. Second strip begins laterally, crosses instep, and goes under arch.

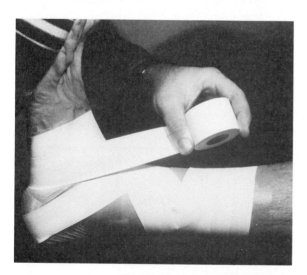

Fig. 9-40 ■ Lateral support. Give lateral lift while going across instep, and tear.

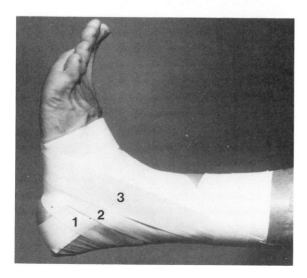

Fig. 9-41 ■ Lateral support. Three checkreins applied laterally.

274

Part two
Principles of rehabilitation, reconditioning,
and athletic training

foot. The more accomplished athletic
trainer will anchor, pull, and tear the
strip in one continuous motion.

Do not apply the tape above the base of
the fifth metatarsal. However, one can go
as high on the anchor strip in front of the
ankle as necessary. Notice the gap in Fig.
9-42 and how this is closed down by applying an opposite angle checkrein (Fig.
9-43) anchored on the heel and coming
across the instep (Fig. 9-44). This in effect
"kicks" the ankle into eversion, preventing
inversion. Following this, apply shingles,
figure-8s, and heel locks as described earlier.

The heel locks and figure-8s should be
applied snugly but not too tightly, especially across the Achilles tendon. It is also
imperative that there be no wrinkles in
the heel (Achilles tendon) and lace (instep)
areas. It is not necessary in preventive
taping to always attach the anchor portion of the tape to the skin or use prewrap; it depends on the activity, the level
of competition, and similar factors. It is
recommended to anchor the tape to the
skin when applying injury strappings. A
heel lift and lateral wedge constructed of
¼- or ½-inch orthopaedic felt and beveled
medially will also help force eversion and
should be applied when the injury strapping is not sufficient alone (Fig. 9-45).

Elastic tape application

Strapping with elastic tape is done in
the fashion of the old "Louisiana Wrap."
This technique has been done for years
with non-elastic cloth wrap. I feel that
cloth wrap does very little to protect the
ankle adequately. It may be better than
nothing, but not by much. Elastic tape, on
the other hand, is useful and can be applied over prewrap or even over a sock. If
lace and heel pads are available, they
should also be used. Generally, the tape is
started across the arch (Fig. 9-46, *A*), goes
under the foot around and across the
malleoli, and back to the instep (Fig. 9-46,
B). This is a figure-8. The next step is to
apply a heel lock to one side (Fig. 9-46, *C*).

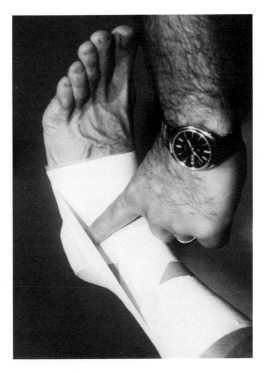

Fig. 9-42 ■ Lateral support. "Gap" formed by
three lateral checkreins.

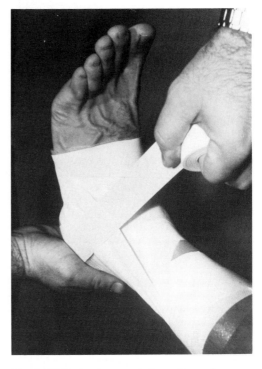

Fig. 9-43 ■ Lateral support. Opposite angle
checkrein anchored on heel.

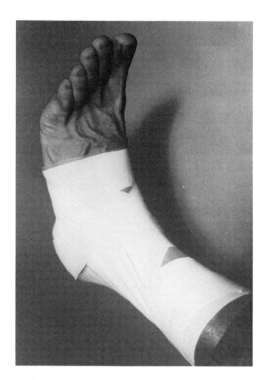

Fig. 9-44 ■ Lateral support. Opposite angle checkrein closing gap and "kicking" ankle into eversion.

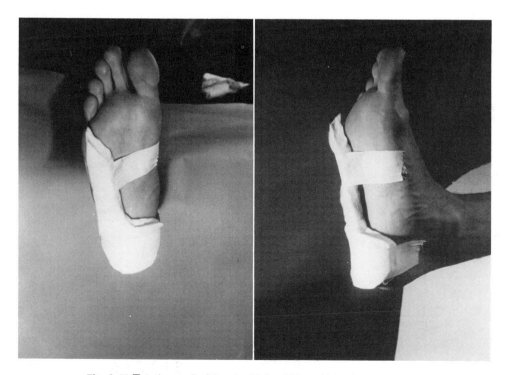

Fig. 9-45 ■ Orthopaedic felt cut with heel lift and lateral wedge or bar.

276

Part two
Principles of rehabilitation, reconditioning,
and athletic training

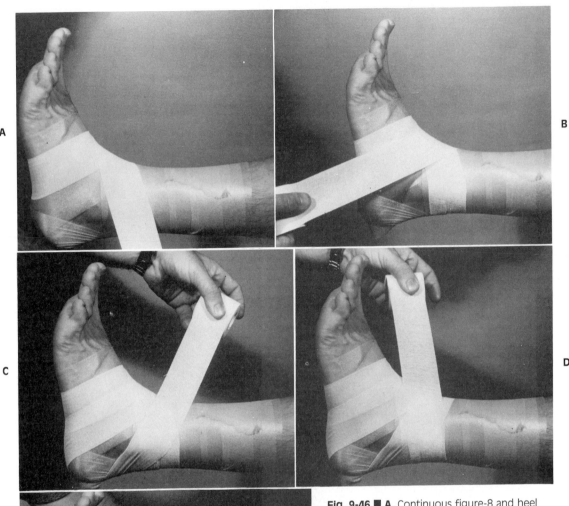

Fig. 9-46 ■ **A,** Continuous figure-8 and heel lock. **B,** Instead of tearing at end of figure-8, continue under foot and begin loop of heel lock. **C,** Continue heel lock around shaft of leg. **D,** Descend beginning a second looping of heel lock. **E,** Continue heel lock up ankle.

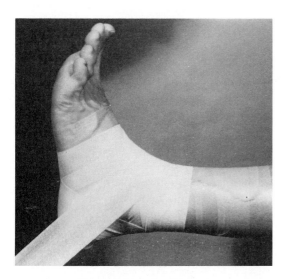

Fig. 9-47 ■ "Split" the heel.

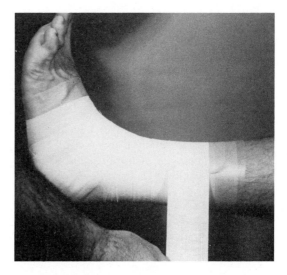

Fig. 9-48 ■ Continue tape up lower leg.

Continue with a circular motion around the top of the lower leg above the malleolus resulting in the proper angle to come back down and lock the opposite side (Figs. 9-46, *D* and 9-46, *E)*. This is the same as the continuous figure-8 and heel lock described earlier. For any level of competition higher than youth league, at least *two* figure-8s and heel locks are necessary when using elastic tape. After the two continuous heel locks and figures are applied, "split" the heel with the tape (Fig. 9-47) and then continue the tape up (Fig. 9-48) the lower leg to the base of the gastrocnemius, and tear or cut the tape. The elastic tape should always be anchored with adhesive tape (Fig. 9-49). The elastic tape job may be strengthened by placing an adhesive tape figure-8 or a figure-8 with heel locks over the top of the elastic tape. The elastic tape provides a great deal of forefoot freedom while giving adequate, firm compression and support to the ankle joint.

Combination strapping

The most common preventive and basic strapping used today is a combination of elastic and adhesive tape strapping. The anchor on the lower leg is applied with adhesive tape and this is followed by three

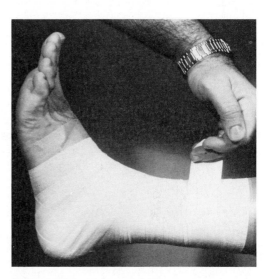

Fig. 9-49 ■ Adhesive tape anchor on elastic tape.

adhesive stirrups. As always, fan the stirrups out proximally. Elastic tape is then applied as figure-8s and heel locks as described on p. 276. Finish off by circling up to the base of the gastrocnemius and anchoring at the top with adhesive tape. A figure-8 and heel lock with adhesive tape is then applied.

Many variations of ankle taping can be created. Remember that the basis for all injury taping is to determine what motion needs to be prevented, what motion needs

278

Part two
Principles of rehabilitation, reconditioning,
and athletic training

TAPING VARIATIONS

Elastic tape figure-8s/heel locks	= Greater mobility
Moleskin stirrups	= Stronger strapping
Moleskin figure-8	= Stronger strapping

---

to be accented and then to take the necessary steps to satisfy those goals.

For a stronger strapping that can be used on a relatively acute injury, moleskin is used for the stirrups (Fig. 9-50) and occasionally for the loop figure-8 (Fig. 9-51). This adds much greater support and has excellent adhesive ability. It should be placed at the end of injury strapping.

Anterior tibiofibular sprain

Injuries of the distal tibiofibular joint present a difficult taping problem. The most effective method uses a light tape cast applied with two or three layers of shingles on the posterior aspect of the an-

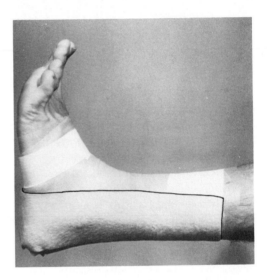

Fig. 9-50 ■ Moleskin stirrup.

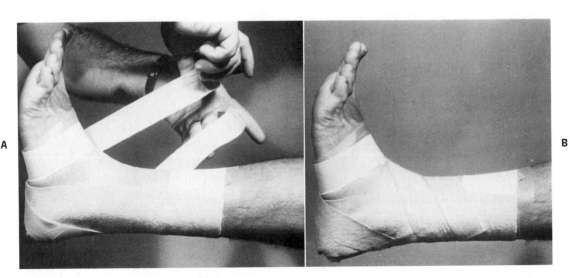

A

B

Fig. 9-51 ■ **A,** Moleskin "loop" heel lock. **A,** Measured. **B,** Applied.

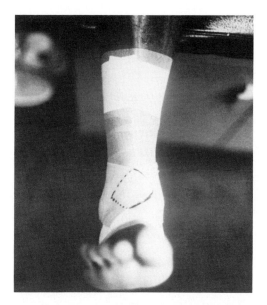

Fig. 9-52 ■ Moleskin shingle overlapping and adhering to itself for anterior tibiofibular support.

kle. The tension at which the tape is applied is critical. If too much pressure is used, the tape irritates the injury and the athlete experiences increased pain. If insufficient tension is applied, the bone will have a tendency to "spread." The goal therefore is good support without undue pressure. An alternate strapping technique for this injury uses a 3-inch-wide moleskin strip applied as a shingle, overlapping and adhering to itself on the anterior aspect of the ankle (Fig. 9-52).

Plantar flexion prevention

Sometimes it is necessary to prevent or limit plantar flexion. This can easily be accomplished by placing a series of 1-inch checkreins between the two anchors (Fig. 9-53). Overlap approximately one half (Fig. 9-54), and remember to let the tape follow (Fig. 9-55) the contours of the foot and ankle (Fig. 9-56). Cover with elastic tape if this is the only support needed, or proceed with other strappings with the plantar flexion strap as a base.

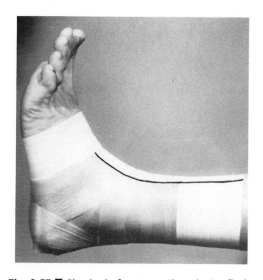

Fig. 9-53 ■ Checkrein for preventing plantar flexion.

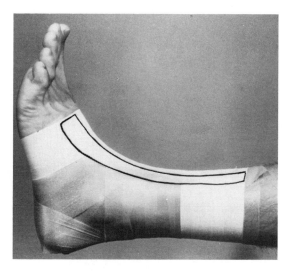

Fig. 9-54 ■ Checkreins overlapping.

Part two
Principles of rehabilitation, reconditioning,
and athletic training

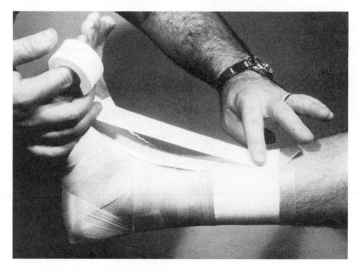

Fig. 9-55 ■ Checkrein application.

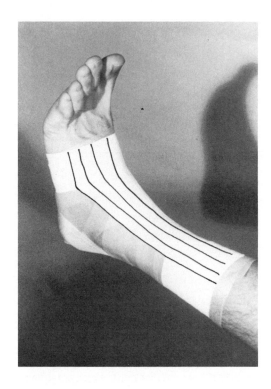

Fig. 9-56 ■ Checkreins anchored at top and
bottom.

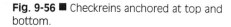

■ FOOT
Sprains of the great toe

One of the most common injuries of the foot is the so-called turf toe or Astrotoe. The diagnosis of this metatarsophalangeal (MTP) joint injury is easily made by noting the mechanism of injury. Usually a player overloads the foot and hyperextends the great toe, spraining the ligaments of the first MTP joint. In some cases the sesamoepicondylar ligaments and the flexor hallucis brevis muscle are also injured.*

Initial treatment

Initial treatment is with ice and light compress wrap. Subsequently ice baths and range of motion exercises as tolerated are employed. It is important to maintain the range of motion of the ankle and the flexibility of the heel cords so as not to create "big toe pain" because of improper gait.

Taping

When preparing to apply tape for athletes with turf toe, the hair on the dorsum of the foot and toe should be shaved, then sprayed with pretape spray. An anchor strip is placed around the great toe, approximately three fourths of the way toward the end of the toe. Occasionally a small Telfa pad is placed over the toenail to prevent irritation when removing the tape. Next an anchor strip is placed around the arch at the midportion of the

---

*Editors' note: It is always important to assess the anatomic alignment of the foot when evaluating chronic great toe problems. Also, the overall flexibility and pliability of the foot should be noted. Presence of a hallux rigidus, a relaxed medial capsular ligament structure, and power of the big toe flexor, adductor, abductor, and extensor muscles should all be checked. Correction for any muscular deficits must be made, as well as protection of the affected joints from overload with pain using orthotics and supports. These can be used not only in the athletic shoe but also in the everyday walking shoe (see Chapter 20).

foot, remembering to spread the foot as it is applied. A doughnutlike hole (Fig. 9-57, A) is then cut in a strip of 1½-inch tape, which is then placed over the toe (Fig. 9-57, B). Plantar flex the foot to help isolate

TURF TOE TAPING	
Objective:	Limitation of motion at metatarsophalangeal joint of great toe
Technique	Telfa pad over toenail
	Shave
	Prewrap
	Anchor strip
	Doughnut-shaped tape strip
	Checkreins
	Elastic tape cover layer
Variations:	Moleskin strip on plantar aspect to supplement tape
	Proximal metatarsal pad to move area of weight bearing proximal to metatarsal head
Additional measure:	Steel plate in shoe to give forefoot support and rigidity

and relax the MTP joint. The toe itself is immobilized by a series of overlapping checkreins of 1-inch tape. The checkreins reduce the stress borne by the metatarsophalangeal and interphalangeal joints by limiting motion. These checkreins are placed with the foot at 90 degrees and the great toe in anatomic neutral position. It is important not to flex or extend the toe at the metatarsophalangeal joint as the taping proceeds.

The strips extend from the anchor strip at the tip of the toe to the anchor strip around the midarch and are put on with minimal force. They are simply laid in place, overlapping halfway over the previous piece and fanning out as a large anchor around the arch (Fig. 9-58). Application of these checkreins continues from the sole around to the dorsum of the foot.

282
Part two
Principles of rehabilitation, reconditioning,
and athletic training

The tape is then reanchored twice around the toe. Anchor strips are now placed starting from the lateral border of the tape at the bottom of the foot (Fig. 9-59). They are pulled around the ball of the foot (Fig. 9-60), giving a lift to the metatarsophalangeal joint (Fig. 9-61), and are finally anchored on the dorsum of the foot above the fourth metatarsal. On the sole of the foot the strips will begin at the fourth metatarsal and go around to the top. This process is continued until midarch is reached (Fig. 9-62). When anchoring at the bottom, starting at the fourth metatarsal, come immediately across the arch to provide a lift as the tape comes across the arch. However, do not entirely encapsulate the foot with one-inch adhesive tape.

The taping procedure is completed by anchoring a light elastic tape around the foot to keep the tape from curling or rolling up. Apply the elastic tape from mid-foot toward the toes to avoid ridges when a sock is put on.

Additionally, moleskin may be used in place of several layers of the tape to supplement the tape and save time. For serious sprains, or if the tape provides insufficient support, a piece of orthopaedic felt can be cut and fitted to isolate and alleviate pressure from the metatarsophalangeal joint (Fig. 9-63). This treatment provides added weight bearing area proximal to the metatarsal head during gait. Hence when the athlete pushes off or goes up on the toes, the weight bearing area is proximal to the first MTP joint and motion at the sprained joint is limited. The metatarsal pad should be skived, or beveled, down toward the lateral edge and made larger beneath the arch so that the weight bearing portion of the foot is now proximal to the metatarsal heads. This pad is placed in position after the ankle has been taped

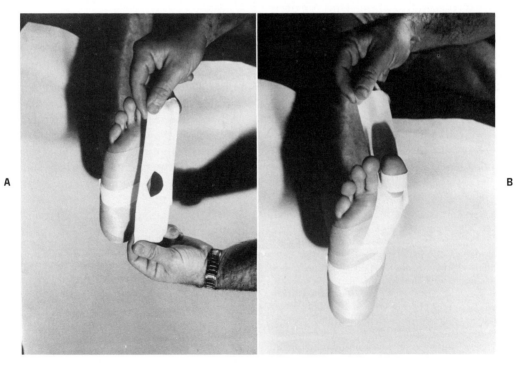

A
B

Fig. 9-57 ■ **A,** Doughnut hole cut in tape. **B,** Doughnut hole placed over toe with equal force on dorsal and plantar sides of foot. This helps immobilize joint.

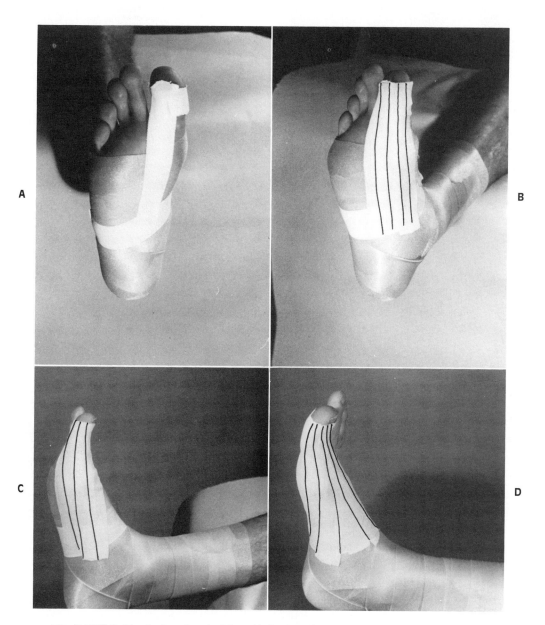

Fig. 9-58 ■ **A,** Checkreins placed while ankle is at 90 degrees and toe is in neutral. **B** to **D,** Overlap 50% near toe and "fan out" while anchoring.

Part two
Principles of rehabilitation, reconditioning,
and athletic training

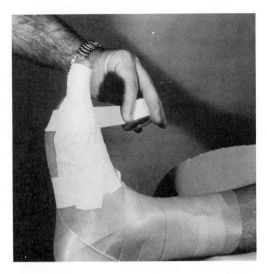

Fig. 9-59 ■ Anchor strips starting laterally across sole.

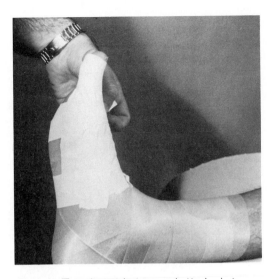

Fig. 9-60 ■ Anchor strip torn and attached at approximately the fourth metatarsal.

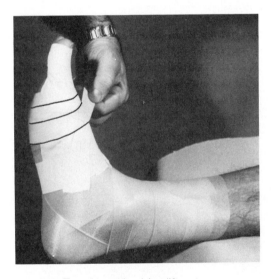

Fig. 9-61 ■ Anchor strip giving lift as tape crosses metatarsophalangeal joint.

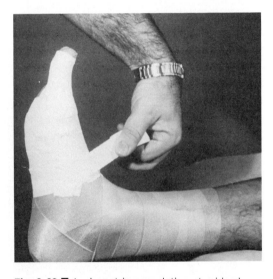

Fig. 9-62 ■ Anchor strip completion at midarch.

and can be used several times. To conserve the felt pad, cut the tape around the pad rather than peel the tape off the felt. Once the felt loses its effectiveness after repeated use, a new pad is required.

Generally, start treatment using the complete pad and checkrein taping of the toe. As symptoms ameliorate, gradually wean the athlete from the pad. Next the doughnut-type taping over the toe joint is discontinued. Last, eliminate the checkrein taping of the toe. This sequence may take several weeks, depending on the position played, the activity level of the sport, and the severity of the injury.

Another valuable technique is the use of

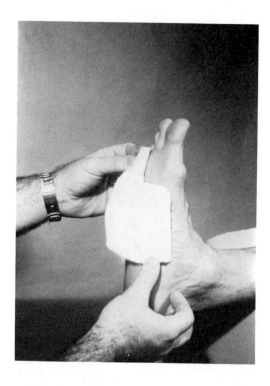

Fig. 9-63 ■ Orthopaedic felt pad cut to support arch and alleviate pressure on metatarsophalangeal joint.

a half steel plate placed between the inner and outer soles of the shoe to give good forefoot support and prevent further hyperextension of the toe.

Prevention of toe injuries

Turf toe and flexor strains can best be prevented by specific attention to proper footwear. The forefoot of the shoe should provide fairly rigid support. It should not bend or twist too easily. An added steel plate allows adequate room and prevents hyperextension and hyperflexion of the joints of the great toe. It does not, of course, provide any additional cushioning or weight distribution.

Longitudinal arch

Prevention of longitudinal arch problems or plantar fascia injury is best accomplished by good heel cord flexibility and the use of proper footwear. Heel cord flexibility can be tested by the trainer while the athlete is on the taping table by pushing the foot back and noting the flexibility of the heel cord. With the knee extended and the foot dorsiflexed, acute plantar fascia injuries can occur that are very painful and debilitating. Treatment should begin promptly. Ice baths, compression, and support are all indicated. After 2 or 3 days, contrast treatments are sometimes used. A very effective program at this point is the "ballerina treatment" (p. 305). Gentle heel cord and plantar fascia stretching is begun, within pain tolerance limits, in conjunction with a contrast therapy program. Arch taping and a heel lift are often used to provide support during the entire convalescence.

Taping of the longitudinal arch

Taping of the longitudinal arch begins with preparation of the bottom of the foot. The athlete should be seated on the training table. The foot and ankle are held in the neutral position. After cleansing the skin and spraying with a tape preparation spray, the first anchor strip (Fig. 9-64) is placed across the sole of the foot along the base of the toes from the fifth metatarsal to the first metatarsal. A second an-

Part two
Principles of rehabilitation, reconditioning,
and athletic training

LONGITUDINAL ARCH TAPING

Indications:	Plantar fasciitis/resolving plantar fascia strain or rupture
Objective:	To support longitudinal arch and reduce tension on plantar fascia
Technique:	Anchor strips
	Checkreins
	Circumferential strips
	Elastic tape anchor
Variation:	Moleskin to supplement longitudinal tape

---

chor strip (Fig. 9-65) is applied extending from the head of the fifth metatarsal to the head of the first metatarsal with the tape passing around the back of the heel. The purpose of this taping technique is to create an artificial arch with checkreins applied to prevent tension on the plantar fascia. Therefore start at the base of the great toe, come across the midsole of the foot, around the back of the heel, and attach the tape on top of the initial strip (Fig. 9-66). Pull snugly so that there is a gap between the tape and the longitudinal arch. The next strip should be started about a ½ inch over, gently following the same angle and again attached on top of itself (Fig. 9-67). This process should be continued completely across the sole of the foot until the head of the fifth metatarsal is reached (Fig. 9-68). An anchor strip from the fifth metatarsal to the first metatarsal is again applied. Then, using 1½-inch tape, start at the base of the heel (the beginning of the arch) and place a strip along the edge of the fifth metatarsal on the sole of the foot, coming along the arch (Fig. 9-69). Provide lift to the longitudinal arch by attaching the tape around to

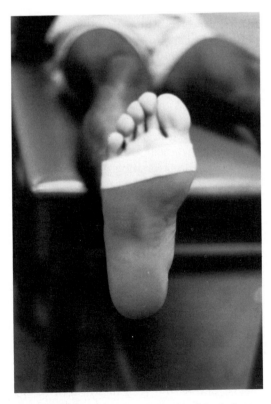

Fig. 9-64 ■ Anchor strip across sole of foot along the base of the toes.

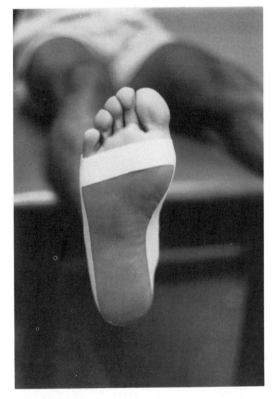

Fig. 9-65 ■ Second anchor strip extending from head of fifth metatarsal to the head of the first metatarsal.

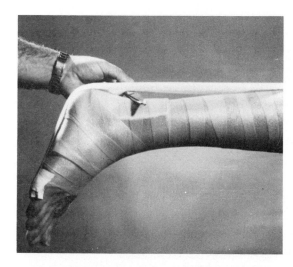

Fig. 9-85 ■ "Gap" formed when tape is applied properly.

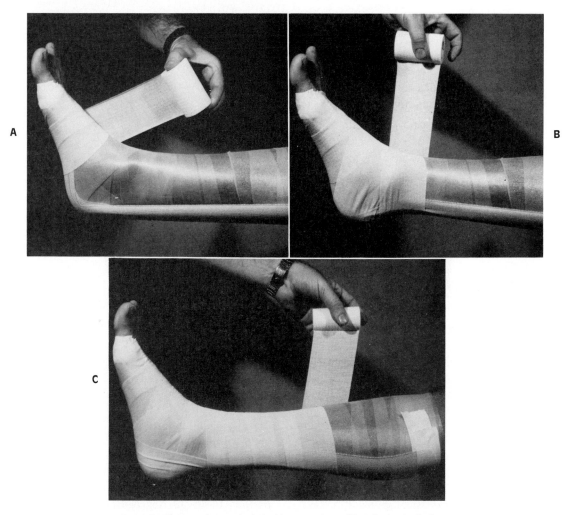

Fig. 9-86 ■ Strapping completed by covering with 3-inch elastic tape.

302

Part two
Principles of rehabilitation, reconditioning,
and athletic training

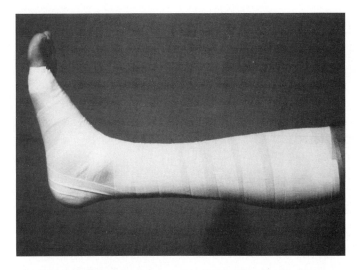

Fig. 9-87 ■ Anchor at top and bottom with adhesive tape.

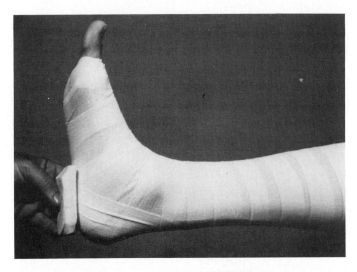

Fig. 9-88 ■ A ½-inch heel lift is taped directly to heel.

team, Eddie Abramoski. It is said that Dr. Godfrey devised the incline board for children with spastic cerebral palsy who had tight Achilles tendons or clubfeet. To effectively stretch the muscles, a child would receive physical therapy once a day. However, Dr. Godfrey felt that the best relief of the pain associated with this condition could be accomplished with multiple treatments throughout the day. For young patients, shoes were fixed to

the incline board he designed. The patients were then placed with their feet in the shoes and allowed to stand on the incline board for the appropriate length of therapy. This technique, of course, has been modified and applied to athletics.

An incline board should measure 1 foot wide, 18 inches deep at the base, 6 inches high, and create an incline of approximately 15 to 18 degrees. Incline boards can easily be made in any woodworking

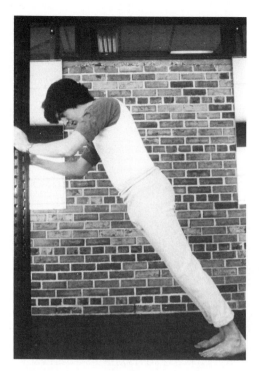

Fig. 9-89 ■ Most common heel cord stretch.
Leaning against wall, keeping knees straight and
heels flat on floor.

shop. Portable incline boards are commercially available and are most useful for athletes who travel extensively.

The most common stretch for the heel cord complex is performed by facing and leaning against a wall with the feet approximately 3 feet from the wall, keeping the knees straight and the heels on the floor (Fig. 9-89). This is an excellent stretch but is usually not done for the length of time required to effectively stretch the heel cord complex. As described in most of our treatment regimens, we feel that small doses of treatment many times a day are more effective than one large dose. This is also true for heel cord stretching in the prevention or treatment of Achilles tendinitis. Heel cord stretching also has value in plantar fasciitis, arch problems, and shin splints.

The incline board is used as follows. The athlete stands near the top of the board, making sure at all times that the heels are flat and touching the board (Fig. 9-90). As stretching or flexibility is achieved, the athlete moves down toward the base of the board while leaning against the wall (Fig. 9-91). The knees are kept in full extension. The stretch should be felt in the proximal gastrocnemius area and not in the tendinous portion of the heel cords. Recommended treatment time is 3 to 5 minutes for six to eight times a day. For early Achilles tendinitis the number of repetitions remains the same; however, the amount of time spent on the board should be increased to approximately 5 minutes per session. As treatment continues, the number of times that the exercise is done during the day can be increased to 10 to 12. Thus with a 5-minute session carried out 12 times a day, an hour is spent on the incline board. This approach is more beneficial than standing on the board for 10 to 15 minutes each session. Stretching of one muscle tendon unit for an extended time can lead to overuse syndrome, soreness, and increased symptoms of tendinitis. During early treatment on the incline board, active exercises such as toe raises should not be performed.

Standing on the incline board for 15 minutes, pain free, during a preparticipation screening before an athletic season is a useful test to determine flexibility of the heel cord complex.

In the training room situation, one helpful method of stretching is to have several boards around the training room so that as the athletes await their turn to get taped, they can stand on the Achilles slant boards in a rotation fashion. Any player with tight heel cords or undergoing treatment for Achilles tendinitis should be given an incline board to take home.

The advantage of the incline board for heel cord stretching is its ease: the athlete can talk, read a play book, do homework, or watch TV while accomplishing the stretching program.

When an athlete feels that he or she is

304

Part two
Principles of rehabilitation, reconditioning,
and athletic training

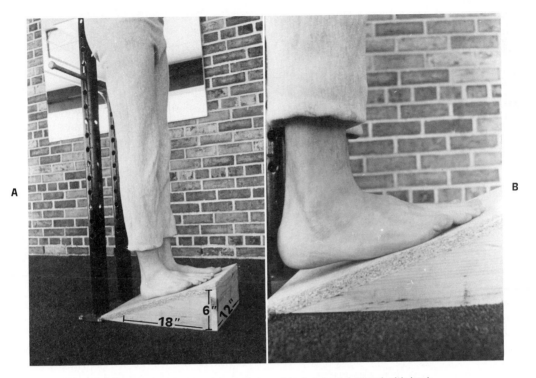

Fig. 9-90 ■ **A,** Dimensions and correct use of incline board. Stand with back against wall and feet on board near the top. **B,** Incorrect method of standing on board. Heels must be touching board so that Achilles tendon is not under too much tension.

Fig. 9-91 ■ Feet gradually worked to base of incline board. Stretch should be felt in calf (gastroc) muscle, *not* in Achilles tendon.

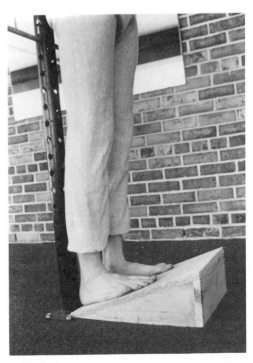

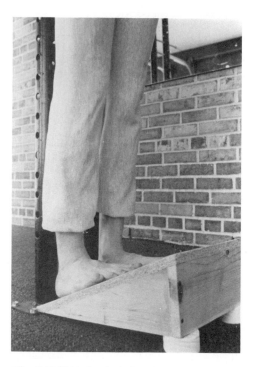

Fig. 9-92 ■ Method of elevating incline board.

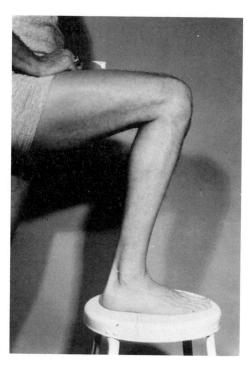

Fig. 9-93 ■ Foot placed flat on chair.

not gaining any further flexibility on the incline board, added elevation can be placed under the board to create more tilt and hence more stretch (Fig. 9-92). The athlete can also try to flex the toes up while keeping the heels down and knees straight. When athletes become sufficiently "stretchable," other exercises or accentuations of the range of motion can be performed on the incline board. Calf or toe raises can be performed in conjunction with stretching, as long as athletes remember to always try to stretch twice as long as they exercise.

Foot-on-chair method of heel cord stretching

Another effective technique for stretching heel cord is the "foot-on-chair" method.* The athlete places the affected

foot on a chair, keeping the heel touching the chair and the entire foot flat (Fig. 9-93). The knee is then brought forward as far as possible, still keeping the heel flat on the chair (Fig. 9-94). Since the knee is flexed, the stretch will be concentrated in the area of the soleus.

This stretching technique is also useful as a guide to the flexibility of the soleus. With the knee in the most anterior position, drop a plumb line from the patella down to the chair (Fig. 9-95, *A*). The measurement may be taken between the end of the toes and the plumb line. This distance can be compared between affected and unaffected legs to determine progress in the stretching program (Fig. 9-95, *B*).

"Ballerina" treatment

Another technique is called the "ballerina treatment" because it was shown to Dr. James A. Nicholas by a prominent ballerina in the New York City area. It is a very effective method of treating musculotendinous injuries, particularly those chronic tendinitis problems that one of-

---

*Editors' note: This is an effective test of and treatment for soleus contracture and posterior compartment pain from tightness. When evaluating an athlete with leg pain, this test should be performed. It should be included as a part of flexibility programs for the heel cords.

Part two
Principles of rehabilitation, reconditioning,
and athletic training

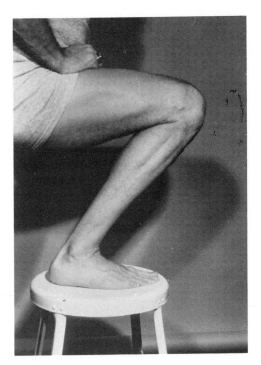

Fig. 9-94 ■ Knee is brought forward as far as possible while keeping heel flat on chair.

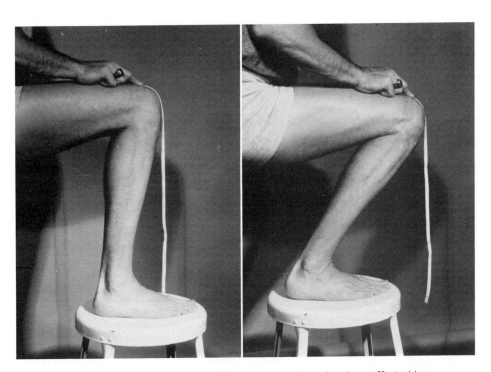

Fig. 9-95 ■ Plumb line for comparison between affected and nonaffected legs.

ten encounters. It is very simple to apply; all that is needed for the treatment is a hand towel, a plastic bag, a common electric heating pad, and an elastic bandage.

The hand towel is soaked with warm not excessively hot, water, since the towel will be next to the skin. The towel is wrung out so it remains quite moist. The warm wet towel is placed next to the affected area. A plastic bag is placed on top of the hot towel, and the electric heating pad is placed on top of the plastic bag. The plastic bag forms a barrier between the wet towel and the electric heating pad. Finally, the elastic bandage is wrapped around the towel and heating pad to hold everything in place. The heating pad is turned to a medium setting. It is left on from 3 to 5 hours or even overnight. The temperature setting should never be higher than medium. During the treatment, the affected area should be elevated higher than the heart.

This treatment is very effective and convenient. The athlete can easily do it at home during the evening and night. The ballerina treatment is also useful during travel, since the modality takes up very little space. The athlete can carry the heat-

ing pad, elastic wrap, and plastic bag in a kit and use the hand towels available at the hotel while on the road.*

Peroneal tendon strains

Strains of the peroneal tendons may occur in association with inversion ankle sprains or as an isolated injury. Treatment following the injury is identical to that for an ankle sprain. Ice bath treatment is often very successful in ameliorating early symptoms with this injury. Application of tape for peroneal tendon strains is often beneficial; the taping technique is identical to that for ankle sprain taping. Eversion is stressed, inversion is limited, and a lateral heel wedge or heel lift is placed in the shoe (see section on outside injury strapping). An L-shaped or horseshoe-shaped pad is placed around the lateral malleolus to help maintain pressure over the peroneal sheath (Fig. 9-96).

---

*Editors' note: Where there is swelling it is useful to elevate the foot of the bed about 6 to 8 inches with books or blocks. This is easier than keeping a leg elevated on a pillow all night. Elevating the foot of the bed keeps the leg elevated whether the patient sleeps on the side or the stomach, and it is not dangerous.

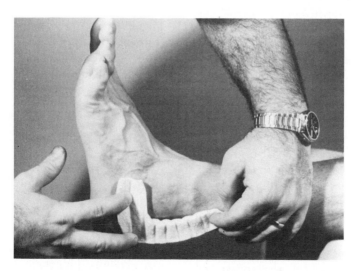

Fig. 9-96 ■ L-shaped pad placed around malleolus to maintain pressure on peroneal tendons.

308

Part two
Principles of rehabilitation, reconditioning,
and athletic training

With complete disruption of the peroneal sheath and displacement of the peroneal tendons, cast immobilization may be
required. Following the removal of the
cast, taping as just described is generally
indicated to provide support during the
rehabilitation phase.

Rarely, a player may strain a longer
portion of the peroneal tendon or the musculotendinous junction. Treatment for this
injury is similar; however, the taping is
extended proximally up the lower leg. In
this case taping would include application
of elastic tape on the lateral border of the
tibia, across the instep, and then a lift
"outside" and anchoring the tape just below the knee at the head of the fibula.

Shin splints*

Prevention is the best cure for shin
splints. This includes careful planning of
training techniques, use of appropriate
footwear, and avoidance of training on
hard surfaces. Heel cord tightness may
contribute to shin splints. If the heel cord
is tight, when fatigued the heel cord muscles will shorten and the anterior compartment muscles will have to work over-
time when dorsiflexing the foot. Therefore,
an adequate heel cord stretching program
is certainly included in the overall program to prevent shin splints. Stretching of
the anterior compartment muscles can be
achieved by sitting on the heels or by
stretching the dorsum of one foot while
standing normally on the opposite foot
with a bent knee.

Ice baths and ice massage are effective
treatments for shin splints. If possible,
eliminate practice sessions and active
work for the athlete when a severe case of
shin splints has occurred. Immediate
treatment includes ice, ice massage, ice
baths, and aggressive stretching on the incline board. Heel lifts and orthotics are
occasionally effective during the practice

---

*See Chapter 21 for a discussion of the various causes
of leg pain, including tendinitis, compartment syndrome, stress fracture, and so on.

session. If the shin splints are so severe
that the athlete cannot participate, rest
for 3 to 5 days is prescribed to allow the
inflammation to resolve. Ice treatments,
along with ballerina-type heat treatments
are also recommended. Stretching on the
incline board should be performed 10 to
12 times each day, 5 minutes per session
for a total of 1 hour. It should always be
borne in mind that this problem is usually
brought on by overuse. Therefore, players
returning from a rest period created by
shin splints should be allowed to practice
when they are asymptomatic but be ex-
cused in the early going from all agility
drills.

Taping of shin splints

Taping for shin splints is occasionally
effective. For a single-event exercise other
than football, taping may allow an athlete
to participate for a short time. If the pain
is on the lateral border of the tibia, then
tape should be started laterally, pulled
across with a downward angle medially,
and circle below the calf muscle, and reat-
tach the tape at the top using 1½-inch
tape (Fig. 9-97). In effect, the taping is attempting to pull the anterior muscles toward the tibia to relieve tension. These
strips should be overlapped and continued down to the top of the malleoli. They
may be anchored with elastic tape or elastic bandage. Arch taping and arch supports sometimes can be of value when
taping for shin splints. Prevention by early
vigilant diagnosis and adequate rest and
exercise treatment is still the best cure.

■ KNEE TAPING AND SUPPORT

Assuming that a knee injury or instability has been accurately diagnosed and a
nonoperative course is indicated, effective
use of taping techniques may help a
player to return to participation. This is a
very common practice for chronic medial
collateral ligament laxity, and some lateral
collateral ligament laxities, with or without rotational instability. Taping can be
especially effective on "skill" people who

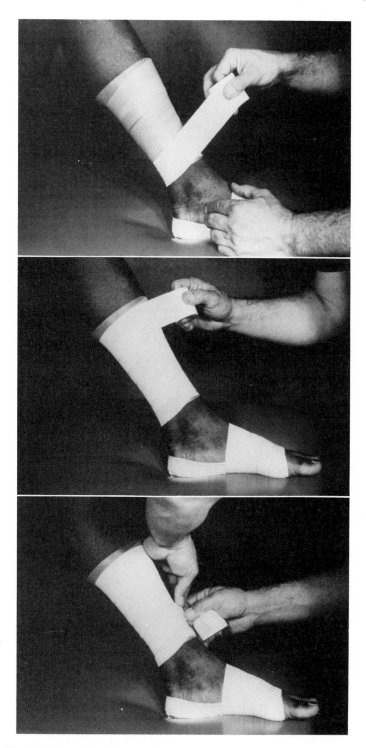

Fig. 9-97 ■ Lateral skin splint taping. Tape started laterally, pulled downward and across and reattached on lateral border. Continue on down to just above the malleoli.

Part two
Principles of rehabilitation, reconditioning,
and athletic training

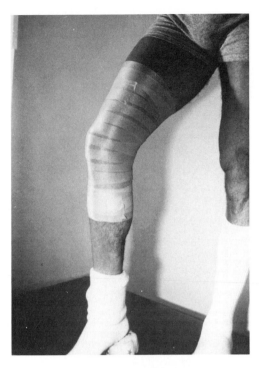

Fig. 9-98 ■ Application of prewrap. Note that athlete is standing with knee slightly flexed. A small object beneath the heel is useful in helping relax the athlete's leg.

require a lot of freedom of movement and where bracing may detract from the freedom of movement that they must enjoy to compete effectively (e.g., football wide receivers, running backs, and defensive backs).

When taping the knee, stretching of the quadriceps, hamstrings, and gastrocnemius is essential. The taping somewhat constricts the bellies of the muscles, creating increased workload on the muscles and perhaps making them more prone to strains late in the contest or practice session.

Preparation

The knee should be shaved from below midcalf to above midthigh, then cleaned and sprayed with tape adherent. A lubricated pad is placed behind the knee to prevent friction burns. An underwrap should then be applied, making sure there is room at midthigh and midcalf lev-

els to allow for anchoring of tape directly to the skin (Fig. 9-98).

One-plane instability

Apply anchor strips with 3-inch elastic tape, preferably heavy elastic of the Elasticon variety or high tensile strength thin elastic tape (Fig. 9-99). The elastic tape anchor should be applied snugly but not too tightly. The anchor strips should have about 2 inches of direct skin contact around the circumference of the thigh and calf. For the standard taping and general support, Xs should be made, crossing the medial and lateral joint lines (Fig. 9-100). They are applied distally and proximally, starting posteriorly at the gastrocnemius, coming across the knee joint and anchoring anteriorly on the thigh. The next strip goes in the opposite direction, from anterior tibia to posterior thigh. These strips may be applied from proximal to distal as opposed to distal to proximal to aid in cutting the tape. Approximately 95% of the "stretch" should be taken out of the X strips. Next alternate strips should be placed on the outside (Fig. 9-101). The X strips should be alternated medially, then laterally, so that they overlap, first the medial, then the lateral, providing opposite forces so that the tape is working against itself. At least two full Xs should be placed medially and laterally (Fig. 9-102). We feel that if support is to be achieved and maintained, it is necessary to tape both the medial and lateral side of the knee regardless of whether the injury is isolated on the medial or lateral side. The best support is achieved by having the tape work against itself.

If there is no patellar involvement, the tape may be anchored top and bottom and finally cut (Fig. 9-103). The anchor strips are applied snugly to provide strength and integrity to the taping. They should not constrict the thigh muscles or the gastrocnemius. An anchor with adhesive tape must follow on the elastic tape. If possible, do not encircle the calf or thigh with the adhesive tape (Fig. 9-104). If circular tape is necessary because of

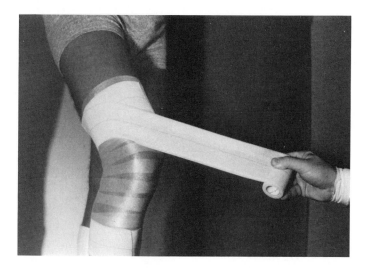

Fig. 9-108 ■ Start laterally and cross medially across the joint line.

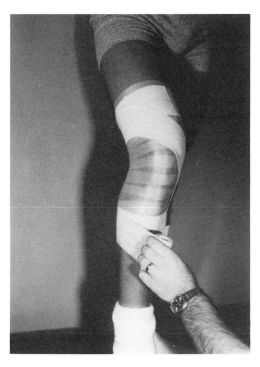

Fig. 9-109 ■ Continue around behind
gastrocnemius and attach anterolaterally.

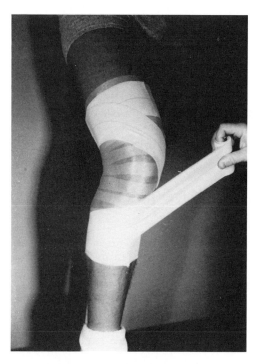

Fig. 9-110 ■ Begin posterolaterally, pulling tape
around, crossing the medial joint line, and
continuing up and around.

316

Part two
Principles of rehabilitation, reconditioning,
and athletic training

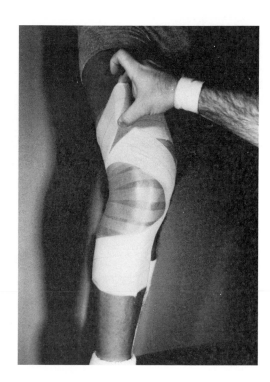

Fig. 9-111 ■ Cut and attach on the anterolateral aspect of the thigh.

should then be anchored as previously described with concentric spirals placed lightly around the knee. Taping for various other rotatory instabilities is easily created using the principles described previously. Adjust where the tape begins and the torsion of the tape to fit the rotatory instability present. A horseshoe felt can be placed on top of this taping if patellar restraint is also required.

Hyperextension

The knee is prepared in the usual manner. The basic hyperextension knee taping is applied with the athlete prone on the training table. Less prewrap is used but is still applied 4 to 6 inches above and below the knee joint. Several lubricated pads behind the knee are necessary. The knee is then flexed to 20 degrees or just short of where the pain begins on terminal extension. With a relatively acute injury, less extension is allowed. As the injury heals, less pain is present and the danger of reinjury is diminished, so more extension is permitted. The common method of taping is

to anchor at the top and bottom midthigh and midcalf areas as before. Strips are then applied in a crisscross butterfly fashion, overlapping each strip by approximately half (Fig. 9-113). This is done twice so there is a wide base of support on the anchor crossing to give good firm support

HYPEREXTENSION TAPING	
Objective:	Limited terminal extension
Indications:	Hyperextension injury
Position:	Patient prone with knee flexed 15 to 20 degrees
Technique:	Lubricated pads behind knee
	Prewrap
	Anchor strips on thigh and calf
	Crisscross butterfly taping with gap between tape and knee (knee slightly flexed)
	Concentric anchor tape taking longitudinal strips flush to prewrap
	Heel lift in shoe
Variation:	Moleskin longitudinal strips

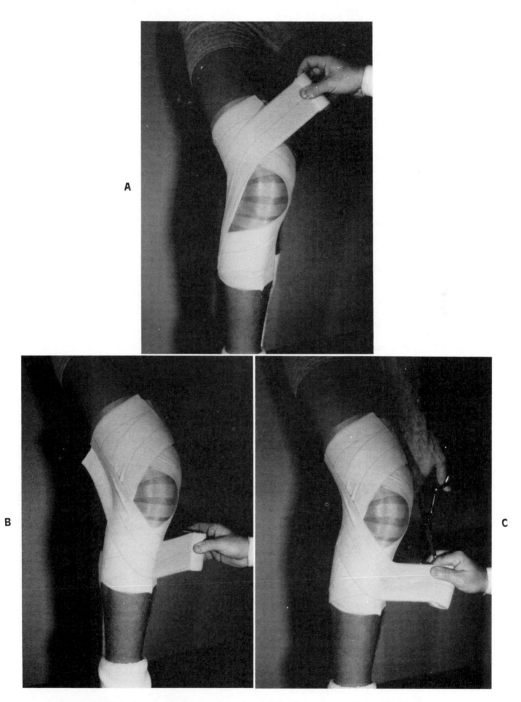

Fig. 9-112 ■ **A,** Opposite strips are begun below the knee and anteromedially to cross the lateral joint line and cut. **B,** Then strip is brought above the knee laterally, pulling gently medially, and **C,** cut.

318

Part two
Principles of rehabilitation, reconditioning,
and athletic training

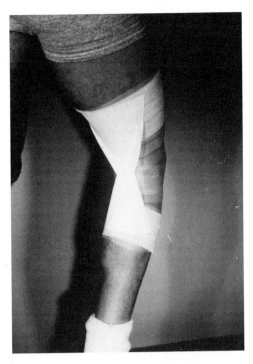

Fig. 9-113 ■ ''Butterfly'' used for hyperextension strapping.

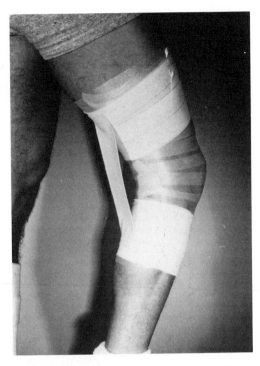

Fig. 9-114 ■ Moleskin used in straight strips for hyperextension strapping.

across the joint line. The strips are placed in a fashion that leaves a gap between the posterior crease of the knee and the tape. This creates a bridgelike formation of tape lying above the popliteal crease. The crossing strips are then anchored down with concentric elastic tape from distal to proximal. At this time, the gap at the flexion crease is eliminated by taking the tape flush to the posterior aspect of the knee.

Another worthwhile method uses moleskin adhesive tape. Moleskin is stronger than regular adhesive and provides greater resistance to extension. Simply use several strips of moleskin as the checkrein (Fig. 9-114). It may be applied from proximal to distal in two or three strips running parallel. It can also be applied in a crossing or butterfly fashion (Fig. 9-115). Since moleskin is stronger and less tape is required, the entire taping technique is less time consuming and less bulky. If taping for a chronic injury, a single strip of moleskin may be all that is

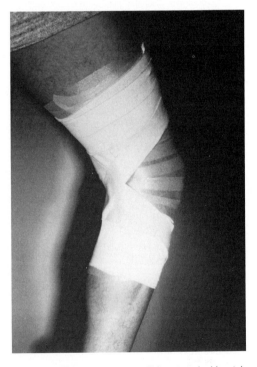

Fig. 9-115 ■ Xing or ''butterflying'' moleskin strips for hyperextension.

necessary to prevent hyperextension. Too much "accented" flexion may not allow sufficient function for the athlete to perform.

During hyperextension taping, the integrity of the tape may be maintained by applying an elastic bandage or a cohesive elastic bandage on top of the taping. This is particularly beneficial if the tape is applied well before the contest. The other elastic bandage is removed before the contest.

When taping the extremity to prevent hyperextension, a ¼- to ½-inch heel lift should be placed in the shoe of the affected leg to reduce the tension on the anchored areas of the strapping. A disk or bar should replace the rear cleats for natural turf football shoes (see Fig. 9-183).

■ MUSCLE STRAINS—A TRAINER'S VIEWPOINT
Hamstring injuries

Strains of the hamstring may be graded as first, second, and third degree, or mild, moderate, and severe. Treatment varies in aggressiveness, depending on the severity of the injury. Early recognition and diagnosis of the degree of injury is a primary concern, but sometimes this is very difficult to determine. It should always be noted whether the injury was an actual first-degree strain or a cramp resulting from fatigue or dehydration.* The only way to be absolutely sure of this differentiation is the length of time the symptoms are present. If simply a cramp, symptoms will resolve within 2 to 3 days. If the symptoms last longer, then the injury is most likely a first degree strain.

The athlete should be questioned about the mechanism of injury. It should be determined whether the athlete was in full stride, whether he or she felt the pain coming on, whether it started out as an ache, or whether it suddenly "grabbed" the player.

To diagnose the degree of injury, place

the player prone, off of the field, either on the bench or in the training room. Have the athlete gently flex the knee to approximately 15 degrees and ask the athlete to point to the area that is most sore. If the athlete points to a large area with the entire hand, as is the case most of the time, have the athlete indicate the injured area with just one finger. When this is done, begin gentle palpation, noting whether there is a defect in the area. Also, note the degree of pain on palpation. If there is no obvious defect or mass, have the athlete actively flex the knee against resistance at about 15 degrees of flexion. Then again palpate the area to note whether a defect is now present.

A good knowledge of the anatomy of the hamstrings is vital to isolate the three different muscles and their various segments. Determine whether the strain is in the belly of the muscle, at the muscular tendinous junction in the tendinous portion, or in the proximal origin of the muscle. A third degree strain or complete rupture of one of the hamstring muscles will be very evident on palpation. Occasionally it may be obvious with just visual examination of the hamstring area. In this case there will be a large defect present, with a proximal mass representing the "balling up" of the muscle tissue. If the athlete is severly disabled, ice and compression should be immediately applied. Third degree strains are serious injuries, and rest, ice, and compression are the main treatments for 4 to 6 weeks. Crutches are mandatory. Fortunately, this is a rare occurrence.

A second degree or moderate strain may or may not have a palpable defect. A first degree strain will have no palpable defect and will have less pain than the second degree strain. One key in recognizing the degree of injury is that in a second degree strain, a wider area of pain is generally found. Many times a first degree strain can be pinpointed by one finger. First and second degree strains are treated identically.

---

*See p. 46 for a discussion of muscle cramps.

Part two
Principles of rehabilitation, reconditioning,
and athletic training

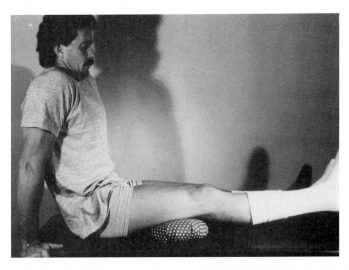

Fig. 9-116 ■ Athlete sitting on ice bag with leg in extension for hamstring injury.

Once the injury has been documented as a first or second degree strain, the athlete is removed from competition and placed on the training table sitting up with his or her back against the wall and the leg held with the knee as close to full extension as possible (Fig. 9-116). The affected area is rested on an ice bag. The heel of the foot is supported with a pillow or a block to maintain the knee in extension. Thus the muscle strain is being iced in extension. This is the opposite of the most common method of cryotherapy, which is done with the player prone, the knee flexed, and the ice resting on the affected area. Icing the muscle in extension provides early stretching of the muscle injury. Even though this may be somewhat more uncomfortable in the early stages of treatment, the ice will provide an anesthetic effect after 7 to 10 minutes, which allows the treatment to continue at a tolerable pain level. All further static ice treatments are administered in this fashion.

After the injury site has been iced for approximately 20 minutes, the athlete is permitted to shower. A compression bandage of Webril and cohesive bandage is applied. Remember to spray several areas with pretape spray to keep the Webril

from slipping. This will keep the bandage in place overnight if necessary. Depending on the time of day that the injury occurs, the ice in the static stretch position should be applied two or three more times. No other stretching should be performed on the first day of injury.

On the second day after injury, an examination is performed after removal of the compression bandage. Again, palpate the area, have the athlete explain where it hurts, and gently test the strength of the muscle and range of motion. Depending on the amount of pain exhibited and the amount of strength present, more aggressive treatment can be initiated at this time. If the site is very tender and the athlete has trouble flexing the knee, another day of static icing and stretching should be performed before initiation of aggressive treatment. When sufficient healing has taken place, aggressive treatment can be begun. This program includes repeated icing, ice massage, and stretching. First, ice the hamstrings for 10 to 15 minutes with the knee extended. The athlete should be sitting back against a wall with the foot placed on a block to maintain knee extension. After the area has been iced, the athlete is then rolled onto the stomach. The leg is over the edge of the

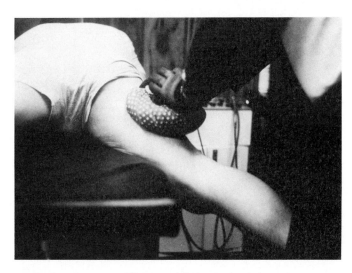

Fig. 9-117 ■ Deep ice massage begun while hamstring is in eccentric contraction.

table so that the hamstrings can eccentrically contract during application of deep ice massage (Fig. 9-117). The deep ice massage is administered for 12 to 15 minutes with a good deal of pressure. Throughout the ice massage time, the athlete maintains an eccentric contraction in the hamstrings. Following the deep ice massage, modified Williams flexion exercises (p. 323) are performed to gently stretch the hamstrings and low back. The modified Williams exercises are performed every hour on the hour if possible. The goal is to achieve 10 repetitions of the five different exercises in a 12- to 18-hour period. It should be remembered that it is preferable to perform the exercises for a short duration many times during the day rather than performing one long bout of exercise once a day. The entire aggressive treatment program is administered three to four times a day, depending on the amount of time available. No heat is used during the first 3 or 4 days of treatment.

When the athlete can perform the modified Williams flexion exercise of the bent knee to straight leg raise and have the leg raised beyond a 90 degree angle from the perpendicular while keeping the knee perfectly extended and the toes dorsi-

flexed, activity can be begun. At this point, therapy includes stationary bicycle riding for 7 to 10 minutes, followed by ice and compression modality treatment. Immediately following this treatment, the modified Williams flexion exercises are again performed. Stationary bicycle riding is done two to three times a day as pain permits. Generally, for a first degree strain, this point will come on the third or fourth day after injury. For a second degree strain, this point is usually reached on the seventh to tenth day. Once bike riding is well tolerated, the athlete is instructed in the technique of the striding exercises. Striding is performed following a good warm-up on the bicycle. The striding exercises are performed as tolerated with the goal being ten 100-yard strides (p. 328).

Deep ice massage technique

Deep ice massage is usually performed with an English ice bag rather than an ice cup. However, the injured area may be prepared for the deep ice massage with an ice cup. Preparation consists of local cooling by direct application of ice either with an ice cup or ice bag for 10 to 15 minutes. Following this cooling process, ice massage is performed by hand by the trainer. It is a tiresome but effective mo-

Part two
Principles of rehabilitation, reconditioning,
and athletic training

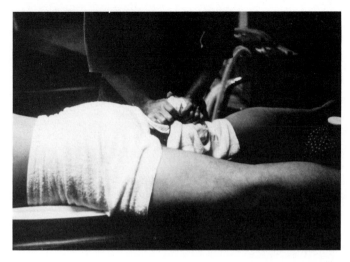

Fig. 9-118 ■ Using a wet towel when administering deep ice massage to aid in preventing skin abrasion.

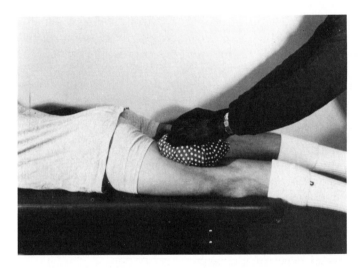

Fig. 9-119 ■ Trainer using neoprene gloves to protect hands from cold.

dality. When necessary, two trainers can take 10-minute shifts applying the ice massage. The ice massage is applied to the effected muscle with the muscle in an eccentric contraction if possible.

It has been found that ice massage is generally most affective when applied for between 12 and 15 minutes. Mild frostbite can result from more than 20 minutes of application. When working on an individual with low body fat and well developed musculature, the kneading process can also lead to abrasion of the superficial skin. If this occurs, massage is temporarily suspended. If resumed at a later date, precautions, such as a wet towel over the affected area between the ice and skin, are applied during deep ice massage (Fig. 9-118). To protect the trainer who administers the deep ice massage, it is suggested that neoprene gloves be worn while performing the massage (Fig. 9-119).

sleeve, especially in hot weather. If warmth is needed in the injured area, a piece of neoprene may be cut and placed over the area with an analgesic balm. It is then lightly secured with Webril and elastic tape or cohesive bandage.

When the athlete is returning to activity, heel lifts should be placed in each shoe to take a small amount of stress off the hamstring. This is particularly necessary in defensive backs. Make sure that the Williams flexion exercises are continued eight to ten times per day.

When athletes are returning to activity, the athlete is permitted to use the hydrocollator pack or warm moist heat to warm the muscle up before activity.

On the first several days, only the actual movements of the sport should be performed. Agility drills and conditioning drills are not carried out to avoid muscle fatigue. When an athlete is returning to action after a muscle strain, the first several days are spent at less than 100% full capability. While returning to activity, the athlete must maintain over 90 degrees of hip flexion with the knee extended on the extension portion of the modified Williams flexion activity exercises. When activity is begun, an aching similar to a toothache in the damaged muscle is normal. As long as the athlete maintains flexibility and does not overstretch or overstride, the muscles should not be reinjured.

After every bout of exercise, the injury site should be iced with the athlete in the seated leg-extended position. Depending on the symptoms and activity level, the deep ice massage can be continued. Once the athlete has reached full activity level, the deep ice massage is discontinued. Warm-up before activity is always continued as are icing the leg after activity and working on flexibility exercises.

Note that any player recovering from a strained muscle should definitely maintain the adequate hydration level. A problem with dehydration may have contributed to the initial strain and if not corrected will continue to aggravate the condition.

Hamstring taping

I feel that if a muscle is taped or strapped too tightly, the athlete cannot feel the painful warning of impending reinjury. Furthermore, with taping, the sensation that the muscle is fatiguing or shortening may be lost, leading to reinjury. When a damaged muscle is wrapped tightly, tied down, or placed in a neoprene sleeve, the muscle must work harder against the constriction of the bandage and is more likely to fatigue earlier. Fatigue will lead to muscle shortening and cramping, and reinjury will follow.

Taping for hamstring strains should be done only for a single-event contest or near the end of the season, when the athlete will have time to recover and rehabilitate fully in the off-season.

When it does become necessary to tape a hamstring injury, the accepted taping technique includes application of anchor strips immediately proximal to the posterior crease of the knee, at the fold of the buttocks, and just below the waist. The site of the injury is located by palpation. A hard foam rubber or felt pad is taped in the area of the strain, immediately proximal or distal to the strain, depending on the location of the injury (Fig. 9-125). If the injury is proximal, the pad is placed proximal to the injury. An alternative method of pad placement may be attempted if the injury is in the midportion of the muscle. This is especially effective on a strain in the muscular portion of the biceps femoris. With this technique, two pads are placed on the leg (Fig. 9-126). The first long thin pad (1½ inches wide by 8 inches long) is placed medially along the edge of the muscle. Next a wider pad (4 inches wide by 8 inches long) is placed laterally along the edge of the muscle. The bars are applied in a manner that "squeezes" the muscle and makes it "thicker" (Fig. 9-127). With padding and taping, one is shortening the working por-

330

Part two
Principles of rehabilitation, reconditioning,
and athletic training

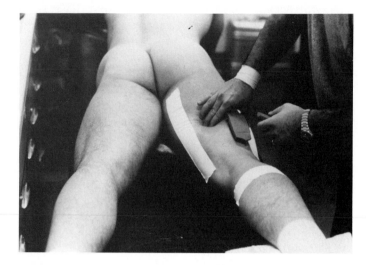

Fig. 9-125 ■ Anchor strips and placement of foam pad to shorten muscle.

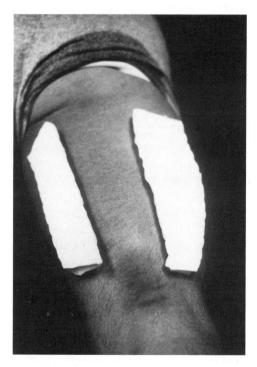

Fig. 9-126 ■ Alternate method of pad placement.
Pads placed on either side of working muscle.

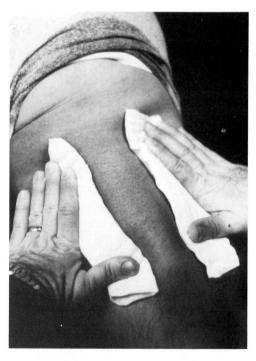

Fig. 9-127 ■ Alternate method of pad placement.
Graphic squeezing of muscle.

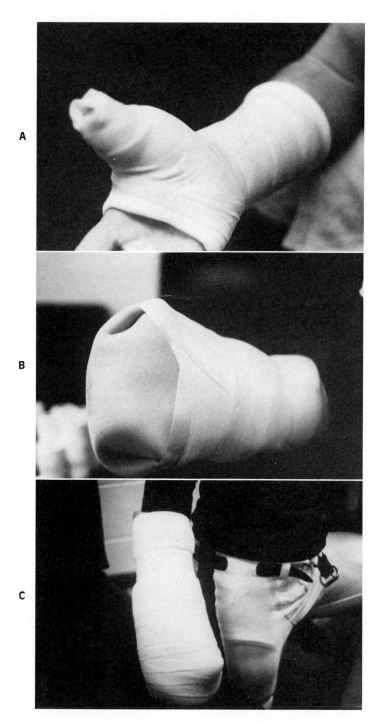

Fig. 9-136 ■ **A,** Unprotected cast. **B,** One-half inch foam wrapped around cast. **C,** Tape securing foam. Athlete is ready for competition.

342

Part two
Principles of rehabilitation, reconditioning,
and athletic training

What is protective equipment?

Protective equipment can be anything from a simple elastic wrap to a rigid cast, as long as it serves a purpose—mechanical, psychological, or otherwise. It can be a simple Ace elastic wrap, adhesive tapes, neoprene wrap and sleeve, synthetic cloth, foam, plastic, casting material, brace, orthotic, or any combination of some or all of these products. Protective equipment must protect the body part and allow function but also keep from injuring the athlete, his teammates, or opponents, by the nature of the device's exposed rigid surfaces or sharp, unprotected protrusions.

Stock vs. custom items

Stock items are prefabricated and packaged, ready for immediate use. Custom-made items are constructed individually for a given athlete and a particular injury (Fig. 9-137). These two forms can be combined by taking a stock item and customizing it.

Stock items

Stock items have many attractive features. Materials and methods of manufacture not readily accessible to the trainer or team physician are made available. Stock items are ready for use with enough straps and sleeves to fully use the piece as it is intended. Some problems are associated with stock items: cost, sizing, and public awareness of their availability. Cost can be either an asset or a detriment to a stock item. Products made in mass quantities tend to be available at attractive prices, whereas innovative products with a unique attribute tend to be very expensive, sometimes too expensive for some athletic programs.

Sizing can be a factor with stock items because of uncertainty or inconsistency about what is small, medium, or large. One company's small certainly may vary from what another manufacturer deems small. Often the various products and their sizes are not on hand to permit di-

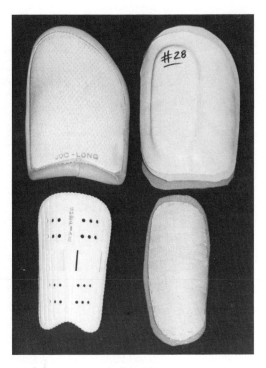

Fig. 9-137 ■ Stock vs. custom pads. Stock *(left)* and custom *(right)* thigh and shin pads.

rect comparison of one product with another.

Awareness of product availability is sometimes a problem. Not all weekend athletes, neighborhood programs, or even physicians and trainers read all the literature and advertisements that promote specialized protective equipment. An often-heard comment is, "I didn't know this pad even existed." Many small neighborhood surgical supply houses or local sporting goods stores cannot stock a full array of pads. They may carry only one manufacturer's product line or not have the room to stock the item. Also, infrequent demand may not mandate the need to stock such items.

Custom items

Custom items have characteristics all their own. Two of the advantages of custom-made items are sizing and specificity of purpose. If a pad is customized, it should fit exactly as intended and provide

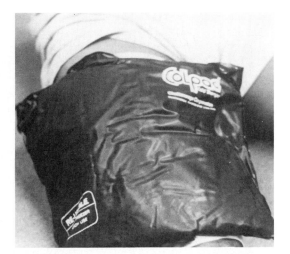

Fig. 9-157 ■ Cooling process sped up with cold pack.

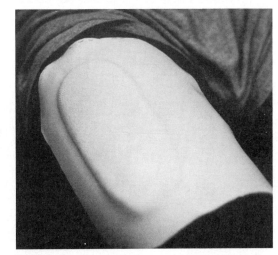

Fig. 9-158 ■ Untrimmed shell.

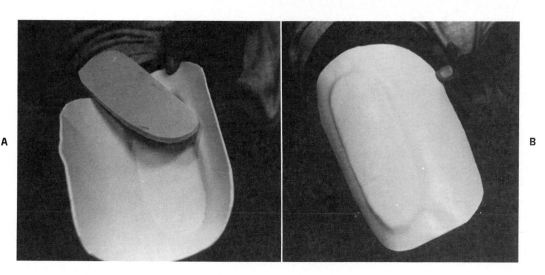

A

B

Fig. 9-159 ■ **A,** Foam used to create "bubble" is removed. **B,** Trimmed shell.

354

Part two
Principles of rehabilitation, reconditioning,
and athletic training

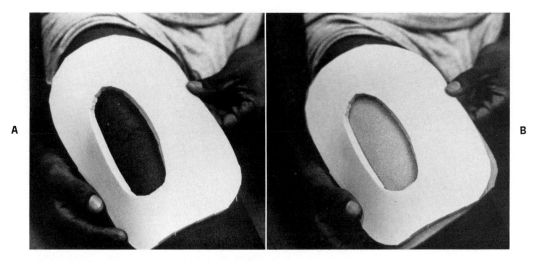

Fig. 9-160 ■ **A,** Doughnut-shaped foam lining. **B,** Doughnut combined with softer foam.

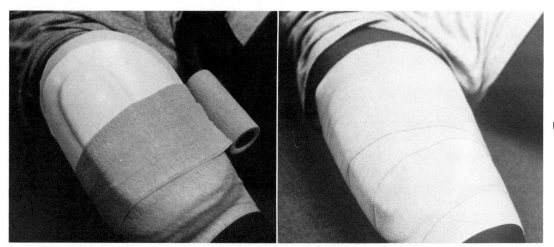

Fig. 9-161 ■ **A,** Trial fitting of pad with elastic wrap. **B,** Complete pad wrapped in place.

relief to the tender area (Fig. 9-160). A trial fitting is advised before joining all the materials using tape or adhesives (Fig. 9-161). Additional padding may be required for the outside surface of the pad to protect teammates and opponents from the hard surface. Finally, allow the athlete to fully evaluate the device to avoid disturbing performance in competition (Fig. 9-162).

Specific protective equipment
Trunk and thorax

The trunk and thorax need to be protected in collision sports. Shoulder pads, such as used in football, may suffice, depending on how far the anterior and posterior trim line of the pad covers the thorax. Many extra pads and belts are available for protection of the thorax and rib cage. The most popular in football are the

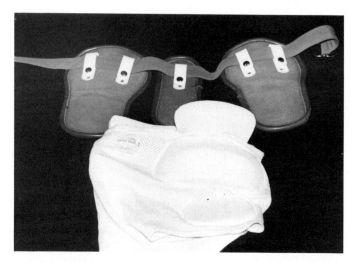

Fig. 9-166 ■ Belt-type and girdle-style hip pads.

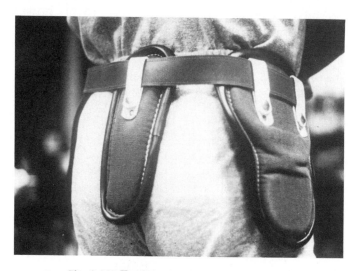

Fig. 9-167 ■ Belt-type hip and coccygeal pads.

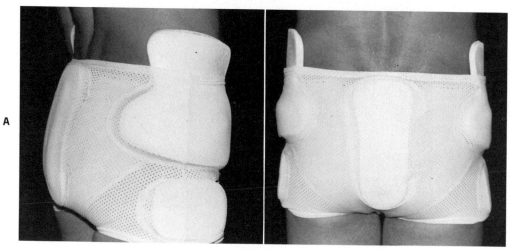

Fig. 9-168 ■ Girdle-style hip and coccygeal pads. **A,** Side. **B,** Back.

Part two
principles of rehabilitation, reconditioning,
and athletic training

(Fig. 9-168). The main shortcoming of this type of pad is that the athlete feels bound down and thinks this padding is too bulky. This area of the body tends to be neglected in some collision sports, and athletes often do not wear appropriate padding until they receive an injury and realize they should have worn pads. Many times football players will cut foam rubber and slip it into their pants over the iliac crest to protect against lateral blows. Such pads are marginally effective compared to more rigid hip pads.

Groin and genitalia

In dealing with sports that involve high velocity projectiles, such as hockey, lacrosse, and baseball, some form of cup protector for male athletes should be used. This type of protective equipment is a commonly stocked item and is held in place by a jock strap support.

Thigh and upper leg

Participation in collision-type sports requires thigh protection, or thigh boards, as they have been called in the past (Fig. 9-169). These pads are generally slipped into pockets sewn into the pants (Fig. 9-170). Hockey and football players commonly use such

pads, and many times, in the case of an injury, pads are custom-made to cover an even wider area of the leg. One situation faced with these pads is the tendency to shift from side to side, especially in a collision, exposing areas that were originally intended to be protected. This problem must be addressed when selecting and fitting pants and protective pads. Often custom alteration provides the best solution. Different thigh boards and thigh pads are commercially available in varying thicknesses, widths, and heights (Fig. 9-171). Thigh pads were once made of small, inflatable air bags, but these tended to have too much bounce and are not used much today (Fig. 9-172). Athletes want to wear the thinnest and smallest pads, thinking larger ones will slow them down. As sports medicine practitioners, we must encourage athletes to wear the padding that is best suited to protect them.

Knee

There are many protective pads available for the knee, but generally they fall into two categories, either basketball-style or football-style (Fig. 9-173). The basketball- and wrestling-style knee pad is a pad within a sleeve that can be slipped over

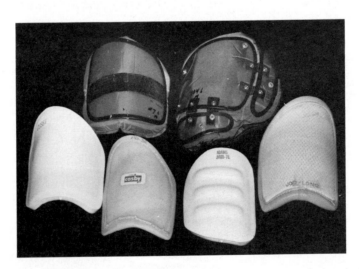

Fig. 9-169 ■ Various thigh pads, including Donzis style *(top),* now manufactured with a black polymer shell.

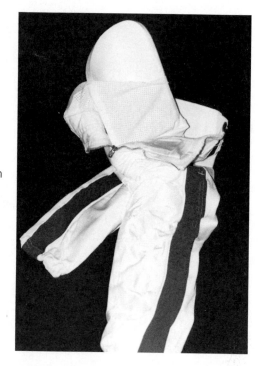

Fig. 9-170 ■ Slipping thigh board into mesh pocket of football pants.

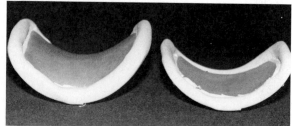

Fig. 9-171 ■ Side view of thigh pad thickness.

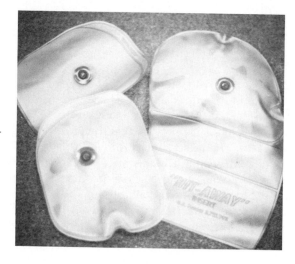

Fig. 9-172 ■ Airpads.

Part two
principles of rehabilitation, reconditioning,
and athletic training

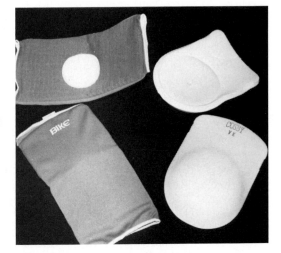

Fig. 9-173 ■ Basketball/wrestling-style knee pad
(left) and football-style *(right)*.

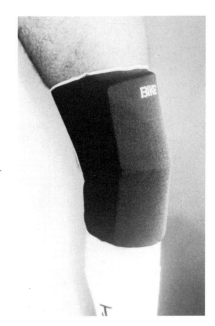

Fig. 9-174 ■ Basketball/wrestling knee pad.

the knee area with some form of strapping behind the popliteal area. These pads differ in the trim line, the area they cover, and the type of strapping behind the knee (Fig. 9-174). The main-shortcoming of this type of pad is that athletes tend to feel that in an extremely flexed knee position, the webbing or strapping behind the knee is limiting. Certainly the knee is one of the areas for which neoprene sleeves have become popular. This type of pad does provide a little bit of protection from concussion, but again more support is afforded from compression and the warmth that the insulating rubber provides.

The football- and hockey-type knee pad is held in place by the pants in a pocket sewn into the pant leg. This type of pad tends to be displaced easily in a collision when the pants leg shifts from side to side. They do afford a certain amount of comfort from the fact that there are no

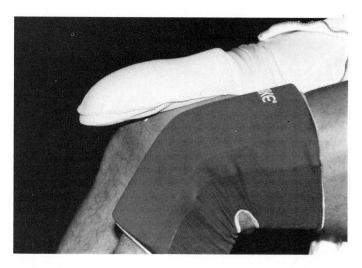

Fig. 9-175 ■ Both different pads shown in place with mesh pocket of football pant exposed.

binding straps that go behind the knee*
(Fig. 9-175).

Shin and lower leg

Protection of the shin and lower leg is
commonly neglected in most sports. In
those sports involving hard projectiles or
extensive collision, it is advisable to provide some type of protection to this area.
There are hard-shell molded shin guards
available, such as those manufactured by
Casco. Soccer shin guards, which simply
slip down into knee-length socks and are
held in place by the elastic of the sock,
are convenient and readily available (Fig.
9-176). Different types and grades of foam
can be used inside the sock to provide tibial protection and one is limited only by
one's materials and imagination.

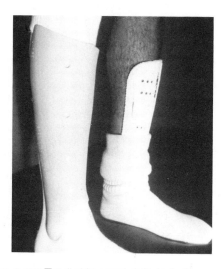

Fig. 9-176 ■ Full shin guard *(left),* including
protection over malleolus and slip-in soccer-style
pad *(right).*

---

*Editors' note: Not to mention the use of various
braces first popularized at Lenox Hill Hospital with
the development of the Lenox Hill derotation brace
in 1965 and the two-piece patella restraining brace at
that time. Now, two decades later, over 20 knee
braces are used with varying acceptance and wide
appreciation of the need for protection. This market-
place requires a thorough scrutiny as to the value of
current braces compared with the rigid tests that we
used together with Jack Kennedy and Stan James on
the Lenox Hill brace leading to 7 years of trial before
publication of value.

Ankle

This area of the lower extremity is not
commonly padded but is more commonly
protected with athletic tapes and wraps.
The upper last of footwear affords protection to much of the ankle, such as in
hockey and football, where high-top
skates or shoes are worn. Certainly in the
case of goalies and catchers, special pads
exist that cover the whole extremity including the knee, shin and ankle. If the

Part two
principles of rehabilitation, reconditioning,
and athletic training

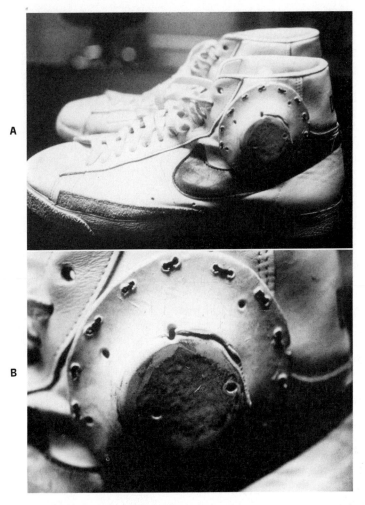

Fig. 9-177 ■ **A,** Plastic shell attached to basketball shoe. **B,** Close-up of plastic shell "sewn" to basketball shoe.

ankle needs further protection, custom hard shells can be fabricated from casting material attached to the outside of the shoe, providing additional protection to the bony protruberances of the ankle (Fig. 9-177).

Foot and forefoot

If the foot and forefoot require extra protection in addition to that afforded by the shoe (Fig. 9-178), a hard shell can be manufactured to go over the outside of the shoe. Occasionally an injury to a toe requires relief directly over the area. A hole can be cut in the shoe, and a protec-

tive shell can be made to protect the exposed toe (Fig. 9-179). A fiberglass cast can be molded over the shoe, using a temporary foam insert to provide a "bubble" of relief directly over the injured area. Care must be taken to allow the cast to contact the shoe all around the sensitive area and allow for support from direct blows (Fig. 9-180). The bottom is cut away from the cast to expose the bottom of the shoe, and the shell is attached using tape and/or hardware (Fig. 9-181).

The foot and arch can be protected by a number of different products, and a whole array of custom-made orthotics are

375

Section 1 FOOT AND ANKLE
Chapter 10 Anatomy and physical
examination of the foot and ankle

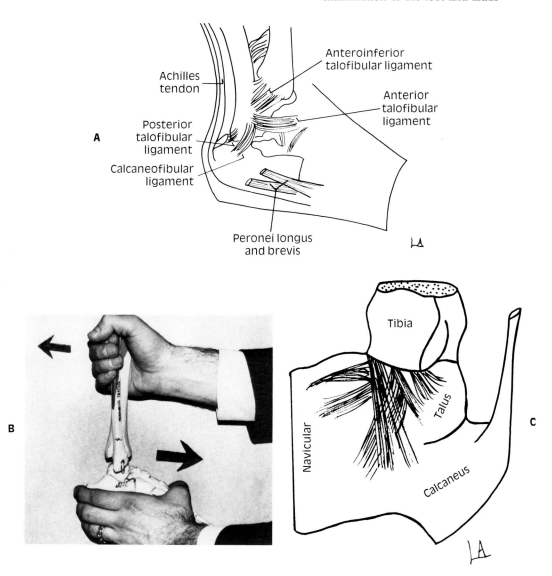

Fig. 10-4 ■ **A,** Lateral ligamentous stability of ankle is afforded by anterior talofibular, calcaneofibular and posterior talofibular ligaments. **B,** Anterior drawer test. **C,** Deltoid ligament may be seen spanning medial aspect of ankle joint, taking origin from distal medial malleolus and inserting onto navicular, talus and calcaneus.

rupture the calcaneofibular ligament and the lateral ankle capsule will allow contrast material to exit the ankle joint and enter the interior of these tendon sheaths. Because of the spontaneous closure of capsular rents, the ability to visualize the interior of the peroneal tendon sheaths may be lost by 24 hours after injury.

The third lateral ligament is the **posterior talofibular.** It is the smallest of the lateral ankle ligaments and lies deep to the soft tissues of the posterolateral ankle. It originates from the posteromedial surface of the lateral malleolus and serves as a weak restraint against posterior displacement of the talus within the ankle mortise.

Medially, ligamentous support of the ankle is provided by the **deltoid ligament.** The deltoid ligament is the largest of the ankle ligaments by virtue of its breadth. It extends as a broad fanlike structure

---

DELTOID LIGAMENT

- Largest ankle ligament
- Composed of two layers
- Prevents abduction-eversion of ankle and subtalar joint
- Prevents eversion-pronation and anterior displacement of talus

---

PRIMARY FUNCTIONS OF THE FOOT

Provide a stable platform of support
Attenuate impact loading
Assist in efficient forward propulsion of body

---

across the medial ankle (Fig. 10-4, C). It originates from the inferior aspect of the medial malleolus and has two layers. The superficial layer inserts anteriorly onto the navicular, inferiorly onto the sustentaculum tali of the calcaneus, and posteriorly onto the talus. The deep layer inserts onto the medial body of the talus. The purpose of this ligament is to prevent abduction/eversion of the ankle and subtalar joint. It also prevents eversion, pronation, and anterior displacement of the talus.

Rupture of the deltoid ligament together with compromise of the tibiofibular interosseous syndesmosis will result in widening of the ankle mortise. Functionally this will create mediolateral instability within the ankle mortise. Such instability is poorly tolerated. In almost every patient, it will result in the rapid development of osteoarthrosis of the ankle joint. Clinical assessment of such a disruption of the mortise can be obtained by manual mediolateral stress testing and appropriate roentgenographic studies, including the **mortise view.** This view is obtained by an anteroposterior projection of a 15-degree internally rotated lower extremity. Normally the "cartilage space" of the ankle mortise surrounding the medial, lateral, and superior aspects of the talus should appear of equal dimension (Fig. 10-5). Increase in the medial and/or lateral "joint space" should be interpreted as pathologic widening of the ankle mortise.

Foot

The primary functions of the foot are to provide a stable platform of support, to attenuate impact loading of the extremity during locomotion, and to assist in the efficient forward propulsion of the body. To accomplish these tasks the foot is made up of a multiplicity of semirigid articulations that afford conformity with varying surface topographies. The bony elements are arranged in longitudinal and transverse arches. These are spanned on the planter aspect by soft tissue tension bands to provide impact load attenuation.

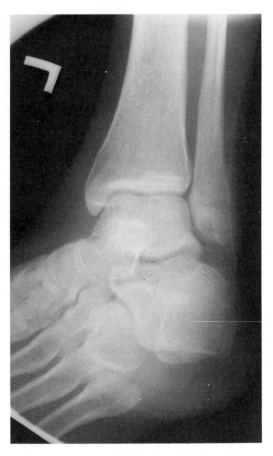

Fig. 10-5 ■ Normal ankle. Note congruity of talar and mortise articular surfaces.

383

Section 1 FOOT AND ANKLE
Chapter 10 Anatomy and physical
examination of the foot and ankle

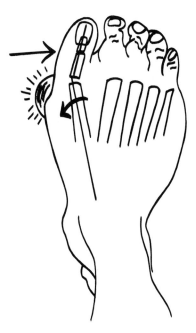

Fig. 10-14 ■ Hindfoot pronation may result in valgus stressing of first metatarsophalangeal joint. Chronic valgus stress may result in inflammation and swelling (bunion), and angulation at this joint (hallux valgus deformity).

valgus) and resultant medial inflammation and soft tissue swelling (bunion formation) at that articulation (Fig. 10-14).

At the distal end of the column are the five digits of the foot. The base phalanx of each digit is a miniature long bone that articulates proximally as a shallow-dished articular surface onto the spherical head of its respective metatarsal. As such the MTP articulations can accommodate up to 90 degrees of both plantar flexion and dorsiflexion together with 20 degrees of medial and lateral rotation about the longitudinal axis of the digit. Each digit is composed of three phalanges except the first digit, which, although more massive than the remaining digits, contains only two phalanges. Unlike the disklike MTP articulations, those between the phalanges are ginglymal (hinged). They are stabilized by collateral ligaments that restrict these articulations to flexion-extension motion.

The terminal phalanges are dorsally protected by a specialized cornified dermis, the nail. However, repetitive blunt trauma (i.e., against the toe box of a running shoe) to this region may give rise to subungual hematomata ("runner's black toes"). Angular conformations or deformities of the MTP or interphalangeal (IP) joints result in bony prominences, which are subject to increased frictional pressure with development of thickened overlying soft tissue (corns and calluses). These deformities have a specific terminology. Those in which there is fixed flexion contracture of the IP joints are **claw toes.** Deformities in which there is extension at the MTP joint with flexion at the IP joints are called **hammertoes.**

The sesamoid and accessory bones of the foot. The sesamoid bones of the foot represent bony inclusions within certain tendons. Their purpose is to reduce frictional stress as those tendons pass over bony prominences and to increase by pulley action the mechanical efficiency of given tendon structures. The most common of these sesamoid bones are the medial and lateral sesamoids, which are found within the flexor hallucis tendon. They are located at the plantar aspect of the MTP joint of the great toe.

Other sesamoid bones may be found within the posterior tibialis tendon (accessory navicular bone), at the medial aspect of the tarsal navicular, or within the peroneus longus tendon (os peroneum) as it passes laterally to the cuboid.

Additionally, an accessory ossicle may be observed at the posterior lip of the talus (os trigonum). This is not truly a sesamoid bone within a tendon but a bony process, likely to be a secondary center of ossification, that has failed to unite with the body of the talus.

Articular function of the ankle-foot mechanism

Earlier it was mentioned that there is an intimate structural mechanical interrelation between the ankle and foot. The talus holds the key to this relationship. As

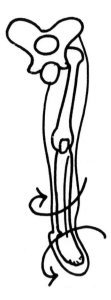

Fig. 10-15 ■ Pronation of talus results in internal rotational torques throughout remainder of the lower extremity.

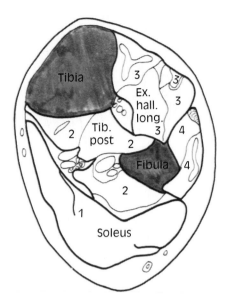

Fig. 10-16 ■ Cross-section through middle one third of leg demonstrates four compartments. *1,* superficial posterior; *2,* deep posterior; *3,* anterior; *4,* lateral.

a part of the ankle joint held within a rigid mortise, the talus is limited to flexion-extension motion. As a part of the foot responsible for pronation, the talus must perform medial rotation as well as plantar flexion. Efficient locomotion requires the simultaneous occurrence of both these talar functions. Therefore the lower extremity must accommodate the internal rotational torque that talar pronation creates and transmits proximally through the rigid ankle mortise during gait. Excessive torque is most efficiently accommodated by a complex combination of knee flexion and internal rotation of the entire lower extremity (Fig. 10-15). Such compensatory motions may place excessive stress at the more proximal structures of the lower extremity, which may in turn result in chronic overuse syndromes at these sites. However, full discussion of this entire pattern of events is beyond the scope of this chapter.

Musculotendinous structures of the distal leg, ankle, and foot

The muscles of the leg (with the exception of the popliteus at the proximal leg)

function as both motors and dynamic stabilizers of the ankle and foot. Those passing from the leg into the foot make up the **extrinsic musculature of the foot.** The muscles of the leg are divided into four compartments: the anterior, lateral, superficial posterior, and deep posterior (Fig. 10-16) (Table 10-3).

The **anterior compartment** contains the dorsiflexors of the ankle, foot, and digits. They are the anterior tibialis, extensor hallucis longus, extensor digitorum longus, and peroneus tertius. These muscles lie along the anterolateral aspect of the leg. Their tendons pass anteriorly to the ankle mortise. Each tendon is protected by a synovial sheath as it passes beneath the fibrous retinaculum, which secures the tendons against the dorsum of the ankle and foot. The major extensor retinaculum is called the **crural ligament.** The name describes its shape as a medially opened V. It consists of two bands that meet, cross, and coalesce at the dorsum of the proximal lateral foot. It functions to prevent bowstringing of the tendons across the anterior aspect of the ankle during active dorsiflexion. The anterior tibi-

385

Section 1 FOOT AND ANKLE
Chapter 10 Anatomy and physical
examination of the foot and ankle

Table 10-3 ■ Musculotendinous compartments of distal leg

Compartment	Muscle	Insertion	Function (primary)*
Anterior	Anterior tibialis	Inferomedial medial cuneiform and first metatarsal	Dorsiflexion and supination of foot
	Extensor hallucis longus	Dorsal base of first distal phalanx	Dorsiflexion of hallux
	Extensor digitorum longus	Dorsal base of second through fifth distal phalanges	Dorsiflexion of digits
	Peroneus tertius	Dorsal base of proximal shaft of fifth metatarsal	Dorsiflexion of foot
Lateral	Peroneus brevis	Dorsolateral base of fifth metatarsal	Eversion and plantar flexion of foot
	Peroneus longus	Plantar-lateral base of first metatarsal and medial cuneiform	Plantar flexion, eversion, and pronation
Superficial posterior	Gastrocnemius	Posterior calcaneus	Plantar flexion and supination
	Soleus	Posterior calcaneus	Plantar flexion and supination
	Plantaris	Posterior calcaneus	Plantar flexion and supination
Deep posterior	Flexor hallucis longus	Plantar base of first distal phalanx	Plantar flexion of hallux
	Flexor digitorum longus	Plantar bases of second through fifth distal phalanges	Plantar flexion of digits
	Posterior tibialis	Plantar medial navicular, medial cuneiform, lateral cuneiform, second and fourth metatarsal bases	Supination and adduction of foot

*Motor functions (primary and secondary) can be determined by examination of the muscle-tendon unit's excursion (origin to insertion) relative to the fulcrum on which it acts.

alis is the largest of these tendons. It inserts onto the medial aspect of the midfoot at the navicular and medial cuneiform. Its function is to dorsiflex and supinate the foot. It is antagnostic to the peroneus longus. The extensors of the digits insert onto the middle phalanges of the toes (terminal phalanx of the great toe). They are supplemented by the short (intrinsic) extensors of the digits (Fig. 10-17).

The **lateral compartment** of the leg contains the peroneii longus and brevis (Fig. 10-18). Their tendons are easily palpated as they pass posteriorly and inferiorly to the lateral malleolus. They insert onto the plantar aspect of the first metatarsal and medial cuneiform and the lateral base of the fifth metatarsal, respectively. The peroneal tendons are stabilized in fibroosseous tunnels superiorly and inferiorly to the ankle to retinacula. The synovial sheaths of these tunnels are intimately bound to the calcaneofibular

ligament (mentioned previously). The peroneii are responsible for eversion and plantar flexion. By concentric and eccentric contraction, the peroneal muscle-tendon units stabilize the foot and ankle against excessive inversion, supination, and adduction. The peroneus longus courses beneath the cuboid and across the midfoot, passing deep to the long plantar ligament. As such, it has great mechanical advantage as a plantar flexor–evertor of the foot.

Injury caused by excessive inversion (classic lateral ankle sprain) may involve the peroneii as well as lateral ligament structures. Clinically this may easily be determined on physical examination. Inspection will demonstrate swelling, erythema, and ecchymosis at the tendon sheaths or the base of the fifth metatarsal. (The latter may indicate an avulsion fracture-sprain of the base of the fifth metatarsal at the insertion of the peroneus

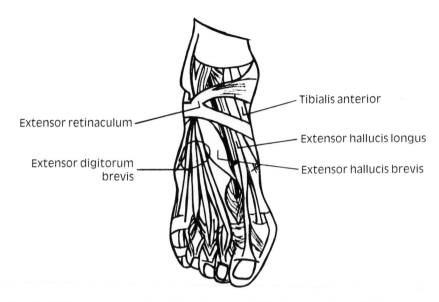

Fig. 10-17 ■ Anterior compartment tendons are stabilized against "bowstringing" during dorsiflexion by crural retinaculum.

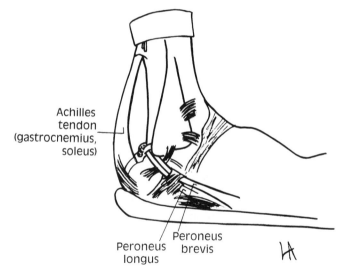

Fig. 10-18 ■ Lateral compartment tendons pass from leg into foot posterior and distal to lateral malleolus.

brevis tendon.) These tendons are readily palpated because of their subcutaneous course at the ankle. Fixed planovalgus foot alignment has been attributed to spastic contracture of the peroneii. Allegedly, this is the result of peroneal depression of the first metatarsal and the medial arch of the foot together with abduction eversion of the midfoot. In fact, the term "peroneal spastic flatfoot" is a misnomer. It is most commonly the consequence of a subtalar coalition. This, rather than peroneal contracture, is responsible for the reduced subtalar mobility and planovalgus attitude of the foot.

Posteriorly the musculature of the distal leg is divided into two compartments, superficial and deep (Fig. 10-19). The **su-**

387

Section 1 FOOT AND ANKLE
Chapter 10 Anatomy and physical
examination of the foot and ankle

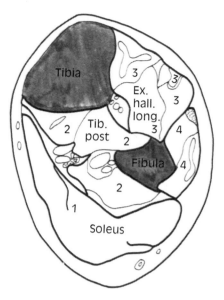

Fig. 10-19 ■ Posterior musculature is divided into deep and superficial compartments.

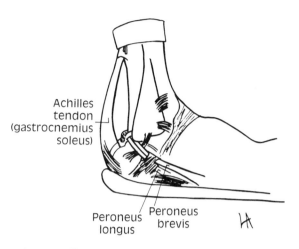

Fig. 10-20 ■ Achilles tendon represents coalescence of gastrocnemius, soleus, and, when present, plantaris tendon.

perficial compartment contains the massive gastrocnemius and soleus and the smaller tendinous plantaris muscles.

Distally the gastrocnemius and soleus muscles coalesce to form the Achilles tendon (Fig. 10-20). The structure of this tendon undergoes a slight internal rotation before its insertion onto the posteromedial aspect of the calcaneal tuberosity. As a result, this tendon serves to ensure heel plantar flexion–supination on contraction of the posterior musculature. The insertion of the Achilles tendon is distal to the peak of the calcaneal tuberosity, necessitating a tendocalcaneal bursa between these structures to reduce frictional stresses. Inflammation of this region caused by anatomic anomalies in the site of the calcaneal projection of excessive frictional stress on the bursa will result in swelling, erythema, and painful thickening of the surrounding soft tissues. This syndrome has been called **Haglund's disease.** Superficial frictional irritation caused by excessive shoe pressure on the posterior aspect of the calcaneus and Achilles insertion may give rise to inflammation and thickening of the subcutaneous calcaneal bursa (**pump bump**).

The superficial posterior muscles are direct antagonists of the anterior compartment. Decreased flexibility in the posterior muscles will therefore demand increased effort on the part of the anterior musculature, as the anterior muscles attempt to effect dorsiflexion of the ankle and foot against both gravity and the increased resistance of the "tight" posterior muscles. This demand for increased effort may result in overexertion of the anterior compartment musculature during cyclic activities (i.e., distance running or walking). The resultant increased blood flow, tissue damage, and swelling caused by overexertion may lead to the development of increased interstitial pressure and an **anterior compartment syndrome.**

Evaluation for posterior compartment tightness will afford an individual the opportunity to anticipate the occurrence of this series of events, thereby providing a rational basis for the inclusion of appropriate flexibility exercises in the preparticipation program of those individuals at risk. Posterior tightness is assessed clinically by passive dorsiflexion of the ankle with the knee both extended and flexed. In these positions the ankle should easily accommodate 30 degrees of dorsiflexion.

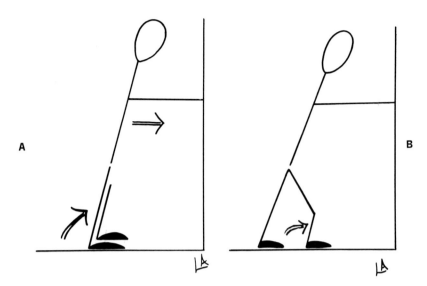

Fig. 10-21 ■ **A,** Tightness of gastrocnemius muscle is best determined by positioning individual facing a wall, heels flat, knees straight, and leaning forward, keeping heels on floor. **B,** Inflexibility of soleus musculature is best assessed by positioning individual with foot to be examined forward, patient facing a wall, heels flat on floor, and ipsilateral knee flexed forward while heel is maintained in contact with floor. Degree of knee flexion is then an accurate indication of tightness or suppleness within soleus muscle.

This is most conveniently measured with the patient leaning forward against a wall with feet flat, knees extended, and lower extremities slightly internally rotated (Fig. 10-21, *A*). This will assess gastrocnemius tightness, because this muscle crosses posterior to both the knee and ankle. Soleus tightness is best assessed by advancing the extremity to be examined toward the wall with the heel flat on the floor. The ipsilateral knee is then flexed forward while the heel is maintained on the ground (Fig. 10-21, *B*). This manuever relaxes the gastrocnemius while maintaining stress on the soleus tendon unit.

The **deep compartment** contains the posterior tibialis and long toe flexors (hallucis and digitorum). Although deepest at the leg, the posterior tibialis becomes the most superficial and anterior of these three tendons in the distal third of the leg. A mnemonic for the position of these three tendons, anterior to posterior at the posteromedial ankle, is "*T*om, *D*ick, and *H*arry," representing the posterior *t*ibialis, flexor *d*igitorum, and flexor *h*allucis, respectively.

The posterior tibial tendon, by far the largest of these three tendons, inserts as a broad expanse onto the plantar-medial and plantar aspects of the midfoot. Specifically, it inserts onto the navicular, medial and middle cuneiforms, and second, third, and fourth metatarsal bases. It dynamically inverts and supinates the foot. Eccentric contraction of this muscle serves to modulate subtalar pronation.

Activities that create cyclic pronation loading (i.e., distance running) may give rise to chronic overuse syndromes involving the posterior tibialis muscle and its tendon (posterior tibial tendinitis). Clinically this condition causes tenderness at the medial midleg along the tibia on both exertion and palpation. It has been referred to as **shin splints.** Shin splints have been demonstrated to occur with greater frequency in individuals with certain predisposing factors. These factors are (1) inadequate posterior tibialis strength and endurance conditioning and (2) insufficient ligamentous and/or bony support of the talus to resist excessive pronation. The latter condition has been

aft shear reflects both the backward pressure of the foot against the ground at the time of toe-off, as well as the resultant of the forward lean of the body at the same time (see Fig. 11-8, *B*). Note the force involved is only about one third of the body weight as compared to the greater force observed for the vertical force. For running, the force is approximately one half of the body weight.

The medial and lateral shear force demonstrate that at the time of initial ground contact there is a force directed medially or towards the midline of the body (see Fig. 11-8, *C*). Following this, there is a lateral shear, away from the midline. The magnitude of this force again is less and represents about 10% of body weight.

The torque measurement reflects the rotation of the lower extremity that occurs during walking (see Fig. 11-8, *D*). As pointed out previously, there is internal rotation at the time of initial ground contact, following which there is progressive external rotation until the time of toe-off. This torque measurement reflects this motion. Unfortunately, torque measurements are not available for running.

Based on the measurements of the vertical force, an individual weighing 150 pounds who walks with a step length of 2½ feet for a mile takes approximately 2110 steps. He absorbs at initial ground contact, considering an impact of 80% of

---

**CUMULATIVE VERTICAL FORCE AT
GROUND CONTACT**

Walking	63.5 tons/foot/mile
Running	110 tons/foot/mile

(See text for calculations.)

---

body weight, a total of 253,440 pounds (127 tons) or 63.5 tons per foot. If the same individual runs a mile, with a step length of 4½ feet, he takes approximately 1175 steps and absorbs at initial ground contact, considering an impact of 250% of body weight, a total of 440,625 pounds

(220 tons) or 110 tons per foot. What needs to be further considered is the fact that the individual who walks a mile does so over about 20 minutes, whereas the individual who runs a mile does so in approximately half that time or less. It becomes readily apparent that one of the main functions of the foot and lower extremity during walking and running is that of force dissipation.

Ankle joint motion

The ankle joint plays a very vital role during running in the absorption of the impact against the ground. At the time of initial ground contact during jogging and running, the foot goes into a moderate degree of dorsiflexion during the first half of the stance phase. This dorsiflexion at the ankle is controlled by an eccentric or lengthening contraction of the posterior calf muscles. During walking, plantar flexion occurs following ground contact, following which dorsiflexion occurs. However, during jogging, running, and sprinting, dorsiflexion occurs on ground contact. In the limited studies that have been carried out regarding sprinting, it appears that although the sprinter initially contacts the ground with the foot in plantar flexion, a moderate amount of dorsiflexion occurs. Although the ankle joint may not pass into dorsiflexion per se, it moves through a range from approximately 45 to 60 degrees of plantar flexion to almost neutral position. In this manner the absorption of energy is occurring.

By the midstance phase in jogging and running, when maximal dorsiflexion has occurred, rapid plantar flexion begins and continues through toe-off. Following this dorsiflexion occurs once again.

The movement that occurs about the ankle joint consists mainly of dorsiflexion and plantar flexion, and little or no transverse rotation occurs within the ankle joint. The transverse rotation that occurs in the lower extremity above the ankle joint is transmitted across the ankle joint into the subtalar joint.

The exact force exerted across the ankle joint during walking and running has been estimated to be between four and six times the body weight. Needless to say, this calculation is difficult to make with great assurance, and in part it is based on a mathematic model.

■ SAGITTAL PLANE MOTION OF THE LOWER EXTREMITY

I have previously discussed the transverse plane rotation that occurs in the lower extremity. Motion also occurs in the sagittal plane, as illustrated in Fig. 11-9. The sagittal plane motion remains rather constant for walking, jogging, and running, but is altered to a certain extent during sprinting, which is beyond the scope of this chapter. It is interesting to note that the configuration of the curve is essentially the same as that for the transverse plane, except that both the magnitude and inclination are changed with increasing speed. These changes in mag-

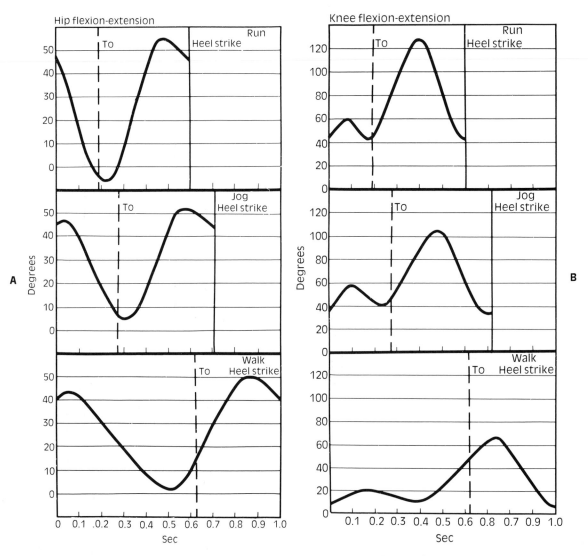

Fig. 11-9 ■ Sagittal plane motion of lower extremity during walking, jogging, and running. *to,* Toe-off; *hs,* Heel strike. **A,** Hip joint. **B,** Knee joint. **C,** Ankle joint.
From Mann, R.A. Biomechanics of running. In American Academy of Orthopaedic Surgeons: Symposium on the Foot and Leg in Running Sports, St. Louis, 1982, The C.V. Mosby Co.

chapter 13

Roentgenographic techniques

David L. Milbauer

Shashikant Patel

■ THE FOOT

Standard views

The **dorsoplantar** (anteroposterior) projection of the foot permits visualization of the tarsal bones anterior to the talus, the metatarsals, and the phalanges (Fig. 13-1). This projection is obtained with the entire plantar surface of the foot resting on the film holder with the x-ray beam directed perpendicular to the film and centered at the base of the third metatarsal. Coned views may afford greater detail of a suspected lesion.

Various oblique projections have been employed in conjunction with the dorso-plantar projection to visualize the osseous structures and their relationship to each other in the foot. The medial and lateral oblique projections are obtained with the x-ray beam passing in a dorsoplantar projection, having the patient rotate the foot either medially or laterally approximately 30 degrees, depending on the views desired. The **lateral** oblique projection demonstrates the interspaces between the first two cuneiforms as well as the first and second metatarsals (Fig. 13-2, *A*). The **medial** oblique projection shows the interspaces between the cuboid and adjacent calcaneus, fourth and fifth metatarsals, and third cuneiform as well as the talonavicular articulation (Fig. 13-2, *B* and *C*). Numerous other oblique views for better visualization of the tarsus have been described, and these views can be tailored to the individual clinical setting.

The **lateral** views of the foot may be obtained in either lateromedial or mediolateral projections. With the medial aspect of the foot in contact with the film holder, the foot usually assumes a true lateral position, and therefore the lateromedial projection is the desired view (Fig. 13-3, *A*). A true lateral position may be difficult to obtain in this way when there is a prominent medial malleolus, hallux valgus or other deformity, or severe patient discomfort. In such cases the mediolateral projection is obtained (Fig. 13-3, *B*).

The calcaneus, which is well visualized on a coned-down lateral view (Fig. 13-4), can also be imaged with a semiaxial pro-

Text continued on p. 424.

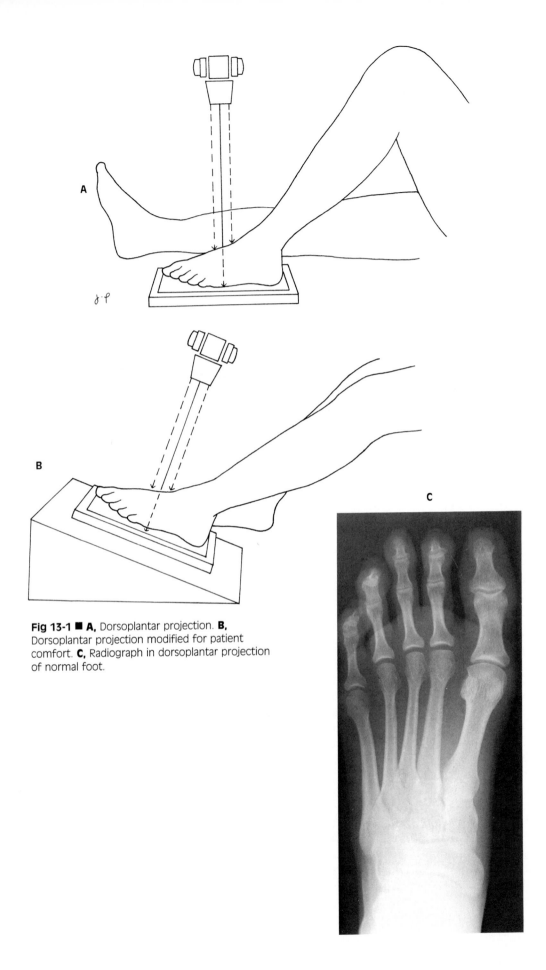

Fig 13-1 ■ **A,** Dorsoplantar projection. **B,** Dorsoplantar projection modified for patient comfort. **C,** Radiograph in dorsoplantar projection of normal foot.

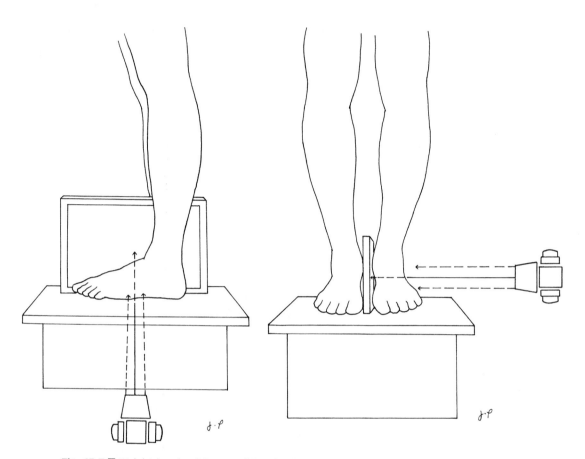

Fig. 13-7 ■ Weight-bearing lateromedial projection of the foot. Film cassette is held in place by both legs, as shown.

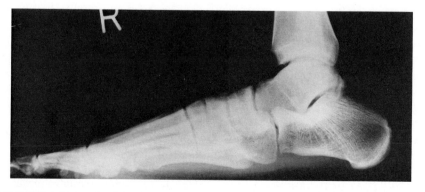

Fig. 13-8 ■ Weight-bearing lateral roentgenograph. There is flattening of longitudinal arch with slight malalignment of tarsus and early degenerative changes.

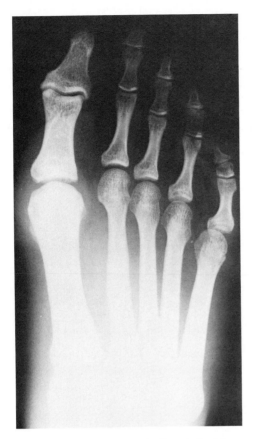

Fig. 13-9 ■ Dorsoplantar projection. Early changes in turf toe (hallux rigidus) are present at first metatarsophalangeal joint.

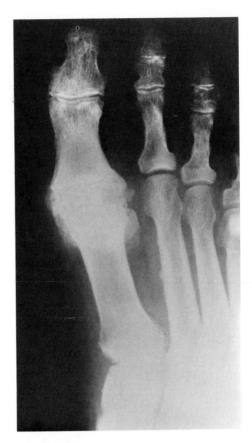

Fig. 13-10 ■ Coned-down radiograph. Late changes in turf toe (hallux rigidus) are present. There is obliteration of first metatarsophalangeal joint with alignment maintained.

ment.[13,25,26] The metatarsals, especially the second and third, and the calcaneus seem particularly prone, although any bone in the foot may be susceptible, including the other tarsal bones, the sesamoids, and even accessory ossicles.[25] Similar roentgenographic changes are observed irrespective of the site of involvement. The initial roentgenograms are often normal. Serial studies may reveal subtle blurring of the trabecular margins and fluffy densities that represent new bone formation.[26] Later, sclerotic bands at the fracture site in trabecular bone and periosteal new bone at cortical sites are demonstrated (Figs. 13-11 to 13-13).

Stress fractures of the tarsal navicular bone may be difficult to demonstrate on routine roentgenograms and even standard tomograms. The fracture is usually linear in the sagittal plane and therefore may only be seen on dorsoplantar views or coned-down dorsoplantar views (Fig. 13-14). Associated plain film findings have been summarized by Pavlov[28] and include sclerosis of the proximal articular borders of the tarsal navicular, a short first metatarsal, metatarsus adductus of the first through fourth rays, and hyperostosis or stress fractures of the second, third, and/or fourth metatarsals[28] (Fig. 13-15). On the lateral view, especially in the standing position, there is tarsal malalignment with the talus and navicular dorsal to the cuneiforms (Fig. 13-16).

Radionuclide bone imaging may be very

of the ankle in the anteroposterior, lateral, and mortise views are sufficient to evaluate ligamentous problems. However, tomography or in some instances CT scanning may assist in further evaluation of the intraarticular structures. Roentgenograms of the ankle in the anteroposterior projection following medial and lateral stress of the ankle would further help to determine the integrity of the ligaments.

In a normal arthrogram of the ankle, as seen in Fig. 13-38, the articular surface of the ankle appears smooth, and the contrast is contained within the synovial cavity. There is no contrast present outside the ligamentous attachment on the frontal projection. A small amount of contrast material extends normally between the distal tibia and fibula to a distance of about 2 to 2.5 cm. Any extension of contrast beyond this limit suggests partial or complete diastasis of the distal tibiofibular syndesmosis. On the lateral projection there is some bulging of the capsule anteriorly as well as posteriorly, more so in the case of the latter. The synovial surface appears smooth anteriorly, but posteriorly the outpouching is normally somewhat irregular in outline. In approxi-

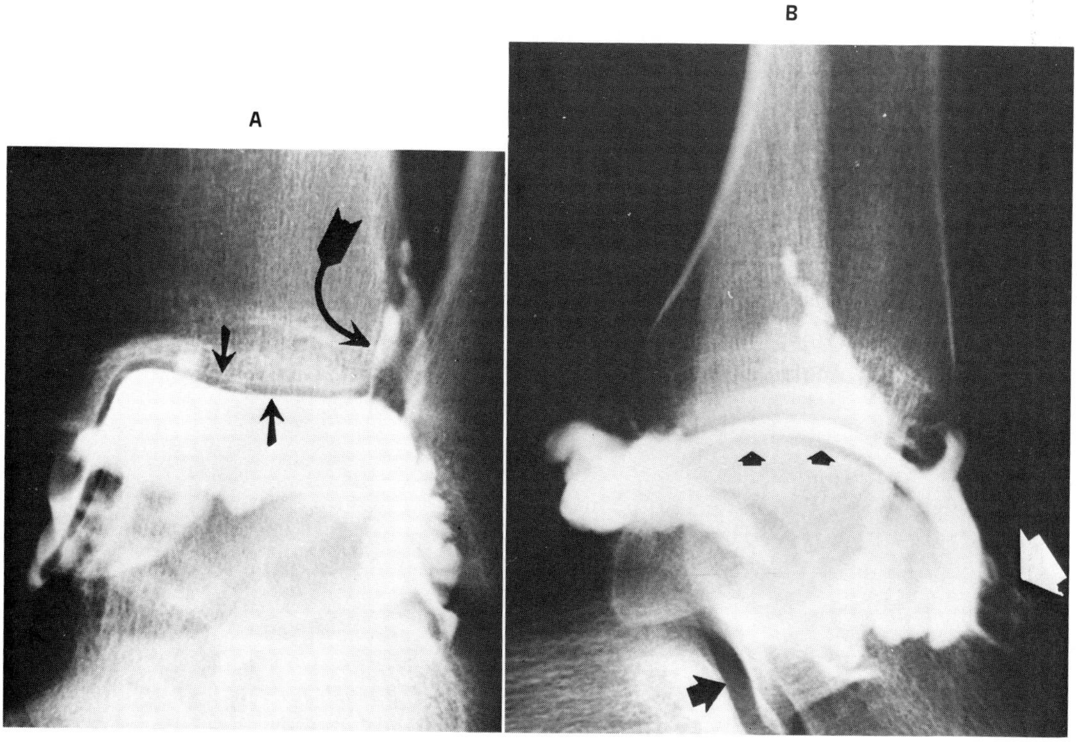

Fig. 13-38 ■ Normal ankle arthrogram. **A,** Anterior view of ankle arthrogram (single contrast) reveals that contrast agent is confined within joint capsule, inside synovial lining. Articular cartilage of distal tibia *(straight black arrows)* is clearly outlined and is normal. Distal tibiofibular syndesmosis is outlined with contrast. This recess usually extends for 2.5 cm. or less and is a normal finding. **B,** Lateral view of ankle. Anterior and posterior joint recesses are well seen, posterior being larger of the two. Articular surface *(small black arrows)* of talus is seen in its entirety and appears normal. Slight leakage of contrast at needle puncture site is indicated by white arrow. Posterior subtalar joint contains no contrast medium, because 90% of these joints do not communicate with ankle joint. Small amount of contrast projected on distal tibia is contrast in distal tibiofibular syndesmosis.

Continued.

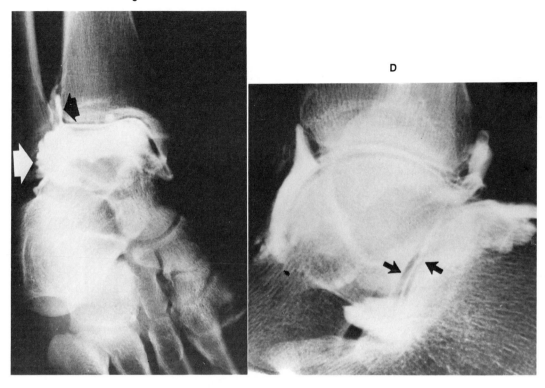

Fig. 13-38 ■ cont'd. C, Mortise view demonstrates distal syndesmosis fully and articular area more clearly without any overlap by fibula *(black arrow).* White arrow points to synovial surface along lateral aspect of ankle. This "fimbriated" appearance is a normal finding and is partly attributed to various ligamentous and capsular fibers in this region. **D,** Close-up of another ankle arthrogram in lateral projection reveals presence of contrast in posterior subtalar joint. Ten percent of these joints communicate with tibiotalar joint.

mately 10% of cases, the subtalar joint communicates with the ankle joint. This is well shown in Fig. 13-38, *D.*

The most common ligamentous injury of the ankle involves the calcaneofibular and the anterior and posterior talofibular ligaments. The anterior talofibular ligament is closely applied to the joint capsule. A tear of this ligament is revealed by contrast that leaks out of the joint anteriorly and laterally to the distal fibula. Fig. 13-39 reveals this clearly, both on the anteroposterior and mortise views.

Because of the close proximity of the calcaneofibular ligament to the peroneal tendons and their synovial sheaths, a tear of the calcaneofibular ligament is usually associated with opacification of the syno-

vial sleeves surrounding the peroneal tendons (Fig. 13-40). This appearance can be seen in both acute as well as chronic injury of the calcaneofibular ligament. Fig. 13-41 is a good example of such an injury; the tear of the calcaneofibular ligament is very clearly visualized on the frontal, mortise, and the lateral views of the ankle.

Injuries of the less commonly torn deltoid ligament of the ankle can also be detected by arthrography. Fig. 13-42 reveals leakage from along the medial aspect of the joint from rupture of the deltoid ligament. There is also slight widening of the medial joint space. Arthrography of the ankle proper, subtalar arthrography, and talocalcaneonavicular arthrography are commonly employed to evaluate the sub-

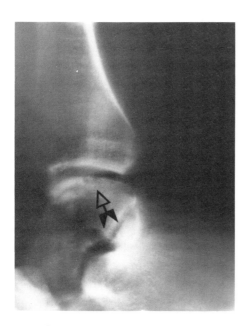

Fig. 14-8 ■ Osteochondritic lesions of the talus are generally located medially and in the anterior portion of dome.

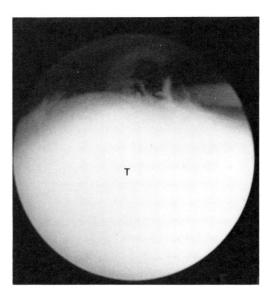

Fig. 14-9 ■ The fibrillated appearance of talar articular surface overlying an osteochondritic lesion can be appreciated arthroscopically.
From Drez, D., Guhl, J.F., and Gollehon, D.L.: Clin. Sports Med. **1**:35, 1982. Reproduced by permission.

vage and debridement using the intraarticular shaver. Also, direct joint surface observation will provide a more accurate assessment of actual cartilage destruction than roentgenograms, thus directing further care.

Osteochondritis dissecans. Osteochondritis dissecans of the talar dome may be followed arthroscopically. Articular surface integrity can be assessed by palpation with a probe, and, if needed, debridement, drilling of the defect, and loose body removal can be done[4,5] (Figs. 14-8 and 14-9).

Visible osteochondral fractures and loose bodies. Visualization of osteochondral fragments and loose bodies can be obtained arthroscopically, and removal or replacement done with triangulation of appropriate instruments into the ankle joint (Fig. 14-10).

Vague complaints and symptoms. Occasionally, when clinical examination and all other tests are negative yet the athlete

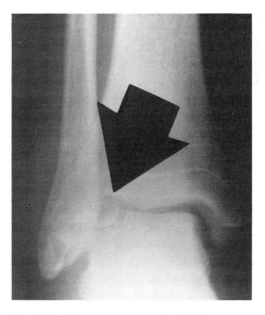

Fig. 14-10 ■ The appearance of a typical osteochondral fracture that could benefit from arthroscopic evaluation and surgery.

has persistent vague complaints, arthroscopic examination may be helpful. If pathologic lesions are found, they may be rectified; if none are found, the patient's worries may be alleviated, thus allowing return to a normal level of activity.

Approaches

Five portals can be used for arthroscopic examination and surgery of the ankle. The ankle joint is separated for arthroscopic purposes into anterior and posterior cavities, with three portals located anteriorly and two posteriorly.[4]

Successful examination of the joint depends on knowledge of the intraarticular anatomy and organization of the procedure, both of which are facilitated by division of the joint into logical sections that are studied in order.

Anterior portals. In general, the anterior portals are most useful because the patient is examined in the supine position. There is also increased versatility for triangulation along with a larger area of view when compared with the posterior portals.

Despite these obvious advantages for anterior approach, the posterior portals

---

ANTERIOR PORTALS

- Anteromedial
- Anterocentral
- Anterolateral

---

will be needed when examination of the posterior joint cavity cannot be carried out from an anterior portal or when strictly posterior injury exists.

There are advantages and disadvantages with each of the portals. Because of the shape of the ankle joint (Fig. 14-11), advance of the arthroscope sleeve and trocar over the talar dome into the posterior joint cavity is usually impossible from the anteromedial or anterolateral portal. As a result, the anterocentral portal (Fig. 14-12) has a great advantage for more complete

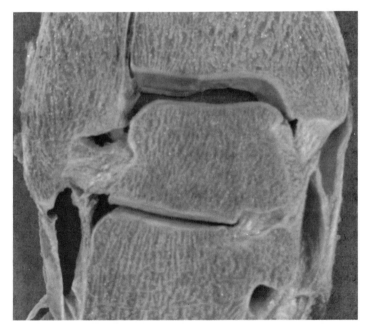

Fig. 14-11 ■ Barring ligamentous injury, normal articulation of the talus with the tibia will generally permit advancement of the arthroscope only over the concave central portion of the dome.

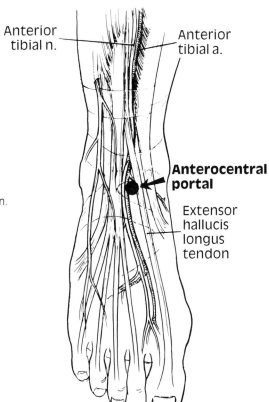

Fig. 14-12 ■ Location of anterocentral portal is shown.
From Drez, D., Guhl, J.F. and Gollehon, D.L.: Foot Ankle
2:138, 1981.

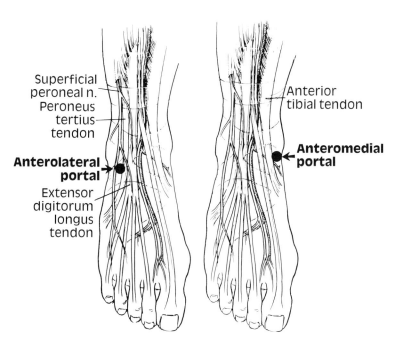

Fig. 14-13 ■ Locations of anterolateral and anteromedial portals are shown.
From Drez, D., Guhl, J.F., and Gollehon, D.L.: Foot Ankle **2:**138, 1981.

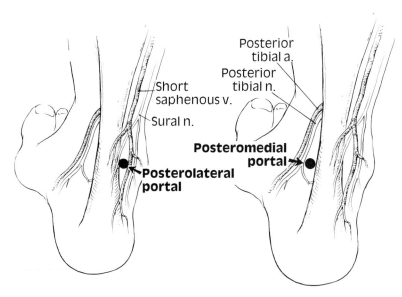

Fig. 14-14 ■ Posterolateral and posteromedial portal locations are shown.
From Drez, D., Guhl, J.F. and Gollehon, D.L.: Foot Ankle **2:**138, 1981.

intraarticular visualization. A disadvantage is proximity to the dorsalis pedis artery. As long as care is taken in placement of the sleeve and trocar, this should not be an overriding concern. The anterolateral and anteromedial portals (Fig. 14-13) allow the best view of the articular surfaces on their respective sides of the joint; however, if abnormalities of the anterior synovial wall or talar neck need to be examined, the anteromedial portal is best used for lateral visualization and vice versa.

When intraarticular surgery is needed, instruments may be triangulated from the anterocentral portal, or the arthroscope may be changed to this portal for triangulation through the anteromedial or lateral portal.

Posterior portals. The posterior arthroscopic portals—posterolateral and posteromedial (Fig. 14-14)—are generally used only when symptoms are well localized to the posterior aspect of the ankle. If, for example, loose bodies are known to be present in the joint and are not located with anterior approaches, an examination from posterior is mandatory. In addition,

---

POSTERIOR PORTALS
■ Posteromedial
■ Posterolateral

posterior portals will occasionally be needed to evaluate osteochondral fractures or osteochondritic lesions located far posterior on the talar dome.

Because the posterolateral space is larger and easier to enter than the posteromedial, nearly all posterior evaluation should be done from this portal. The posteromedial portal will be needed only if there is difficulty entering laterally, such as in the presence of postoperative scarring or injuries to the lateral side of the ankle posteriorly.

Technique

As with knee arthroscopy, ankles are examined in the operating room with full sterile preparation. An uninflated tourniquet is placed about the thigh for use should excessive bleeding into the joint be encountered. In practice, inflation of the tourniquet is seldom necessary.

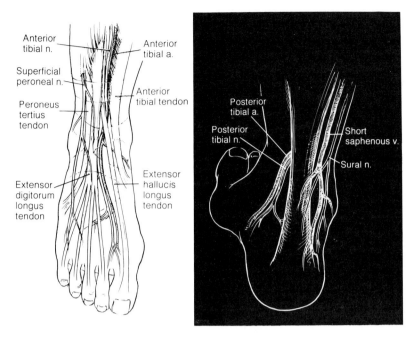

Fig. 14-15 ■ Anterior and posterior extraarticular structures should be reviewed along with their relationship to arthroscopic portals.
From Drez, D., Guhl, J.F. and Gollehon, D.L.: Foot Ankle **2:**138, 1981.

Local, spinal, or general anesthetic may be used; however, adequate visualization of the joint will often be impossible without the complete muscle relaxation afforded by spinal or general anesthesia.

Because extraarticular anatomic structures are more compactly arranged at the ankle than at knee level, it is mandatory that additional care be taken in placement of arthroscopic portals. Extraarticular anatomy anteriorly and posteriorly (Fig. 14-15) should be reviewed before each examination and the important structures marked before starting the procedure. For examination using anterior portals, positions of the anterior tibial, extensor hallucis longus, and extensor digitorum communis tendons and the dorsalis pedis artery are marked (Fig 14-16). For posterior portals the medial and lateral borders of the Achilles tendon, the peroneal tendons, and the posterior tibial artery are located and marked (Fig 14-17).

Diagnostic examination is best carried out using the anterocentral portal because of the increased area of view afforded by this approach. The technique of arthroscopic examination by this portal will be described, as will the intraarticular structures visualized (see boxes, p. 470).

A bolster is placed under the hip on the involved side. After standard skin preparation, the procedure is begun by flexing the foot plantarward and dorsally to locate the anterior edge of the tibia (Fig. 14-18). A 1½-inch, 18-gauge disposable needle is placed in the anteromedial or anterolateral portal position and a section of sterile extension tubing is attached. The joint is aspirated of effusion, then distended using a 60-cc syringe to inject saline solution through the tubing. Intraarticular needle placement is confirmed by the ease of saline injection and return of fluid with aspiration. A number 11 scalpel blade is

ARTHROSCOPICALLY VISIBLE STRUCTURES OF THE ANTERIOR JOINT CAVITY

- Anterior compartment
  Anterior synovial wall
  Anterior aspect of proper tibiotalar joint
- Anterolateral compartment
  Anterior synovial wall
  Anterior talofibular ligament
  Anterior aspect of distal tibiofibular joint
  Anterior aspect of lateral talomalleolar articulation
    Anterolateral articular surface of talus
    Anterolateral articular surface of tibia
    Anterior articular surface of lateral malleolus
- Anteromedial compartment
  Anteromedial synovial wall
  Anterior aspect of medial talomalleolar articulation
    Anteromedial articular surface of talus
    Anteromedial articular surface of tibia
    Anterior articular surface of medial malleolus

From Drez, D., Guhl, J., Jr., and Gollehon, D.L.: Foot Ankle **2**:138, 1981.

ARTHROSCOPICALLY VISIBLE STRUCTURES OF THE POSTERIOR JOINT CAVITY

- Posterior compartment
  Posterior synovial wall
  Posterior and superior aspect of proper tibiotalar joint
- Posterolateral compartment
  Posterolateral synovial wall
  Posterior talofibular ligament
  Posterior aspect of distal tibiofibular joint
  Posterior aspect of lateral talomalleolar articulation
    Posterolateral articular surface of talus
    Posterolateral articular surface of tibia
    Posterior articular surface of lateral malleolus
- Posteromedial compartment
  Posteromedial synovial wall
  Posterior aspect of medial talomalleolar articulation
    Posteromedial articular surface of talus
    Posteromedial articular surface of tibia
    Posterior articular surface of medial malleolus

From Drez, D., Guhl, J., Jr., and Gollehon, D.L.: Foot Ankle **2**:138, 1981.

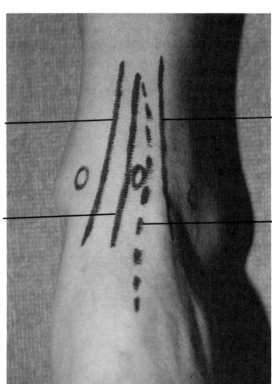

Anterior tibial tendon

Extensor hallucis longus tendon

Extensor digitorum communis tendon

Doralis pedis artery

Fig. 14-16 ■ Anatomic structures about intended arthroscopic portals are marked at start of procedure.

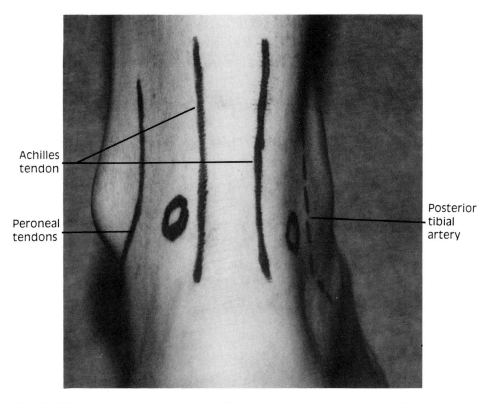

Fig. 14-17 ■ Posteriorly, prominent anatomic structures and portals may be outlined just as for anterior approaches.

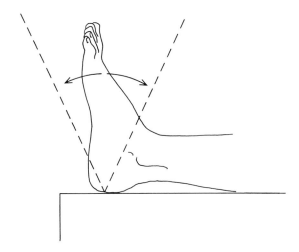

Fig. 14-18 ■ Plantar flexion and dorsiflexion of ankle facilitates locating joint line for needle placement.

then used to make a small incision at the chosen portal site. A hemostat is inserted into the skin incision and used to spread down to the joint capsule, thus moving vital structures out of the path of intended arthroscope insertion. The sheath and sharp trocar are placed into the incision, directed toward the midline, and with a controlled twisting motion are felt to pop through the joint capsule. During this insertion maneuver, joint distention must be maintained with firm pressure on the syringe plunger. Entrance into the joint is confirmed by the rush of saline solution on removal of the trocar from the sleeve. The blunt trocar is next substituted for the sharp one. The sleeve and trocar are advanced carefully but with firm pressure directly over the center of the talar dome into the posterior joint cavity. The telescope is then placed into the sleeve, the needle removed from the joint, the extension tubing attached to the sleeve stopcock, and the light source hooked to the arthroscope.

As examination is begun, the posterior synovial wall and posterior aspect of the tibiotalar articulation are seen (Fig. 14-19). Synovial bands and folds are thin and lightly colored in the normal situation. When a chronic intraarticular problem exists, inflammation will result in thickening and darkening of the synovium. With angulation of the visual field of the 25-degree arthroscope and a gentle move toward the posteromedial aspect of the ankle, the posterior aspect of the medial malleolus will be visualized, along with the capsular thickening of the deltoid ligament (Fig. 14-20). Direction of the field of view inferiorly gives a view of the talomalleolar articulation (Fig. 14-21). Mediolateral force applied at this time will allow assessment of talar motion in the mortise.

The arthroscope is not advanced further anteriorly but is maintained in the posterior cavity, next being directed toward the posterolateral corner, where the posterior talofibular ligament is examined (Fig. 14-22). Inversion stress helps with as-

sessment of ligament competence at this point. The posterior tibiotalar articulation is assessed laterally, which naturally leads to the posterior portion of the tibiofibular joint (Fig. 14-23). Under normal circumstances a synovial fold is present about this joint, and the joint itself does not accommodate the tip of a probe (Fig. 14-24). If the probe fits easily into the joint or if gross widening is observed with mediolateral force, ligamentous incompetence of the tibiofibular articulation exists. If this joint laxity is chronic, synovitis can usually be observed around the articulation (Fig. 14-25).

The arthroscopic field is angled inferiorly to bring into view the full talofibular articulation (Fig. 14-26). With careful advancement of the arthroscope anteriorly, the articular surface of the fibular malleolus and the entire talomalleolar articulation can be examined (Fig. 14-27). Movement toward the tip of the fibula brings the anterior talofibular ligament into view (Fig. 14-28).

The lateral articular surface of the talus can be followed proximally until the anterior tibial articular cartilage can be seen (Fig. 14-29). A thorough examination of the anterolateral tibiotalar joint and the anterolateral synovial wall can be done at this point. A view of the anterior tibiotalar articulation can then be obtained during a sweep from the lateral malleolus to the tip of the medial malleolus (Fig. 14-30).

The anterior aspect of the medial talomalleolar articulation is examined (Fig. 14-31), after which the view is carried to the anteromedial synovial wall and deltoid thickening in the capsule (Fig. 14-32). The view of the capsule naturally moves to the neck of the talus and the anterior recess, which can be viewed from anteromedial to anterolateral in a search for loose bodies or osteophytes (Fig. 14-33).

Because of the narrowness of the ankle joint, continuous injection of saline solution during the procedure is required to maintain distention and minimize the chance of instrument breakage. Extra

Fig. 14-19 ■ Posterior aspect of tibiotalar joint and posterior synovial wall. *t*, tibia.

Fig. 14-20 ■ Posteromedial synovial wall and medial malleolus. *M*, medial malleolus; *T*, talus.

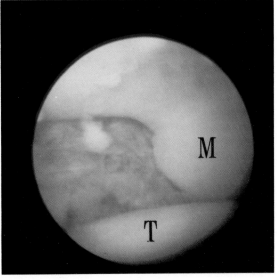

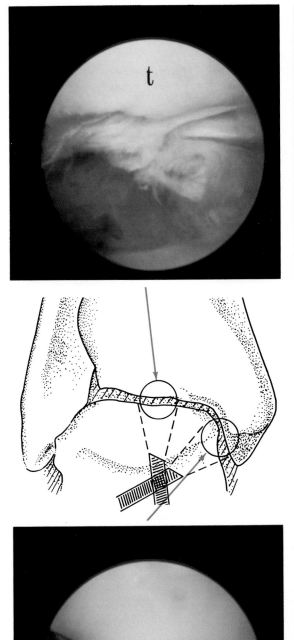

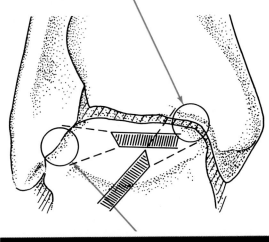

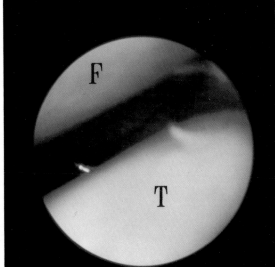

Fig. 14-21 ■ Superior aspect of medial talomalleolar articulation. *M*, medial malleolus; *T*, talus.

Fig. 14-22 ■ Use of probe to spread talofibular joint so visualization of posterior ligaments and capsule can be achieved. *T*, talus; *F*, fibula.

Fig. 14-23 ■ Posterior aspect of the tibiofibular articulation and posterolateral capsular structures. *F*, fibula; *t*, tibia.

Fig. 14-24 ■ Probing of the tibiofibular joint and normal synovial fold about the joint can be done to assess ligamentous stability. *t*, tibia.

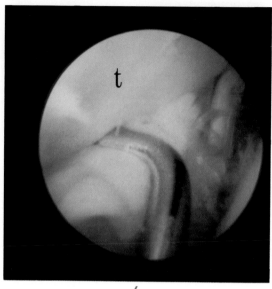

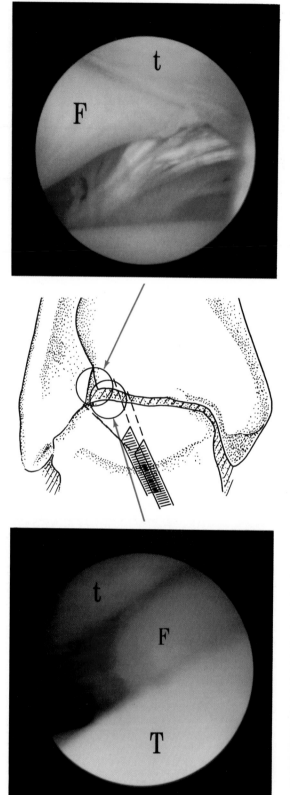

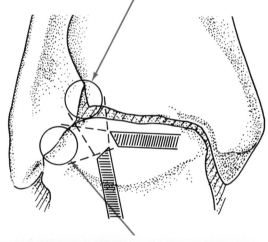

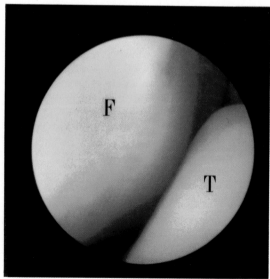

Fig. 14-25 ■ Inflamed synovial tissue may be seen about a chronically unstable tibiofibular joint. *T*, talus; *t*, tibia; *F*, fibula.

Fig. 14-26 ■ Lateral talomalleolar space and articular surfaces. *F, fibula; T, talus.*

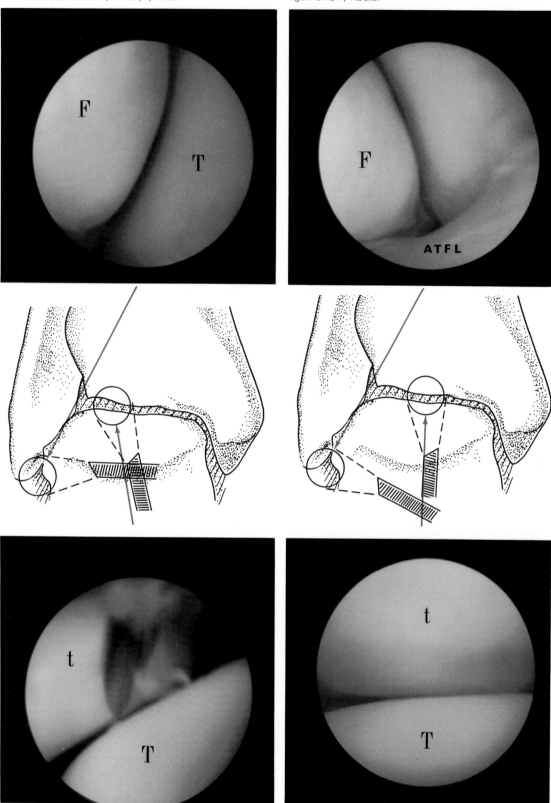

Fig. 14-27 ■ Distal portion of fibular malleolus and lateral flare of talus. *F,* fibula; *T,* talus.

Fig. 14-28 ■ Anterior talofibular ligament and talofibular articulation. *ATFL,* anterior talofibular ligament; *F,* fibula.

Fig. 14-29 ■ Anterior aspect of tibial and talar articular surfaces. *t,* tibia; *T,* talus.

Fig. 14-30 ■ Anterior tibiotalar joint. *t,* tibia; *T,* talus.

Fig. 14-31 ■ Medial talomalleolar articular surfaces. *T*, talus; *M*, medial malleolus.

Fig. 14-32 ■ Medial malleolar surface; deltoid thickening of capsule and anteromedial synovial wall can be seen. *M*, medial malleolus.

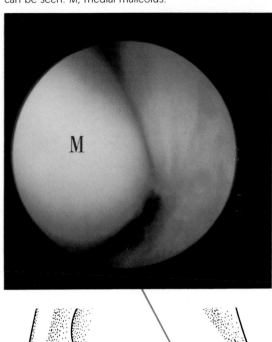

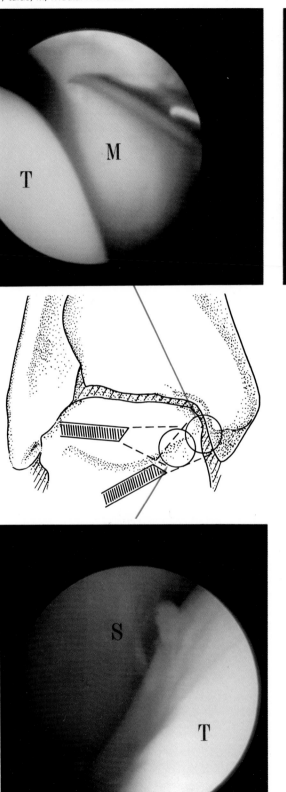

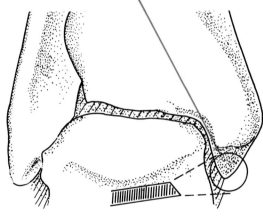

Fig. 14-33 ■ Anterior neck of talus and anterior synovial wall. *T*, talus; *S*, synovial wall.

portals into the joint must be kept small; joint distention and visualization will be lost if fluid pressure is inadequate. At the termination of the procedure the joint is drained, portals are closed with 4-0 nylon suture, and the leg is wrapped in a sterile pressure dressing from the toes to upper calf.

Postoperative regimen

The patient is allowed up on crutches the same day as surgery, with weight bearing encouraged, unless surgical work has been performed on the articular surfaces. In that circumstance, weight bearing is not allowed for 6 weeks. Forty-eight hours after surgery, the pressure dressing is removed, bandages are placed covering the arthroscopic portals, and rehabilitation is begun.

Initially and for the first 7 to 10 days, range of motion of the ankle is emphasized. In those who are allowed weight bearing, excessive standing or walking is discouraged. After the preoperative range of motion has been regained, a lower leg strengthening program is begun, with emphasis placed on the peroneal musculature. The rehabilitation regimen is the same in those who have had articular surface surgery.

Usually discharge from the hospital is on the morning following surgery. Sporting activities can generally be resumed 2 to 3 weeks postoperatively, but not until all ankle swelling with activity has stopped.

Contraindications

As with any major operative procedure, ankle arthroscopy should be postponed if there is any evidence of local or systemic infection. When infection is present, the condition should be evaluated and appropriate therapy begun. The arthroscopic procedure may then be safely done after symptoms have resolved.

Although not often encountered in the active athlete, significant joint stiffness makes manipulation and distraction of the joint difficult. This problem can inter-

fere with and make an adequate examination impossible.

Complications

If the arthroscopic procedure is done under operating room conditions and the ankle is reprepared and redraped before arthrotomy, one should expect no increase in infection rate over other standard arthroscopic procedures.

The danger of injuring vessels, nerves, or tendons is minimal if these structures are palpated and marked and dissection to the joint capsule is carried out carefully. By keeping the joint firmly distended with saline solution and manipulating the foot and instruments carefully, instrument breakage can be minimized.

During extended procedures, saline solution extravasation into the tissues about the ankle could conceivably result in a compartment syndrome; however, we have never seen this complication. With elevation and the standard compression dressing, this fluid generally rapidly resorbs.

■ SUMMARY

Adequate evaluation of ankle problems requires careful collection of data, including history, physical examination, and appropriate roentgenographic testing. Despite thorough evaluation, problems are often encountered that defy precise diagnosis. These problems include the following.

1. Persistent posttraumatic symptoms
2. Acute ankle swelling with hemarthrosis
3. The need for articular surface evaluation before reconstructive procedures or for osteochondritis dissecans, arthritis, or articular fractures
4. Vague complaints and symptoms.

Arthrography and arthrotomy are two methods for more precise interarticular evaluation; however, these procedures have disadvantages that make them less than desirable.

Much broader possibilities for examination and operative correction are afforded by arthroscopy of the ankle. In addition, the morbidity associated with this procedure is comparatively small when the advantages are considered. Arthroscopy of the ankle, when mastered, is an especially helpful additional tool for diagnostic and therapeutic care of the problem ankle.

REFERENCES

1. Burman, M.S.: Arthroscopy or the direct visualization of joints, J. Bone Joint Surg. **13:**669, 1931.
2. Chen, Y.C.: Clinical and cadaver studies on the ankle joint arthroscopy, J. Jpn. Orthop. Assoc. **50:**631, 1961.
3. Chen, Y.C.: Arthroscopy of the ankle joint, Arthroscopy **1:**16, 1976.
4. Drez, D., Guhl, J., Jr., and Gollehon, D.L.: Ankle arthroscopy: technique and indications, Foot Ankle **2:**138, 1981.
5. Drez, D., Guhl, J., Jr., and Gollehon, D.L.: Ankle arthroscopy: technique and indications, Clin. Sports Med. **1:**35, 1982.
6. Eriksson, E., Sebik, A.: Arthroscopy and arthroscopic surgery in a gas versus a fluid medium, Orthop. Clin. North Am. **13:**293, 1982.
7. Gillquist, J., and Lijedahl, S.O.: Arthroscopy of the ankle joint. In Berci, G., ed. Endoscopy, New York, 1976, Appleton-Century-Crofts.
8. Harrington, K.D.: Degenerative arthritis of the ankle secondary to long-standing lateral ligament instability, J. Bone Joint Surg. **61A:**354, 1979.
9. Heller, J.J., and Vogler, H.W.: Ankle joint arthroscopy, J. Foot Surg. **21:**23, 1982.
10. McGinty, J.R.: Arthroscopic removal of loose bodies, Orthop. Clin. North Am. **13:**313, 1982.
11. Mital, M.A., and Karlin, L.I.: Diagnostic arthroscopy in sports injuries, Orthop. Clin. North Am. **11:**771, 1980.
12. Parisien, J.S., and Shereff, M.J.: The role of arthroscopy in the diagnosis and treatment of disorders of the ankle, Foot Ankle **2:**144, 1981.
13. Pritsch, M., Horoshovski, H., and Farine, I.: Ankle arthroscopy, Clin. Orthop. **184:**137, 1984.
14. Rehm, K.E., Schultheis, K.H., and Krauss, R.: Indication, technic and value of arthroscopy of the upper ankle joint, Unfallchirurgie **9:**152, 1983.
15. St. Pierre, R.K.; Velazco, A., and Fleming, L.L.: Impingement exostoses of the talus and fibula secondary to an inversion sprain: a case report, Foot Ankle **3:**282, 1983.
16. Watanabe, M.: Selfoc-arthroscope, Surg. Ther. **26:**73, 1972.
17. Wolin, I., Glassman, F., Sideman, S., et al.: Internal derangement of the talofibular component of the ankle, Surg. Gynecol. Obstet. **91:**193, 1950.

chapter 15

Ligament injuries of the ankle and foot

Kenneth M. Singer

Donald C. Jones

■ THE ANKLE

Ankle injuries are common at the levels of athletic participation. Ankle injuries vary considerably in degree and intensity, depending on the structures involved and the extent of damage to each structure.

Anatomy

There is a discrete capsule attached to the edges of the articular surface of the tibia, fibula, and talus that completely surrounds the joint and imparts stability.[39] However, the majority of the stability is provided by discrete ligamentous structures laterally and medially.

On the lateral side (Fig. 15-1), the **ante-** **rior talofibular ligament** runs obliquely from the anterior aspect of the fibula to the anterior portion of the talus, inserting just superior to the lateral articular facet. The **calcaneofibular ligament** arises at the apex of the lateral malleolus and extends inferiorly and posteriorly to insert in a prominence on the lateral surface of the midportion of the calcaneus. The calcaneofibular ligament is the strongest of the lateral ligaments and is a very discrete structure as opposed to the anterior talofibular ligament, which often occurs as a thick condensation in the capsule. The **posterior talofibular ligament** traverses the posteromedial aspect of the fibula to the posterior surface of the talus, where it inserts in a prominence just distal to the articular surface. This ligament is actually an intraarticular structure. It has no independent stabilizing function and plays only a supporting role in lateral ankle stability.

The medial side of the ankle is covered by the broad **deltoid ligament**, which consists of superficial and deep fibers (Fig. 15-2). The superficial fibers of the deltoid ligament diverge from the medial malleolus distally and extend anteriorly to the neck of the tarsal navicular and posteriorly along the medial aspect of the os calcis to the sustentaculum tali. The deep fibers consist of the anterior talotibial and posterior talotibial ligaments, two structures that originate from the medial malleolus and insert anteriorly along the neck

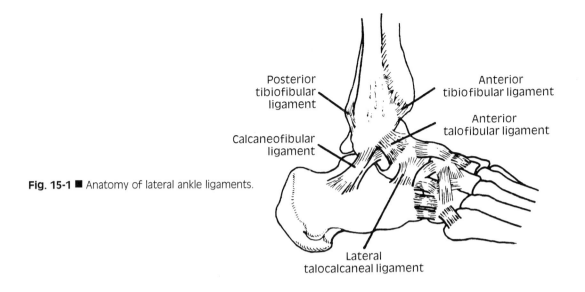

Posterior
tibiofibular
ligament

Anterior
tibiofibular ligament

Anterior
talofibular ligament

Calcaneofibular
ligament

Fig. 15-1 ■ Anatomy of lateral ankle ligaments.

Lateral
talocalcaneal ligament

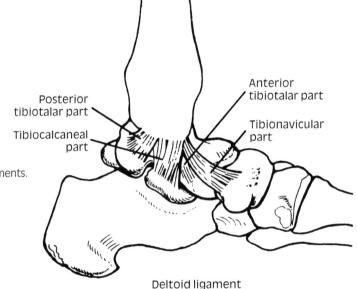

Posterior
tibiotalar part

Tibiocalcaneal
part

Anterior
tibiotalar part

Tibionavicular
part

Fig. 15-2 ■ Anatomy of medial ligaments.

Deltoid ligament

of the talus and posteriorly as far as the posteromedial tubercle of the talus. While the deltoid ligament can be divided anatomically into its component parts, functionally it should be considered as a single structure.

The distal tibia and fibula are attached by the **anterior tibiofibular ligament,** which is very strong, approximately 2.0 cm in width, and quite thick. The **poste-** **rior tibiofibular ligament** is a less discrete structure, connecting the tibia and the fibula posteriorly.

Pathomechanics

The vast majority of ligamentous injuries to the ankle in athletes occur to the lateral structures. With the foot at 0 degrees of dorsiflexion, the calcaneofibular ligament is tight and the anterior talofib-

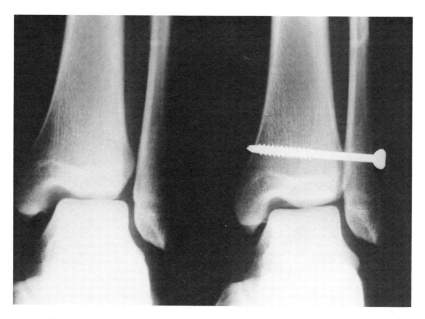

Fig. 15-11 ■ Roentgenograms showing disruption of the distal tibiofibular syndesmosis with widening of ankle mortise, which has been reduced by distal tibiofibular syndesmosis screw.

sition and a short leg cast used for another 3 weeks. During this time partial weight bearing may be instituted, but continued roentgenographic evaluation is necessary to ensure the reduction is well maintained.

Operative reduction is usually indicated for a significant tibiofibular diastasis. The deltoid ligament is repaired and the syndesmosis treated with a transfixion screw (Fig. 15-11). Repair of the deltoid ligament can usually be accomplished by primary sutures. The ligament tear is identified and followed anteriorly, because a portion of the fairly strong anterior capsule is invariably torn in association with this injury. Repair of the deltoid ligament is usually accomplished by primary sutures, and if the distal tibiofibular ligament is repairable it should either be sutured or reattached to bone. Weight bearing is discouraged until the transfixion screw is removed after 4 to 6 weeks. If there is a fracture of the distal fibula, it is treated with open reduction and internal fixation. The deltoid ligament may or may not be repaired, and a transfixion screw may not

be necessary (Fig. 15-10,*B*). Active motion is begun in 2 to 3 weeks, but protected weight bearing should be continued for a minimum of 6 to 8 weeks. Rehabilitation is accomplished as described for lateral repairs.

Sprains of the deltoid and tibiofibular ligaments carry a much longer period of

---

Deltoid ligament sprains
Tibiofibular ligament sprains
↓
Longer morbidity!

---

morbidity in the athlete than do the lateral ankle ligaments.

Late reconstruction of lateral ankle ligaments

Chronic lateral instability of the ankle may result from two situations. Inadequate treatment of a complete lateral ligament tear with early return to sporting activities will allow the ligament to heal in a relaxed position with mechanical instability. Through a similar mechanism, re-

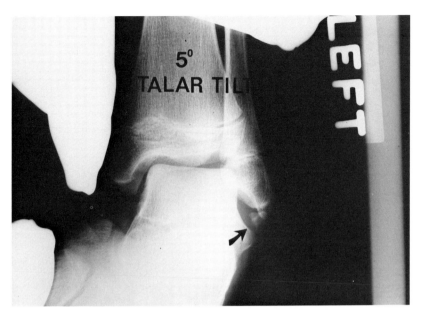

Fig. 15-12 ■ A 14-year-old girl with history of ankle "giving way" on multiple occasions following injury 3 years previously. Roentgenograms show avulsion fracture from distal fibula that has not united and a 5-degree talar tilt, indicating that giving-way symptoms were not related to ankle instability. Excision of distal fibular fragment through short transverse skin incision relieved all symptoms.

peated "sprains," each allowing the lateral supporting structures to stretch a small amount, may produce an incompetent lateral support. The symptoms and disability vary depending on the amount of instability and the demands placed on the ankle.

The individual with chronic instability complains that the ankle gives way or turns over into inversion easily. Usually this occurs during athletic activities

---

CHRONIC ANKLE INSTABILITY

Complaints of giving-way
History of repeated injury
Calf atrophy
Increased laxity ⟶ Anterior drawer
⟶ Inversion
Lateral tenderness
Soft tissue swelling

---

that involve pivoting, twisting, or quick changes in direction, and there generally is a history of repeated injuries. Physical findings are most often easy to demon-

strate and include atrophy of the calf, increased clinically detectable inversion and anterior drawer laxities compared with a normal ankle, and frequently lateral tenderness and swelling if there has been a recent episode.

It is important to document with stress roentgenograms that mechanical instability is indeed present, because Freeman et al.[29] have shown that some ankles exhibit functional instability and yet are mechanically stable. This is attributed to inadequate proprioceptive function and responds well to an appropriate, supervised physical therapy program. A second situation in which the athlete may have symptoms resembling chronic instability, with the ankle giving way and being unreliable with "cutting" activities, is the presence of a separate ossicle in the fibulotalar joint from an old injury (Fig. 15-12). We have seen several such athletes with minor amounts of talar tilt and a small, loose fragment. Removing the fragment without reconstructing the ankle joint relieves their symptoms.

When mechanical instability is present and functional disability results, an extensive education and rehabilitation program should be instituted. This program should aim at maximally strengthening the posterior tibial and peroneal muscles (see p. 176). Heel cord stretching exercises should be performed, and functional activities such as the bongo board, jumping back and forth over a stick placed 1 foot above the ground, single-foot hopping exercises, and jumping up and down a low step should be emphasized. The athlete should be fitted with a supportive device, such as a commercially available ankle lacer, an air stirrup, or Gibney-type strapping (see p. 271). These measures may sufficiently decrease symptoms in some individuals to allow them to return to their preferred activities without surgery. Total limb rehabilitation should not be neglected, because proximal muscle weakness may be present (see pp. 172-175).

If the individual continues to have symptoms of instability and pain following rehabilitation, reconstruction of the lateral ligaments is beneficial. This procedure has a predictable, high success rate.

There have been a variety of methods used for reconstructing the lateral ankle ligaments, employing the peroneal tendon, the fascia lata, or a portion of the Achilles tendon. The most common procedures at this time are the Watson-Jones procedure,[65] the Evans procedure,[23] and the Chrisman and Snook modification of the Elmslie procedure.[15]

These procedures all use either all or a portion of the peroneus brevis tendon as a tenodesis, but they differ considerably with respect to their technical and practical implications.

The procedure described by Watson-Jones used the entire peroneus brevis tendon (Fig. 15-13). It is detached as far proximally as possible, and the peroneus brevis muscle is sewn to the peroneus longus tendon to preserve its function. The peroneus brevis is then brought behind the fibula, passed through a tunnel in the distal fibula that is angled distal-

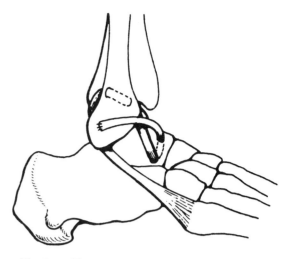

Fig. 15-13 ■ Modified Watson-Jones procedure.

ly from posterior to anterior, passed through a hole in the neck of the talus going from inferior to superior, and then brought back across itself posteriorly and inferiorly. It is then attached to the fibula. There are several reports of good results from this procedure,[3,17,31,65] and in our experience it has also proved satisfactory in eliminating the mechanical talar tilt and providing a very functional ankle without symptoms of instability (Fig. 15-14). The procedure is somewhat difficult to perform, and there is seldom sufficient length of good-quality tendon to complete the entire procedure as described by Watson-Jones. Rather than continue to take the fascia proximally, our procedure is to take as much tendon as possible, and, after bringing the portion of the tendon through the neck of the talus, to sew it back on itself.

From a theoretic standpoint, the Watson-Jones procedure does not adequately replace the calcaneofibular ligament, because the angle of the distal portion of the tenodesis from the base of the metatarsal to the fibula does not parallel the original calcaneofibular ligament. However, with the foot in plantar flexion this portion of the tenodesis would parallel the anterior talofibular ligament, which goes into a vertical position during plantar flexion.

The Evans procedure (Fig. 15-15) is sim-

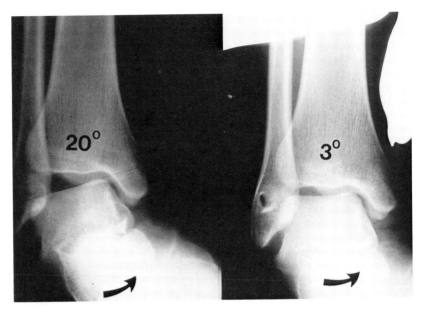

Fig. 15-14 ■ Results of Watson-Jones procedure with reduction of talar tilt from 20 to 3 degrees as demonstrated by inversion stress roentgenograms.

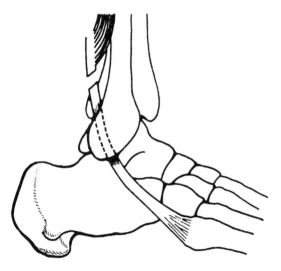

Fig. 15-15 ■ Evans procedure.

pler from a technical standpoint. However, it only provides a tenodesis to the fibula, and the peroneus brevis tendon does not follow the anatomic position of any of the original ligaments.

Chrisman and Snook[15] performed cadaver studies in which they measured the talar tilt following simulation of the Evans, Elmslie,[22] and the Watson-Jones procedures and found that the Elmslie procedure was the most effective in reducing the talar tilt.[15] They subsequently modified the Elmslie procedure, using half of the peroneus brevis tendon instead of fascia lata (Fig. 15-16). The tendon is split from its attachment at the base of the fifth metatarsal proximally, and the anterior portion is brought through a hole in the distal portion of the fibula passing from anterior to posterior just proximal to the joint surface. It then traverses distally to the os calcis, where it is placed into an osteoperiosteal groove and then brought anteriorly to insert into the cuboid. The anterior talofibular ligament is reconstructed by attaching the anterior limb of the transfer to the talus either by suturing it into remnants of the anterior talofibular ligament attachment or by attaching it to bone. The Chrisman and Snook modification of the Elmslie procedure most closely reapproximates the normal anatomy and has provided excellent results.[15,51,56] At present, this is our procedure of choice.

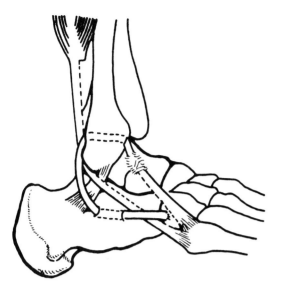

Fig. 15-16 ■ Chrisman-Snook lateral ankle reconstruction.

Some patients with lateral ankle instability also have subtalar instability.[11,15,51] This may explain some of the failures of the Watson-Jones and Evans procedures.

Interestingly, separate investigations of the results of lateral reconstructive procedures have been published fairly recently.[36,55,63] In the study by Horstman et al.,[36] 7 Evans procedures, 30 Watson-Jones procedures, and 17 modified Elmslie procedures, were evaluated. The patients undergoing the Watson-Jones procedure had a much higher incidence of subjective instability. This correlated with talar tilt measurements in that 24% of those in the Watson-Jones group had greater than 5 degrees difference from the normal as compared with 5% in the modified Elmslie group. However, there was a very high incidence of patient satisfaction, well over 90% in all groups. The percentage of individuals returning to preinjury activity level was slightly lower after the Watson-Jones procedure. There was a relatively high incidence of minor postoperative pain in all groups, but a very low incidence of significant pain.

In the review by St. Pierre et al.[55] of the Evans procedure, two modifications of the

Elmslie procedures (that of Chrisman and Snook and that of Goldner), and the Watson-Jones procedure, there was no significant difference in the amount of postoperative pain, swelling, or functional instability. It was their conclusion that over 90% excellent clinical results can be obtained with any of the procedures if performed correctly.

Injuries to the ligaments of the distal tibiofibular syndesmosis

Acute injuries of the distal tibiofibular ligaments are not as uncommon as is often thought. Most often they are incomplete and occur in association with other injuries, and they respond to the treatment instituted for the other soft tissue injuries.

The acute injury with instability often results in ankle diastasis in association with other injuries, as noted previously. Treatment must restore the syndesmosis. Restoring the syndesmosis anatomically with either a distal tibiofibular transfixion screw or repair of the deltoid ligament and the fibular fracture is usually sufficient (see Figs. 15-9,C, 15-10,A, and 15-11,A). If the anterior distal tibiofibular ligament is avulsed with a portion of bone, it should be replaced and internally fixed. Commonly, complete tears of the anterior distal tibiofibular ligament result in considerable attenuation. Direct suturing is not possible in this case and probably is not necessary if the distal tibiofibular joint is reapproximated and allowed to heal.

Isolated injuries to the distal tibiofibular joint usually occur as a result of either external rotation or forced dorsiflexion injuries. If clinical instability is suspected, stress roentgenograms in those positions may be of some value. Ankle arthrography may also be of considerable assistance in evaluating the ankle suspected as having this injury. Dye injected into the joint will escape into the distal tibiofibular syndesmosis if the isolated injury is present.

Because the acute isolated injury to this joint is rare, the literature on the subject is sparse. However, the reader is referred to Chapter 18 for an excellent discussion of this topic. If such an injury is documented, we would advocate exploration of the joint, repair of the anterior distal tibiofibular ligament if possible, and transfixion with a distal tibiofibular screw for 4 to 6 weeks.

Chronic instability of this joint is extremely incapacitating for the athlete. Arthrography will remain positive[42] and assist with the diagnosis. Fixation of the distal tibiofibular joint with the transfixion screw alone is inadequate in patients with chronic instability, and Katznelson et al.[40] have demonstrated satisfactory results with good pain relief and excellent function in 5 of 6 patients treated with distal tibiofibular arthrodesis.

Prevention of ankle injuries

With increasing knowledge on the part of trainers, coaches, and athletes, many ankle injuries can be prevented. Stretching and strengthening exercises of the posterior tibial and peroneal muscle groups (see p. 176), heel cord stretching in an appropriate nonballistic manner (see p. 188), and appropriate footwear (see p. 592) and protective strapping (see p. 271) have all been shown to be efficacious in preventing ankle injuries.

Studies have similarly shown that high-top shoes give an advantage over low-top shoes, particularly in basketball and football, and taping is also effective in decreasing the incidence of ankle ligament injuries.[30,64]

All athletes should be instructed in these exercises. Weekend or middle-aged athletes are particularly at risk, because they are involved in athletic activities on a less frequent basis and therefore do not have the repetitive conditioning and proprioceptive protection of the more frequently involved or younger athletes. Such injuries also seem to be more common in the athlete who is somewhat overweight.

■ THE FOOT
Ligament sprains

Ligament sprains of the foot may be extremely disabling to the athlete, because not infrequently the time required for healing and rehabilitation is far out of proportion to the apparent severity of the injury.

Midtarsal ligament sprain

Injury to the midtarsal ligament is most commonly seen in dancers and gymnasts because of the tremendous demands these athletes place on the midfoot. With this injury, pain may be elicited by forced dorsiflexion and plantar flexion of the midfoot, and tenderness may be noted directly over the area of ligamentous involvement. Roentgenograms are usually negative, although occasionally there will be a small avulsion fracture at the site of injury. Treatment should consist of elevation, rest, analgesics, and midfoot taping. If the recovery is slow, it may be beneficial to place the foot in a firm-soled shoe with a rocker-bottom sole. The shoe is worn during daily activities to decrease the stress across the midfoot and promote healing.

Bifurcate ligament sprain

The bifurcate ligament is situated between the lateral malleolus and the base of the fifth metatarsal with extensions going from the distal end of the calcaneus to the cuboid and navicular. This ligament has classically been considered to be a major stabilizer of the midtarsal (Chopart's) joint. It is subject to injury with inversion injuries to the foot and the ankle, and diagnosis is usually based on the mechanism of the injury and the area of local tenderness. Treatment should be similar to an ankle sprain with local conservative measures and supportive taping. Occasionally a small avulsion fracture will be seen from the calcaneal attachment, and this may remain symptomatic, requiring eventual excision.

Sinus tarsi syndrome

Sinus tarsi syndrome, now a well-recognized entity, was first described by O'Conner in 1958.[12] Since that time, numerous papers have been written on the subject, yet it can be a most difficult problem to treat.

Anatomically, the sinus tarsi is a funnel-shaped tunnel on the lateral side of the foot that has a large opening laterally and a smaller opening medially. The sinus contains the very broad interosseous talocalcaneal ligament and a fat pad. This ligament carries nerve fibers believed to provide proprioception to the hindfoot. It forms a single fibrous band medially, and laterally splits into two separate bands with interposing fibrous tissue containing nerves and vessels.[62]

The mechanism of injury to the sinus tarsi contents is usually forced inversion of the foot. Studies have demonstrated that the talocalcaneal ligament can be torn with forced inversion with the ankle in neutral position. However, this tear will occur only after the sequential rupture of the calcaneofibular and lateral talocalcaneal ligaments.[62] Since this syndrome is most commonly seen in individuals who have a history of multiple ankle sprains, one can theorize that the pathology is caused by repeated microtrauma rather than a single traumatic episode. This concept is supported by Meyer's histologic observation[46] of remodeling of the soft tissue contents of the sinus tarsi.

Symptoms consist of pain and tenderness over the lateral aspect of the sinus tarsi. Inversion forces, even from walking over uneven surfaces, may cause discom-

fort. A subjective feeling of instability is frequently present.

The diagnosis is facilitated by a high index of suspicion in an athlete who has tenderness over the lateral aspect of the sinus tarsi. Temporary relief of symptoms following an injection of local anesthetic into the sinus tarsi is strongly suggestive. Taillard et al.[62] suggested that subtalar arthrography and electromyography are also beneficial in establishing a diagnosis, but we have had no experience with these procedures.

TREATMENT OF SINUS TARSI SYNDROME
Initial

Rest
Antiinflammatory medication
Steroid injection into sinus tarsi
Peroneal strengthening

**Late (unresponsive to initial
therapy program)**

Surgical excision of contents of sinus tarsi

Initial conservative treatment consists of rest, antiinflammatory medication, and steroid injection into the sinus tarsi. Multiple injections may be necessary before the patient becomes asymptomatic. This is facilitated by subsequent peroneal muscle strengthening.[29] The success rate is high. In an unusual series of 116 patients with this relatively uncommon condition, Komprda showed that 73 were completely relieved of all symptoms, and another 25 were markedly improved.[41]

If this treatment regimen is unsuccessful, surgery should be considered. The procedure consists basically of a lateral approach to the sinus tarsi and excision of its contents and is described in detail by O'Connor.[49] This procedure has proved successful in a high percentage of our patients.[49,62] Our very limited experience has been gratifying.

SINUS TARSI SYNDROME

- Pain and tenderness over the lateral aspect of the sinus tarsi
- Subjective feeling of instability
- History of multiple ankle sprains
- Increased symptoms with inversion forces
- Symptoms relieved by local anesthetic injection into sinus tarsi

---

REFERENCES

1. Ala-Ketola, L., Puranen, J., et al: Arthrography and the diagnosis of ligament injuries and classifications of ankle injuries, Radiology **125:**63, 1977.
2. Almquist, G.: Pathomechanics and diagnosis of inversion injuries of the lateral ligaments of the ankle, J. Sports Med. **2:**109, 1974.
3. Anderson, K.J., and LeCocq, J.F.: Operative treatment of injury to the fibular collateral ligament of the ankle, J. Bone Joint Surg. **36A:**825, 1954.
4. Anderson, K.J., LeCocq, J.F., and Clayton, M.L.: Athletic injuries to the fibular collateral ligament of the ankle, Clin. Orthop. **23:**145, 1962.
5. Black, H.M., Brand, R.L., and Eichelberger, M.R.: An improved technique for the evaluation of ligamentous injury in severe ankle sprains, Am. J. Sports Med. **6:**276, 1978.
6. Brand, R.L., and Collins, M.D.F.: Operative management of ligamentons injuries to the ankle, Clin. Sports Med. **1:**117, 1982.
7. Brostrom, L.: Sprained ankles. I. Anatomic lesions and recent sprains, Acta Chir. Scand. **128:**483, 1964.
8. Brostrom, L.: Sprained ankles. III. Clinical observations and recent ligament ruptures, Acta Chir. Scand. **130:**560, 1965.
9. Brostrom, L.: Sprained ankles. V. Treatment and prognosis in recent ligament ruptures, Acta Chir. Scand. **131:**537, 1966.
10. Brostrom, L.: Sprained ankles. VI. Surgical treatment of "chronic" ligament ruptures, Acta Chir. Scand. **132:**551, 1966.
11. Brostrom, L., et al.: Sprained ankles. II. Arthrographic diagnosis of recent ligament ruptures, Acta Chir. Scand. **129:**485, 1965.
12. Brown, J.E.: The sinus tarsi syndrome, Clin. Orthop. **18:**231, 1960.
13. Castaing, J.: Les entorses de la cheville, Conf. Enseignement SOFCOT, Paris, 1968, Expansion Scientifique Francaise, pp. 23-41.
14. Chapman, M.W.: Sprains of the ankle. In American Academy of Orthopedic Surgeons: Instructional Course Lectures, vol. XXIV, St. Louis, 1975, The C.V. Mosby Co., p. 294.
15. Chrisman, O.D., and Snook, G.A.: Reconstruction of lateral ligament tears of the ankle, J. Bone Joint Surg. **51A:**904, 1969.
16. Claustre, J., Simon, L., and Allieu, Y.: Le syndrome du sinus du tarse existe-t-il? Rhumatologie **31:**19, 1979.
17. Coutts, M.B., and Woodward, D.E.P.: Surgery and sprained ankles: lateral ligament tears, Clin. Orthop. **42:**81, 1965.
18. Cox, J.S.: Surgical treatment of ankle sprains, Am. J. Sports Med. **5:**250, 1977.
19. Cox, J.S., and Hewes, F.R.: Normal talar tilt angle, Clin. Orthop. **140:**37, 1979.
20. Debrunner, H.V.: Das Sinus Tarsi Syndrom, Schweiz. Med. Wochenschr. **93:**1660, 1963.
21. Drez, D., Young, J.C., Waldman, D., et al: Nonoperative treatment of double lateral ligament tears of the ankle, Am. J. Sports Med. **10:**197, 1982.
22. Elmslie, R.C.: Recurrent subluxation of the ankle joint, Am. Surg. **100:**364, 1934.
23. Evans, D.L.: Recurrent instability of the ankle: method of surgical treatment, Proc. R. Soc. Med. **46:**15, 1952.
24. Evans, G.A., and Frenyo, S.D.: The stress-tenogram in the diagnosis of ruptures of the lateral ligament of the ankle, J. Bone Joint Surg. **61B:**247, 1979.
25. Evans, G.A., Hardcastle, P., and Frenyo, A.D.: Acute rupture of the lateral ligament of the ankle: "To suture or not to suture?" J. Bone Joint Surg. **66B:**209-212, 1984.
26. Fordyce, A.J.W., and Horn, C.V.: Arthrography and recent injuries of the ligaments of the ankle, J. Bone Joint Surg. **548:**116, 1972.
27. Freeman, M.A.R.: Instability of the foot after injuries to the lateral ligaments of the ankle, J. Bone Joint Surg. **47B:**669, 1965.
28. Freeman, M.A.R.: Treatment of ruptures of the lateral ligaments of the ankle, J. Bone Surg. **47B:**661, 1965.
29. Freeman, M.A.R., Dean M.R.E., and Hanham L.W.F.: The etiology and prevention of functional instability of the foot, J. Bone Joint Surg. **47B:**678, 1965.
30. Garrick, J.G.: Epidemiologic perspectives, Clin. Sports Med. **1:**13, 1982.
31. Gillespie H.S., and Boncher P.: Watson-Jones repair of lateral instability of the ankle, J. Bone Joint Surg. **53A:**920, 1971.
32. Gordon, R.B.: Arthrography of the ankle joint: experience in one hundred seven studies, J. Bone Joint Surg. **52A:**16, 1970.
33. Harrington, K.D.: Degenerative arthritis of the ankle secondary to long standing lateral ligament instability, J. Bone Joint Surg. **61A:**354, 1979.
34. Hauser, E.D.W.: The sinus tarsi syndrome, Ann. Podiat. **1:**11, 1962.
35. Henning, C.E., and Egge, L.N.: Cast brace treatment of acute unstable lateral ankle sprain, Am. J. Sports Med. **5:**252, 1977.
36. Horstman, J.K., Cantor, G.S., and Samuelson, K.M.: Investigation of lateral ankle ligament reconstruction, Foot Ankle, **1:**338-342, 1981.
37. Jackson, D.W., Ashley, R.L., and Powell, J.W.: Ankle sprains in young athletes: relation of severity and disability, Clin. Orthop. **101:**201, 1974.
38. Johannsen, A.: Radiological diagnosis of lateral ligament lesions of the ankle, Acta Orthop. Scand. **49:**295, 1978.
39. Kapandji, I.A.: The physiology of the joints, vol. 2. Lower limb, New York, 1970, Churchill Livingstone.
40. Katznelson, A., Lin, E., and Militano, J.: Ruptures of the ligaments about the tibio-fibular syndesmosis, Injury **15:**170, 1983.
41. Komprda, J.: Le syndrome du sinus du tarse, Ann. Podol. **5:**11-17, 1966.

42. Lauren, C., and Mathieu, J.: Sagittal mobility of the normal ankle, Clin. Orthop. **108:**99, 1975.

43. Lindstrand, A., and Mortneson, W.: Anterior instability of the ankle joint following acute lateral sprain, Acta Radiol. (Diagn.) **18:**529, 1977.

44. Marrero, R.M., and Lopez, A.R.: Tratamiento quirurgico de la lesion cronica del seno del tarso. Nota previa. Actual. Med. Chir. Pied. **11:**173, 1978.

45. Mehrez, M., and el Geneidy, S.: Arthrography of the ankle, J. Bone Joint Surg. **52B:**308, 1970.

46. Meyer, J.M., and Lagier, R.: Post-traumatic sinus tarsi syndrome, Acta Orthop. Scand. **48:**122, 1977.

47. Navarre, M.: A propos du syndrome du sinus du tarse, Acta Orthop. Belg. **32:**743, 1966.

48. Niedermann, B., Anderson, A., et al.: Rupture of the lateral ligaments of the ankle: "operation or plaster cast?" A prospective study, Acta Orthop. Scand. **52:**579, 1981.

49. O'Connor, D.: Sinus tarsi syndrome: a clinical entity, J. Bone Joint Surg. **40A:**720, 1958.

50. Rasmussen, O., Tovborg-Jensen, I., and Boe, S.: Distal tibiofibular ligaments: analysis of the functions, Acta Orthop. Scand. **53:**681, 1982.

51. Reigler, H.F.: Reconstruction for lateral instability of the ankle, J. Bone Joint Surg. **66A:**336, 1984.

52. Roy, S., and Irvin, R.: Sports medicine prevention, Evaluation Management, and Rehabilitation, Englewood Cliffs, N.J., 1983, Prentice-Hall, Inc.

53. Ruben, G., and Witten, M.: The talar tilt angle and the fibular collateral ligament, J. Bone Joint Surg. **42A:**311, 1960.

54. Ruth, C.J.: The surgical treatment of injuries of the fibular collateral ligaments of the ankle, J. Bone Joint Surg. **42A:**229, 1961.

55. St. Pierre, R., Ullman, F., Jr., et al.: A review of lateral ligament reconstruction, Foot Ankle **3:**114, 1982.

56. Savastano, A.A., and Lowe, E.B., Jr.: Ankle sprains: surgical treatment for recurrent sprains. Report of ten patients treated with the Chrisman-Snook modification of the Elmslie procedure, Am. J. Sports Med. **8:**208, 1980.

57. Sellicson, D., Gassman, J., and Pope, N.: Ankle instability: evaluation of the lateral ligaments, Am. J. Sports Med. **8:**39, 1980.

58. Souser, D.D., Nelson, R.C., et al.: Acute injuries of the lateral ligaments of the ankle: comparison of stress radiography and arthrography, Radiology **148:**653, 1983.

59. Spiegal, P.K., and Staples, O.S.: Arthrography of the ankle joint: problems and diagnosis of acute lateral ligament injuries, Radiology **114:**587, 1975.

60. Staples, O.S.: Ruptures of the fibular collateral ligament of the ankle: result study of immediate surgical treatment, J. Bone Joint Surg. **57:**101, 1975.

61. Stover, C.N.: Air stirrup management of ankle injuries in the athlete, Am. J. Sports Med. **8:**360, 1980.

62. Taillard, W., Meyer, J., Garcia, J., and Blanc, Y.: The sinus tarsi syndrome, Int. Orthop. **5:**117, 1981.

63. Vainionpaa, S., Kirves, P., and Laike, E.: Lateral instability of the ankle and results when treated by the Evans procedure, Am. J. Sports Med. **8:**437, 1980.

64. Walsh, W.M., and Blackburn, T.: Prevention of ankle sprains, Am. J. Sports Med. **5:**243, 1977.

65. Watson-Jones, R.: Recurrent dislocations of the ankle joint, J. Bone Joint Surg. **34B:**519, 1952.

66. Watson-Jones, R.: Fractures and joint injuries, ed. 4, vol. 2, Baltimore, 1955, The Williams & Wilkins Co.

chapter 16

Soft tissue conditions of the ankle and foot

Kenneth M. Singer

Donald C. Jones

■ TENDON PATHOLOGY
Tenosynovitis about the ankle

Because the tendons of the foot and ankle have the dual responsibility of providing support and motion, tenosynovitis occurs quite often in athletes. Although seen in all tendons about the foot and ankle, the structures affected most frequently are the anterior tibialis, posterior tibialis, flexor hallucis longus, and Achilles tendons.

Anterior tibial tenosynovitis

The anterior tibialis muscle originates from the proximal two thirds of the tibia, lateral tibial condyle, and interosseous membrane and inserts onto the navicular, first metatarsal base, and medial cuneiform. This musculotendinous unit supplies 80% of the dorsiflexion power of the ankle. Although a very powerful muscle, its straight course under the superior extensor retinaculum results in minimal mechanical demands and therefore less exposure to irritation and inflammation. When localized swelling, tenderness, and crepitance over this tendon indicate a diagnosis of anterior tibial tenosynovitis, rest, ice, and nonsteroidal antiinflammatory medication are very effective. Rupture of the tendon has been reported in older athletes and will present as a relatively painless foot-drop. It must be differentiated from a neurologic deficit such as radiculopathy at the level of L5.

Posterior tibial tenosynovitis

Inflammation of the posterior tibialis tendon is more common than that of the tibialis anterior. As the tendon curves behind the medial malleolus, it functions much as a rope does when going through a pulley, with attrition stresses occurring at the points of contact. During the pronation phase of running gait, the mechanical demands placed on this structure are quite high. Repetitive microtrauma occurs, and the tendon becomes inflamed and may eventually undergo degeneration and rupture. Individuals with more pronation during the stance phase are much more susceptible to this entity.

Posterior tibial tendon tenosynovitis is most commonly seen during athletic activities requiring quick changes in direction, such as basketball, soccer, tennis, and ice hockey. The diagnosis is easily made. There is usually tenderness along

---

POSTERIOR TIBIAL TENOSYNOVITIS

- Tenderness along tendon behind medial malleous
- Crepitus may be present
- Pain with:
  Passive pronation
  Resisted supination
- Associated with hyperpronation

---

the tendon as it courses behind the medial malleolus, and frequently there is associated crepitance. Passive pronation or resisted supination of the midfoot reproduces the symptoms.

In older individuals this tendon can become attenuated and eventually rupture. Observation of the patient from behind will show increased heel valgus and pronation. Asking the patient to stand on tiptoes will demonstrate the absence of heel varus normally seen in this maneuver.

Treatment consists of rest, ice, antiinflammatory medication, and a medially posted orthotic to decrease pronation during the weight-bearing phase. Steroid injection into the tendon sheath should be

---

TREATMENT OF POSTERIOR TIBIAL TENSOYNOVITIS

- Rest
- Ice
- Antiinflammatory medication
- Medial heel wedge
- Short leg non-weight-bearing cast (with foot in inversion) for 10 days (severe cases)
- Rehabilitation program

---

considered, but in most instances will provide only temporary relief and carries a risk of subsequent tendon rupture. In the young athlete with acute tendinitis and crepitance, immobilization and a short leg non-weight-bearing cast with the foot in slight inversion for 10 days to 2 weeks often relieves symptoms dramatically.

If this entity is recalcitrant to the usual methods and swelling and tenderness persist, one should bear in mind that human lymphocyte antigen (HLA) B-27–positive arthropathies may cause chronic proliferative tenosynovitis.

Flexor hallucis longus tenosynovitis

The flexor hallucis longus tendon is lined with a true tendon sheath and courses behind the medial malleolus in a separate compartment. Athletes involved in repetitive push-off maneuvers will transmit tremendous forces across the tendon and its sheath, resulting in irritation and tenosynovitis. This is a common among ballet dancers, and the *sur les pointes* position is frequently implicated (see Chapter 42).

The tendon's course helps to explain the development of this overuse syndrome. The flexor hallucis tendon longus courses behind the medial malleolus in a fibroosseous tunnel on the posterior aspect of the talus (Figs. 16-1 and 16-2). It is bordered anteriorly by the body of the talus, medially by the medial tubercle of the talus, laterally by the lateral tubercle of the talus (the os trigonum if separated), and posteriorly by the flexor retinaculum.

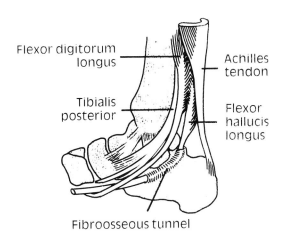

Fig. 16-1 ■ Course of flexor hallucis longus through fibroosseous tunnel behind medial malleolus.

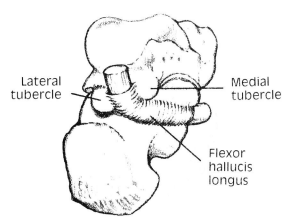

Fig. 16-2 ■ Posterior view of relationship of fibroosseous tunnel to medial and lateral tubercle of calcaneus.

This results in a fairly confined space, which predisposes the structure to mechanical irritation in the presence of inflammation. If the inflammation is prolonged or the fibroosseous tunnel becomes somewhat stenotic, a simple tendon sheath inflammatory response may evolve into a partial rupture of the tendon with snapping or triggering within the tunnel.

If the tendon is inflamed, it is tender along its course posterior and lateral to the medial malleolus. In stenosing tenosynovitis, the signs and symptoms are more dramatic. The patient will complain of pain, tenderness, a snapping sensation posteromedially, and occasionally inability to flex the great toe. Tightness of the flexor hallucis can be observed in many individuals who develop tenosynovitis of this tendon. To check for tightness, note the amount of passive extension of the great toe metatarsophalangeal joint with the foot and ankle in both a neutral and a plantar-flexed position. Inability to extend the joint beyond neutral with the foot and ankle in neutral position, as compared to the passive extension possible with the ankle plantar flexed, indicates contracture of the flexor hallucis longus.

Ice, antiinflammatory agents, and spe-cific strapping or longitudinal arch supports with firm soles will frequently alleviate the pain of tenosynovitis. Surgery is required when the stenotic lesion is present. This consists of release of the flexor retinaculum, although even after surgical release the prognosis is guarded.[64] Frequently the original injury that leads to tenosynovitis is a partial rupture of the central fibers of the tendon. This results in a fusiform enlargement of the tendon itself, so even if the tunnel is decompressed the tendon remains pathologically weakened and may completely rupture.

There is a rarer, more distal form of flexor hallucis stenosing tenosynovitis that occurs where the flexor hallucis longus tendon passes through its sheath between the sesamoids and inserts into the terminal phalanx of the great toe. This is essentially a second pulley system and is very prone to trauma, particularly in runners. The sheath becomes chronically or intermittently inflamed and eventually heals with a constricted area, which impairs passage of the tendon. It often expresses itself with tenderness and swelling in the region of the sesamoids. The diagnostic finding is the patient's inability to flex the interphalangeal joint of the great toe

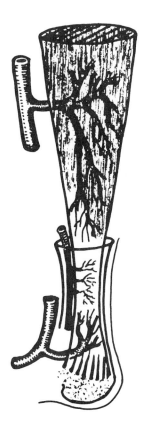

Fig. 16-8 ◼ Blood supply to musculotendinous unit of Achilles tendon. Note where longitudinal vessels supply tendon proximally and distally, while transverse vessels vascularize midportion.

insertion of the tendon and that this is the area of poor vascularity rendered susceptible to chronic inflammation and rupture[28,50] (Fig. 16-8).

One other point concerning the anatomy of the Achilles tendon should be emphasized. The tendon fibers rotate laterally as they descend. Cummins et al.[14] described three patterns of rotation. In the most common, the gastrocnemius contributes two thirds of the fibers posteriorly and the soleus contributes one third. In the second most common, the gastrocnemius and the soleus each contribute one half, and in the least frequent pattern the soleus makes up the posterior two thirds and the gastrocnemius one third. This rotation in the Achilles tendon plays an important part in the development of pathology.

Contributing factors

The terms "tendinitis," "peritendinitis," "tenosynovitis," and "tenovaginitis" have all been used by various authors to describe Achilles tendon disease.[12,13,15] Like Clement, we prefer to use **Achilles tendinitis** and **peritendinitis.** Tendinitis refers to inflammation within the tendon, and peritendinitis describes inflammation

---

CONTRIBUTING FACTORS TO ACHILLES TENDON DISEASE

Training errors
- Increase in training mileage
- Single severe running session
- Increase in training intensity
- Running on hills
- Uneven or slippery terrain
- Recommencement after an extended period of inactivity

Anatomic factors
- Excessive pronation
- Hindfoot varus
- Forefoot varus
- Tight heel cords
- Tibia vara

---

within the peritendon. The etiology of Achilles tendinitis or peritendinitis can be singular or multifactorial. In Clement's study of runners, the primary etiologic factor consisted of training errors, such as a sudden increase in training mileage, a single severe competitive or training session (10 kilometers or marathon), a sudden increase in training intensity, repetitive hill running, recommencement of training after an extended period of inactivity, or running on uneven or slippery terrain.

Excessive pronation of the forefoot has been implicated as an etiologic factor in running-induced injuries.[9,11,13,33] If a runner has hindfoot and forefoot varus, the Achilles tendon is forced to go from lateral to medial as the foot goes from footstrike to midstance. This causes a "whipping" action of the tendon, and, in addition, shear forces are established between the gastrocnemius and soleus portions of the tendon, creating areas of stress concentration. These forces may then compress the vessels in an area that already possesses a tenuous blood supply, establishing the appropriate setting for inflammation and degenerative changes within the tendon as a result of this microtrauma.

Clinical findings

Symptoms of peritendonitis consist primarily of pain in the Achilles tendon area, which is aggravated by activity and relieved by rest. Tenderness will usually be apparent several centimeters proximal to the insertion of the tendon into the calcaneus. Poor flexibility of the gastrocsoleus complex is frequently noted and probably plays a role in the etiology. Less than 25 to 30 degrees of dorsiflexion is likely to increase the tendency of the athlete to develop Achilles tendinitis, as is tibia vara, hindfoot varus, and the tendency toward a cavus foot. One must also examine the feet and legs for alignment problems, and the footwear for external compression areas.

Treatment

Peritendinitis should initially be treated by ice massage, contrast baths, and antiinflammatory medications. If there are alignment problems,[11] orthotics are appropriate. The athlete is usually asymptomatic in a relatively short time.

In more advanced or chronic cases, the pseudosheath of the Achilles tendon will become fibrotic and stenosed and may require surgical decompression. This should consist of excising the entire pseudosheath.[28]

In chronic Achilles tendinitis, the conservative measures just mentioned should be initiated, and rest should be prescribed. It is usually not necessary to immobilize the extremity, but for some patients a 1- to 2-week period in a non-weight-bearing cast will be of benefit. We attempt to provide the athlete with a program of activity that assists him in maintaining cardiovascular fitness, such as use

---

TREATMENT OF ACHILLES TENDINITIS

Ice
Contrast baths
Antiinflammatory medication
Heel elevation
Orthotic (if appropriate)
Stretching
Aerobic, well-leg, and upper body conditioning

---

of the exercise bicycle and swimming. It is particularly important to carefully assess the athlete's alignment, and we frequently treat individuals who have recurrent episodes of acute tendinitis or chronic tendinitis with orthotics. We instruct this athlete to wear the orthosis at all times if he is symptomatic, even during normal daily activities. In all cases, an intensive heel cord stretching program is instituted and continued throughout the athlete's career (see p. 188).

If conservative treatment is unsuccessful after 6 months of extended treatment, surgery is recommended. A posteromedial or posterolateral incision is used to expose the tendon. The peritendon is longitudinally incised to expose the tendon, and if it is thickened, a generous portion of the sheath is excised. If no apparent pathology is noted, one or two longitudinal incisions are made into the tendinous substance. If necrotic tissue is found, it is excised in a wedge-shaped manner. Any incision in the tendon is repaired with absorbable buried sutures. The peritendon is left open and the wound closed in two layers.

In the more advanced cases with chronic long-term symptoms and palpable nodular thickening in the tendon, partial tears may have occurred. The athlete usually has a fairly long history of chronic complaints with shooting or sharp pain in the tendon with activity. There is frequently an area of thickening or induration with an irregular contour in the tendon. Ultrasonography has been helpful in making this diagnosis. Sub-

Pain in this area must be differentiated from tarsal tunnel syndrome or entrapment of the lateral or medial plantar nerves. However, these two entities do not usually exhibit localized tenderness over the plantar fascia and are frequently accompanied by a positive Tinel's sign. One must also be aware of the possibility of an S1 radiculopathy causing this type of pain pattern. But again, there is absence of local tenderness, and stretch signs are present on complete neurologic examination.

It is still a common misconception that the pain of plantar fasciitis is the direct result of the often co-existing anterior calcaneal spur. The calcaneal spur seen on some x-ray is the result of and not the cause of traction, chronic inflammation, and subsequent calcification.[23,37]

The key to effective treatment is early rest. Running is stopped, and the athlete maintains his cardiovascular condition through non-weight-bearing activities such

---

TREATMENT OF PLANTAR FASCIITIS

- Rest
- Ice massage
- Nonsteroidal antiinflammatory medication
- Stretching
- Orthotics (if appropriate)
- Heel lift with cut-out under medial calcaneus
- Aerobic, well-leg, and upper body conditioning
- Steroid injection
- Cast immobilization (rarely needed)

---

as swimming and bicycling. Nonsteroidal antiinflammatory therapy and ice massage (three times a day for 15 minutes) are initiated. Control of excessive forefoot pronation with an in-shoe shock-absorbing medially posted orthosis is often helpful. Gentle stretching of the gastrocsoleus-calcaneous plantar fascia linkage system is instituted.* Plantar fasciitis may take 6

---

*For a discussion of the role of the linkage system in plantar fasciitis, see p. 416.

to 12 weeks to resolve. The athlete must be patient during this period and not return to vigorous activity prematurely, as doing so could convert an acute situation into a chronic one. Running may be resumed when tenderness over the plantar fascia, morning stiffness, and pain with weight bearing have abated.

If the problem continues despite this treatment, steroid injections may be used in a judicious manner. One may also consider the use of cast immobilization in rare resistant cases.

It must be remembered that the majority of cases resolve with conservative care. Patients who remain symptomatic 6 to 9 months after initiation of care may be candidates for surgical intervention. Through a medial longitudinal incision made along the plantar fascial insertion into the calcaneus, the abductor hallucis fascia and the plantar fascia are completely released. A small piece of the calcaneus may also be shaved in an effort to decompress the area. The foot is placed into a bulky dressing with a posterior splint for 2 weeks. Gradual return to activities and stretching are then started and increased for the next 6 weeks.

Baxter and Thigpen[2] feel that recalcitrant calcodynia can be secondary to localized entrapment of the motor branch nerve to the abductor digiti quinti muscle. In their series, 34 feet underwent neuroly-

---

DIFFERENTIAL DIAGNOSIS OF PLANTAR HEEL PAIN

- Plantar fasciitis
- Tarsal tunnel syndrome
- Calcaneal nerve entrapment
- S1 radiculopathy
- Entrapment of abductor digiti quinti motor nerve

---

sis of this nerve with or without minimal plantar fascia release and removal of an impinging heel spur. Of the 34 surgeries, 82% of the patients where satisfied, while 12% were satisfied with reservations.

We attempt to differentiate between nerve entrapment and true plantar fasciitis when possible, and dissect and decompress the branches of the calcaneal nerve before dividing the plantar fascia. At present we are not as certain as Baxter and Thigpen that we can accurately determine which structure is responsible for the symptoms.[2]

■ ENTRAPMENT NEUROPATHIES ABOUT THE FOOT AND ANKLE

Entrapment neuropathies about the foot and ankle may be produced by the compression of the anatomic structures, scar tissue, or external forces caused by the type of footwear.

Sural nerve

Arising from the tibial nerve 3 cm above the knee joint, the sural nerve passes between the heads of the gastrocnemius in 38% of specimens and on the soleus in 40%.[42] Two thirds of the distance to the heel from the knee, the nerve pierces the fascia and gives off cutaneous branches to the distal quarter of the leg, lateral cutaneous branches to the heel, and branches to the dorsum of the foot. The nerve can become entrapped as it exits from the fas-

---

LOCATION OF SURAL NERVE ENTRAPMENT SYNDROMES

- Point of fascial exit (two thirds of the distance between knee and heel)
- Course behind lateral malleolus

---

cia; however, most problems occur where the nerve passes behind the lateral malleous.

Symptoms consist of pain over the lateral aspect of the foot and ankle. The discomfort may be hypesthetic in nature or may rarely have an aching quality. Sensory changes in the distribution of the nerve may be present but often are not. A positive Tinel's sign should be elicited, and symptoms may be produced by plantar flexing and inverting the foot.

The first course of treatment is to determine whether the cause is internal or external. If an offending object such as a stocking or pressure point in a boot or shoe can be identified, this should be padded or removed. Injections of local anesthetic and steroids may be beneficial. Two recent reports review the entity and describe excellent results of neurolysis.

Deep peroneal nerve (anterior tarsal tunnel syndrome)

Emerging from the leg along with the anterior tibial artery at the midanterior aspect of the tibia in front of the ankle joint, the deep peroneal nerve runs lateral to the anterior tibial and extensor hallucis longus tendons and sends a motor branch beneath the long toe extensors to innervate the extensor brevis muscle. It then runs beneath the fascia in the foot to its distal third.

Previous distortions or fractures in the region of the tarsus, osteophytes from osteoarthritis in the region of the medial

---

CONTRIBUTING FACTORS TO ANTERIOR TARSAL TUNNEL SYNDROME

- Osteophytes in medial midtarsus
- Fractures
- Tight shoes
- Space-occupying lesions

---

midtarsus, and any space-occupying lesion may initiate the syndrome. However, Marinacci[55] emphasized the frequency of tight shoes as a cause. Patients complain of pain on the dorsum of the foot that frequently occurs at night and is accentuated by tight-fitting shoes. A sensory deficit in the first web space and atrophy of the extensor digitorum brevis is noted, and occasionally a positive Tinel's sign may be noted over the nerve. Roentgenograms should be taken in hope of identifying a bone spur causing compression. Electromyographic studies demonstrate an increased distal latency of the deep pero-

533

Section 1 FOOT AND ANKLE
Chapter 17 Ankle and foot
fractures in athletics

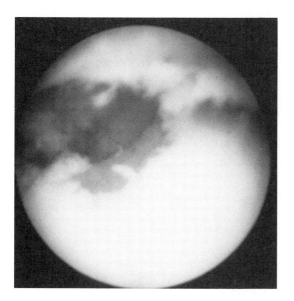

Fig. 17-10 ■ Arthroscopic view of osteochondral defect.

have been small, and removing the fracture fragment and drilling or abrading the base has been successful. Arthroscopy is useful in this condition (Fig. 17-10). Following surgical treatment for an osteochondral fracture, the patient should spend at least 4 weeks without weight bearing or plaster. Early motion is instituted and continued throughout the non-weight-bearing period.

Fig. 17-11, *A*, is a roentgenograph of the ankle of a 50-year-old jogger who suffered an inversion sprain. A mild talar tilt on inversion stress as compared to the opposite side was noted. This injury was treated by strapping and immediate weight bearing. When the patient returned to running 3 weeks later, he experienced continuing discomfort. Repeat roentgenograms of the ankle taken 5 months later showed an osteochondral fracture (Fig. 17-11,*B*). When the later roentgenograms were compared to the

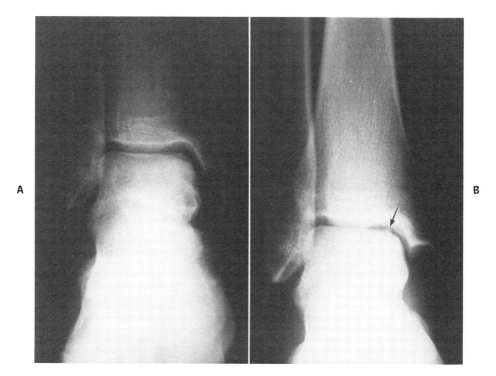

Fig. 17-11 ■ **A,** Inversion sprain in 50-year-old runner. In initial roentgenogram, osteochondral fracture is not appreciated. **B,** Same ankle 5 months later with more apparent lesion.

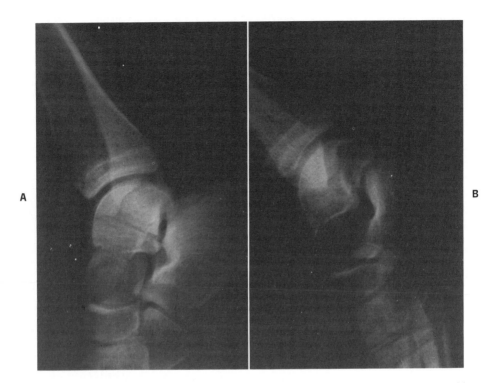

Fig. 17-12 ■ A, Female gymnast with fractured talus. Initial injury. **B,** Female gymnast with fractured talus 4 months later.

original film, this fracture was actually present but was not appreciated originally. An attached loose piece of articular cartilage was removed and the base curetted. The patient returned to jogging 6 weeks after surgery and had no further difficulties.

Fig. 17-12, *A* shows a talar dome fracture in a 20-year-old gymnast who slipped off the edge of a mat while tumbling. She believed that she had sprained her ankle. This fracture was treated for 5 weeks in a short leg walking cast. The cast became soft on one occasion and broke on another. After final removal of the cast, she went back to gymnastics within 1 week, against advice. The fracture went on to heal, but with sequelae (Fig. 17-12, *B*).

Os trigonum fractures

Fractures of the os trigonum have been reported by Ihle and Cochran[22] and Paulos et al.[41] This fracture is often mistaken for an ankle sprain or Achilles tendinitis. The os trigonum is thought to be a supernumerary bone in the posterior part of the talus[13,35,39] (Fig. 17-13). The mechanism of injury is an excessive plantar flexion force on the ankle. It is often associated with injury to the anterior ankle capsule. Ihle and Cochran describe the injury in a professional basketball player.[22] Pain and tenderness are usually located posteriorly in the region of the Achilles tendon. Forced maximal ankle plantar flexion will elicit pain. Paulos et al. describe a 30 degree subtalar oblique roentgenograph as the best way to visualize this area. In a high percentage of cases, a fracture can be differentiated from a normal supernumerary bone. A nuclear bone scan will verify it. Both Ihle and Cochran and Paulos et al. recommend 6 weeks of cast immobilization in acute cases. In chronic cases, a cast will not help, but a period of rest is suggested. If the initial treatment is unsuccessful, the os trigonum should be surgically excised. Surgical excision of a

535

Section 1 FOOT AND ANKLE
Chapter 17 Ankle and foot
fractures in athletics

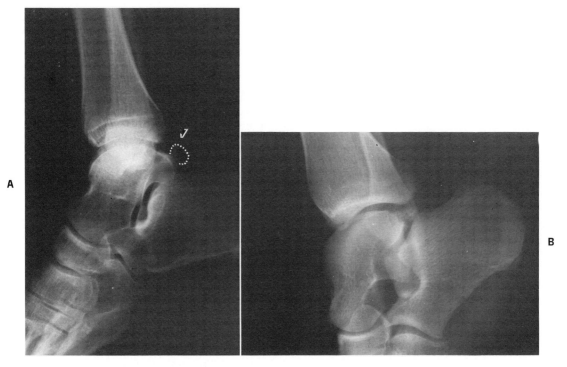

Fig. 17-13 ■ **A,** Os trigonum. **B,** Ballet dancer with posterior ankle pain when en pointe (on the toes). Film taken with patient standing en pointe. Note impingement of os trigonum between posterior tibia and calcaneus. Cystic shanges are visible. The talus is subluxed anteriorly as well, indicating concomitant anterior capsular and ligamentous laxity.

painful os trigonum usually eliminates the problem.

Foot fractures

As they are in the ankle, traumatic fractures of the foot are uncommon. Most of the traumatic fractures that do occur may be treated in a usual orthopaedic fashion. Cast immobilization is not very often indicated for foot fractures, so rehabilitation may be started early. Only specific fractures that require specialized treatment will be discussed in this section. One should never forget the sprain/strain components that may accompany minor foot fractures and should tailor treatment appropriately.

Great toe metatarsophalangeal joint fractures

Fractures about the metatarsophalangeal joint of the great toe are caused by hyperextension, hyperflexion, or abduction forces (the great toe abducts on push-off). This injury occurs most often in football and on artificial turf. The breakdown of the foot support system to emphasize speed appears to be the reason for this injury.[8]

Dancers will occasionally avulse a corner of the base of the proximal or distal phalanx of the great toe.[20] This is associated with capsular tears. Direct violence to the area from a faulty landing when the dancer is fatigued is the most common cause. Rest until the symptoms subside is the treatment of choice.

Fractures in this area are found most commonly in the proximal phalanx, the metatarsal, or the medial sesamoid bone. The medial sesamoid fracture is the most common of the group and the most difficult to treat, and it has the poorest prognosis.

Sesamoid fractures

Fractures of the medial sesamoid can be confused with metatarsalgia or sesamoiditis and in many cases may be a stress fracture. Bilateral foot roentgenograms are of little value, because 75% of individuals with bipartite sesamoids have unilateral involvement.[25] A nuclear bone scan is important to confirm the diagnosis. The majority of these patients will experience pain on hyperdorsiflexing the great toe.[8] Fractures of the medial sesamoid do not heal, but should be treated with rest initially to make sure that the problem is not metatarsalgia or sesamoiditis. Cast immobilization is not indicated. Van Hal et al.[49] suggest repeat roentgenograms at 3-week intervals to look for a spread of the fracture fragments. If there is a spread or if a period of rest does not relieve the symptoms, surgical excision of the entire medial sesamoid will offer variable results.[8,49] Immobilization should be applied for 3 weeks after excision. The average time to return to prefracture status is 10 weeks.

Metatarsal fractures

The most common fracture in the dancer is said to be that of the fifth metatarsal shaft.[17] Metatarsal fractures have been reported from faulty landings by gymnasts.[45]

Whiteside et al.[51] reported on 28 fractures of the fifth metatarsal in intercollegiate athletes. The greatest number were in the proximal portion of the bone. Football accounted for 14 of the fractures, and volleyball accounted for 2. Of the 28 fractures, 26 were treated with crutches and no plaster immobilization. Two thirds of the group were back to work-outs in 6 weeks; all successfully returned to competition. Three of these refractured. The 3 refractures were treated without surgery, and they all went on to heal. Despite the good results with nonoperative treatment in this series, surgical consideration is important initially for fractures of the proximal diaphysis[51] (Fig 17-14, A).

Fractures of the proximal diaphysis of the fifth metatarsal bone are known as **Jones fractures** and should not be confused with a metaphyseal or avulsion fracture of the peroneus brevis. The healing of the proximal diaphyseal fracture is slow, and the fracture union is unpredictable. Return to activity is prolonged and the nonunion rate is high. In the committed athlete, early internal fixation is indicated (Fig. 17-14, B).

■ TRAUMATIC FRACTURES IN THE ADOLESCENT ATHLETE

Fractures of the ankle and foot are rare in the growing athlete. An open physis does not mean that the occurrence of fractures will be greater than sprains. Chambers[6] describes only a few fractures of the ankle and foot in all the children that entered a military hospital for athletic injuries in a 1-year period. There were no fractures of the ankle or foot reported by Nilsson and Roaas[38] in a study of injuries in 25,000 adolescents competing in soccer tournaments. The fractures that do occur usually involve the epiphysis. Treatment is the same as for any epiphyseal separation.

■ STRESS FRACTURES

A stress fracture is the most common fracture in the ankle and foot in athletes.[34,42,49] The most common area for a stress fracture to occur in sports is in the fibula[40] (Fig. 17-15). Stress fractures have been described in all bones of the ankle and foot, including the lateral cuneiform,[32] os calcis,[34] great toe sesamoids,[49] and tarsal navicular.[21]

A stress fracture can be differentiated from a typical overuse syndrome by the fact that pain increases during activity, not following it.[21] Commonly the initial roentgenograms do not show the fracture. A nuclear bone scan has become the most important tool in diagnosing these fractures.[14,31,40,43]

Hunter[21] warns about persistent dorsomedial pain in the foot. This should alert

549

Section 1 FOOT AND ANKLE
Chapter 18 Occult trauma and unusual
injuries in the foot and ankle

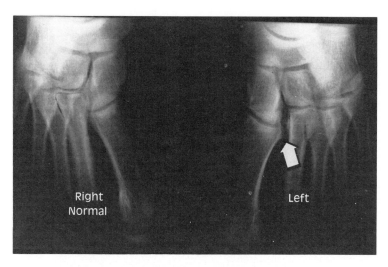

Fig. 18-6 ■ Sagittal diastasis of left foot. Widening of space between first and second tarsometatarsal rays (arrow), compared to normal right foot. Notice normal relationship between middle cuneiform and second metatarsal.

As the athlete falls, forceful rotation of the stabilized forefoot causes a rotational force that results in the diastasis. The absence of abrasions, contusions, or other evidence of crushing injury supports the theory that a forceful forefoot rotation (indirect trauma) rather than a crushing (direct) injury produces sagittal diastasis.

Diagnosis

The diagnosis requires an awareness of sagittal diastasis, an accurate history, clinical examination, and roentgenographic evaluation. Usually these patients complain of immediate severe pain and inability to bear weight. Initially there is no external evidence of trauma, and the pain appears to be far out of proportion to the apparent objective findings. There is no gross swelling or deformity. Swelling develops later and is localized over the dorsum of the foot, which in a day or two develops into an ecchymotic discoloration localized distally between the first and second toes. The distal localization of the discoloration represents dependent drainage from the proximal separation and may distract attention from the site of injury. **The cardinal sign is exquisite point tenderness localized between the first and second metatarsal bases.** Additional areas of tenderness will be noted over associated fractures. Ankle injuries are differentiated by the absence of swelling and tenderness over the malleoli, syndesmosis, and ankle ligaments.

Roentgenographic evaluation

Close scrutiny of the roentgenograms reveals a slight widening of the space between the first and second metatarsal rays. Comparison views are often necessary in the mild separations* (Fig. 18-6). We would like to emphasize that widening of the space between the first and second rays per se is not pathognomonic of traumatic diastasis, because there is wide variation of the normal. Comparison roentgenograms are often necessary to confirm the clinical suspicion, especially in cases of mild separation. An avulsion fracture in the area between the base of the first metatarsal and the medial cuneiform (the region of the Lisfranc ligament)

---

*Editors' note: In mild separations, weight-bearing comparison views are obtained to help determine the extent of injury.

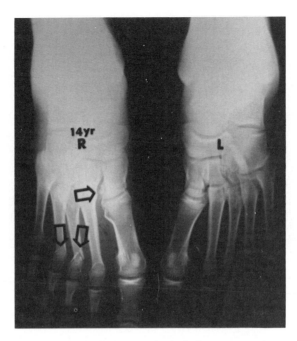

Fig. 18-7 ■ Sagittal diastasis in adolescent. Basketball player "came down on ball of foot." Separation between first two tarsometatarsal rays were unrecognized while attention was focused on fractured metatarsals. This patient was seen because of disability related to diastasis. Pain persisted long after fractured metatarsals were healed and asymptomatic. Notice avulsion fracture in region of Lisfranc ligament—pathognomonic of sagittal separation.

should alert the examiner. It has been noted in some cases that an avulsion fracture of the Lisfranc ligament may not be visible on the initial roentgenograms. In subsequent studies, the fracture becomes clearly evident with localized osteoporosis. The initial roentgenograms are often reported as negative. This diagnosis is missed because comparison films were not made or the injury was overlooked as attention was focused on concomitant fractures. In some cases the ankle instead of the foot is x-rayed. Concomitant fractures we have noted include first cuneiform fractures, fractures of the navicular tuberosity, avulsion fractures in the region of the fifth metatarsal, or fractures of one or more of the the metatarsals (Fig. 18-7).

Medial displacement of the first ray is commonly associated with fractures of the first cuneiform or tuberosity of the navicular; these may not be evident on initial roentgenograms (Fig. 18-8). We feel that some injuries represent spontaneous reduction of lateral subluxations; the four lateral metatarsals move en masse by virtue of the intermetatarsal ligament attachment. Lateral displacement of the metatarsals is usually associated with avulsion fractures in the cuboid–fifth metatarsal area.

Treatment

Recognition and knowledge of the anatomic basis of this injury are prerequisites for treatment. When the diagnosis is made, the foot is immediately immobilized in a well-padded plaster cast with strips of felt applied over the medial and lateral aspects of the foot. The foot is positioned in slight equinus and supination for 5 to 6 weeks. An attempt is made to close the separation by manual compres-

551

Section 1 FOOT AND ANKLE
Chapter 18 Occult trauma and unusual
injuries in the foot and ankle

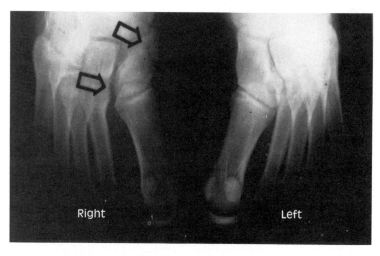

Fig. 18-8 ■ Sagittal diastasis with fracture of medial cuneiform. Diastasis of right foot incurred in diving board injury. Comparison roentgenograms reveal widening between first two metatarsal rays. Fracture of medial cuneiform was not evident in initial roentgenogram.

sion. Usually the initial plaster has to be changed and a new snug-fitting cast applied. In a few cases we were able to elicit a "click" with immediate amelioration of the complaints; this indicates reduction of the medially subluxed first metatarsal. This manipulation is accomplished by pushing the first ray in a lateral direction. When the patient is seen later, after the onset of swelling, a compression dressing is applied and the foot elevated before application of the cast. Open reduction with Kirschner wire transfixion is recommended in wide, unstable separations. To date this has not been necessary in the athletic injuries. In separations greater than 5 mm, open reduction with Kirschner wire stabilization should be considered.

Sagittal separation between the first and second tarsometatarsal rays is usually an unrecognized cause of prolonged unexplained disability. This diagnosis should be considered in the differential diagnosis of occult foot trauma in athletes. Commonly these patients continue to have pain for many months, which gradually subsides. Eventually they accommodate to the discomfort and are able to resume recreational sports. The circumference of the foot remains slightly wider, depending on the amount of separation. However, the prognosis for high-level competition or professional athletics is guarded and depends primarily on the degree of separation and initial treatment. Patients who have an early accurate diagnosis and are treated in plaster are restored to activities sooner. Sudeck's atrophy and months of frustration are avoided because the patient has been forewarned regarding the period of disability. "An informed patient is a happy patient."

■ **TARSOMETATARSAL FRACTURE-DISLOCATION—LISFRANC INJURY**

Fracture-dislocation of the tarsometatarsal region is named after Lisfranc, the surgeon in Napoleon's army who described amputations at the tarsometatarsal junction. Tarsometatarsal fracture-dislocation is an uncommon injury that is notorious for causing prolonged disability and unsatisfactory results. Gross displacement usually occurs in motor vehicle accidents. In athletes, our primary concern is the subtle subluxations that may be overlooked while attention is diverted to a concomitant fractured metatarsal. It is essential to interpret the seriousness of this injury and to realize the importance of prompt reduction and stabilization of the displaced bones.

Mechanism of injury

Cadaver experiments by Jeffreys in 1963[3] and Wilson in 1972[11] confirm clinical impressions regarding mechanism of injury. The ankle is plantar flexed at the time of injury, the hindfoot is locked in the equinus position, and a sudden forceful hyperplantar flexion of the forefoot results in dorsal displacement of the proximal ends of the metatarsals. Sudden forefoot hyperplantar flexion can occur from (a) a fall on the point of the toes, as in the pointe position in ballet, (b) a fall backwards while the forefoot is trapped, as in a stirrup, or (c) sudden high-velocity longitundinal compression. The fall on the point of the toes can occur from stubbing the toes or simply tripping off a step, ladder, or curb. Hyperplantar flexion of the forefoot is produced by "rolling" on the dorsum of the foot—the body weight provides the force that displaces the base of the metatarsals dorsally. Longitundinal compression usually occurs in automobile accidents involving the front seat passenger. The feet are fixed in plantar flexion, and on impact the toes strike the vertical fire wall. This sudden longitudinal compression on impact results in dorsal displacement of the metatarsals. The same longitudinal force is produced when a patient falls backward while sitting on his heel, once again resulting in a hyperplantar flexion of the forefoot while the hindfoot is locked in equinus. A direct crushing injury causes a plantar displacement, in contrast to the dorsal subluxation of the Lisfranc injury. The mechanisms that produce tarsometatarsal dislocations can occur in basketball, a fall from a horse, running sports, tennis, handball, motor bike sports, and others.

Diagnosis

In vehicular injuries with gross displacement, the evidence of serious injury is usually obvious. However, in athletic injuries the findings may be subtle, especially in cases of subluxation. A history of hyperplantar flexion of the forefoot should make the examiner suspect this injury. In mild subluxations, the complaints of pain and inability to bear weight may appear grossly exaggerated. Swelling and tenderness are localized over the dorsum without evidence of trauma to the skin. Concomitant fractured metatarsals occur frequently. A common error is to overlook the serious disruption of the Lisfranc area while focusing attention on a simple metatarsal fracture.

Sprain of the fourth and fifth proximal metatarsal joints without gross displacement is one of the causes of unexplained pain in the foot. This occult trauma, while not a major disability, does cause annoying pain to the athlete. The injury is usually unrecognized and passed off as an ankle sprain with "negative x-rays." With a good history and careful clinical examination pain can be elicited over the dorsolateral aspect of the foot with localized point tenderness and at times slight swelling over the fourth and fifth Lisfranc joints. These are mildly incapacitating but nonetheless disabling to the athlete. Following recognition and explanation of the reason for complaints, these patients gradually are able to resume sports using a protective support. The treatment is essentially recognition, explanation, and reassurance to gradually increase activity to tolerance. The patient usually becomes asymptomatic with the passage of time. The roentgenograms show no abnormality in cases of sprained fourth and fifth Lisfranc joints.

Roentgenographic evaluation

Roentgenograms in cases of subluxation are difficult to evaluate because of the mosaic arrangement, the overlap of articular surfaces, and the wedge-shaped metatarsal bases. Comparison roentgenograms may be necessary. In the anteroposterior view, the medial border of the second metatarsal and the second cuneiform normally form a straight line. A "step off" at this articulation is pathogno-

567

Section 1 FOOT AND ANKLE
Chapter 19 Rehabilitation of the
foot and ankle linkage system

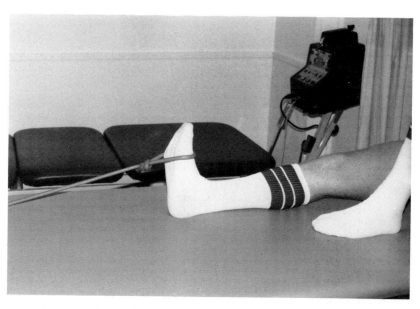

Fig. 19-9 ■ Active-resisted motion should be continued between cryotherapy sessions. These can be performed with surgical tubing.

Table 19-1 ■ Average proximal muscle strength deficits in patients with pathologic conditions of the foot and ankle

Affected body part	Affected versus normal leg deficit
Hip abductors	31%
Hip adductors	30%
Quadriceps	19%
Hamstrings	26%
Total leg strength	26%

From Nicholas, J.A., Strizak, A.M., and Veras, G.: Am. J. Sports Med. **4**:241, 1976. © 1976, American Orthopaedic Society for Sports Medicine.

cluded during this phase. Of course, well leg exercises and aerobic conditioning are continued. One leg stationary bicycling is excellent for aerobic fitness.

Phase III: Intensive rehabilitation

Phase III is a very important part of foot and ankle rehabilitation. It is often omitted or forgotten, because the athlete is now pain free and feels he or she has now fully rehabilitated. Unfortunately, this misconception can lead to many chronic foot and ankle problems. It is in Phase III that the athlete fine-tunes his stretching, strength, and proprioception to a point at which competitive sports may be undertaken without increased risk of reinjury. By Phase III the swelling has resolved, but the athlete should wear a supportive wrap or splint during activity. A Gibney tape wrap with a figure-8 heel lock or a polypropylene splint with a hinge to allow only dorsiflexion and plantar flexion lend lateral stability to injured ankles. An inflatable air stirrup is also useful at this stage (Fig. 19-10). With weight bearing, the medial and lateral air-filled bladders provide intermittent compression above the pressure exerted by inflated bladders without weight bearing. It allows dorsiflexion and plantar flexion and can fit in an athletic shoe.[31] However, all these devices are supplemental supports. The true support will come from proper rehabilitation of the muscle tendon groups of the linkage system.

Stretching

At the present time there are no proven systems for judging the dynamics of a

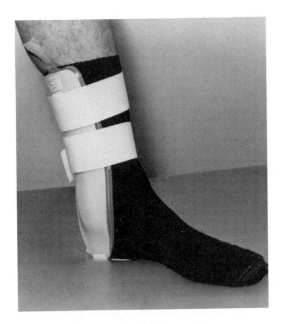

Fig. 19-10 ■ Inflatable air stirrup provides compression and support and allows active dorsiflexion and plantar flexion.

muscle's flexibility or its ability to undergo efficient eccentric contraction. One can easily have the patient keep the affected knee straight and dorsiflex the foot to get a rough idea of the stretch that the gastrocsoleus complex will undergo. However, this is only telling the examiner what the muscle is able to do at absolute rest and has no bearing on how the muscle will function during gait. The goal of stretching is to cause a plastic deformation of the muscle being stretched. To do this effectively, initial muscle stretching should be done before the muscles are warmed up. If the muscle is warm, it will be more likely to undergo an elastic deformation, which is desired before a specific sporting event but not when rehabilitating an injured limb. The quadriceps muscles, gastrocsoleus complex, and hamstring muscles function principally by eccentric contractions. Actually, the hamstring muscles are in eccentric contraction until the end of the swing phase of gait, and then they undergo a sharp, sudden concentric contraction to bring the foot down on the ground. For these muscles to function well, they not only need to be strong, but they must also be well stretched. If the foot is forced into dorsiflexion when the heel cord is tight, the subtalar joint will be forced into supination in an attempt to accommodate the tight heel cord. Unfortunately, this puts the ankle in a most vulnerable position, increasing the possibility of a lateral injury due to inversion. An excellent way to stretch the heel cords is to use a slant board or heel cord stretching box (Fig. 19-11). The slant board can be used in two ways. The vertical end may be placed next to the wall, with the athlete standing with his toes turned inward and heels just touching the floor. The athlete then leans into the wall with the hands, as though doing a push-up. The lean can be held for 20 seconds and then be performed several times, with 10-second resting periods. The stretching can be done without a board by positioning the hands and feet as described above, with the athlete at arm's length from the wall. The distance from the wall can be increased by 1 to 2 feet each week.

The slant board can also be placed with the apex toward the wall, and the athlete may step on the board with the back against the wall and heels flat on the board. The athlete may remain in this position for several minutes to an hour while reading or even doing upper body exercises.

The stretching exercises need to be done at least 3 to 4 times a day; the athlete should rest between stretching sessions. Therefore if the gastrocsoleus complex is to be stretched, the athlete should wear shoes with some heel elevation between stretching sessions to allow the mildly strained muscles to recover from the stress of the stretching exercises before repeating them.

Stretching exercises for the gastrocsoleus, hamstring, and quadricep muscles should be performed as part of the rehabilitation of foot and ankle injuries, so that the entire leg linkage system

575

Section 1 FOOT AND ANKLE
Chapter 19 Rehabilitation of the
foot and ankle linkage system

reached, eccentric exercise may be started. Finally, when 100% of strength at 10 and 20 repetitions per minute has been reached, isokinetic exercise at 40 and 50 repetitions per minute may be started to work the fast-twitch muscle fibers.

Certain activities, such as walking fast, running, performing 45- and 90-degree cuts, and runnning figure-8s of various sizes are allowed once the athlete has reached specific milestones in the rehabilitation of the foot and ankle. It is suggested that the athlete have 100% of strength at 40 to 50 repetitions per minute as compared to the unaffected limb before full competitive activity is resumed.

If additional joint stability is sought from muscle rehabilitation, it is to the athlete's advantage that the muscle fibers that can respond quickest to joint stresses are fully rehabilitated—namely, the fast-twitch muscle fibers. Therefore, it is recommended that this level of rehabilitation be reached before competitive or contact sports are resumed. Exercises will be suggested for the various motions of the foot and ankle complex, such as plantar flexion, dorsiflexion, inversion, and eversion.

Plantar flexion. In performing plantar flexion, the muscles used are the plantaris, posterior tibialis, gastrocsoleus complex, peroneus longus and brevis, and the toe flexors. Isotonic exercises with rubber tubing will have already begun in Phase II. At this point in Phase III, the athlete may begin with exercises that do not require extra weight.

PHASE III: PLANTAR FLEXION STRENGTH PROGRAM

- Toe curling
- Standing toe raises
- Bent-knee toe raises
- Negative repetition work

First, to exercise the toe flexors, the towel curling exercise may be performed. This is easily accomplished by placing a towel on the floor in front of the seated athlete and asking him or her to use only the toes to grasp the towel and pull it toward the body, keeping the feet flat on the ground. This will help strengthen the toe flexors, including the flexor digitorum communis and the flexor hallucis longus.

To work the other muscles of plantar flexion, the athlete may do standing toe raises, with the heads of the metatarsals placed on a 2 to 3-inch block of wood (Fig. 19-19, *A*). This exercise may be modified to isolate the soleus muscle. The athlete will place the heads of the metatarsals on the 2- to 3-inch block of wood, but the knees will be flexed to 90 degrees, and the athlete will hold on to a table or chair. The toe raises will be done in this position with the knees flexed to relax the gastrocnemius muscle while exercising the soleus. (Fig. 19-19, *B*).

Once the athlete can easily perform three sets of 20 repetitions each of these unweighted exercises, weighted exercises may be begun. The standing toe raises may now be modified by having the athlete stand under a Nautilus or Universal machine, with the pressing bar across the shoulders. In this manner, a predetermined weight on the machine will be transmitted to the plantar flexors of the ankle.

To perform the exercise with the knees bent, the athlete should be seated, with the metatarsal heads on a 2- to 3-inch block. A barbell may be rested across the top of the knees, and the toe raises may be performed in this manner, with a fixed, predetermined weight on the barbell (Fig. 19-20).

After the athlete can exercise with both feet for three sets of 10 repetitions each, the exercises should be performed with the affected limb only. After three sets of 10 repetitions each can be performed at a given weight, the weight may be increased by 1 or 2 pounds.

When the strength of the affected leg equals approximately 75% of the strength of the unaffected leg, the athlete may be allowed to begin eccentric work on the plantar flexors of the ankle. This is known to weight lifters as "negative repetitions."

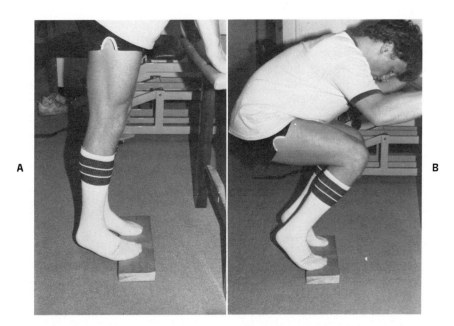

Fig. 19-19 ■ Toe raises can be done with knees straight **(A)** to strengthen gastrocsoleus complex, or with knees bent **(B)** to isolate soleus muscle. These are done with forefoot on 2- or 3-inch block.

This type of exercise can be accomplished easily by using both the uninjured and the injured legs to lift the weight in a concentric contraction. Once the weight is lifted, the unaffected leg is relaxed, and the affected leg is used slowly to lower the weight. In the case of the standing toe raise, the weight would be lifted by both feet, and the unaffected leg would be relaxed, using the affected leg slowly to lower the heel to the floor.

For the bent-knee exercises, a small dumbbell may be placed on the distal thigh of the affected leg, with the metatarsal heads on the wooden block. The concentric lifting of the weight may be assisted by both hands at this time. Once the weight has been lifted, the hands are released, and the weight is slowly lowered during the eccentric contraction of the plantar flexors. This type of exercise maximizes the amount of eccentric work done by the plantar flexors. Since eccentric contractions can accommodate more weight than concentric contractions, the maximal weight desired during the eccen-

tric exercise would be more than the muscle could lift concentrically. For this reason, assistance by the unaffected leg or by the hands is essential in lifting the weight concentrically.

Dorsiflexion. When performing dorsiflexion of the ankle, the muscles used are the anterior tibialis, the extensor digitorum communis, and the peroneus tertius. As mentioned earlier, surgical tubing exercises started in Phase II are now to be supplemented with weighted exercises. The simplest way to exercise the dorsiflexors of the ankle is to strap a free weight of 1 to 2 pounds to the distal portion of the foot. With the knee bent and the lower leg perpendicular to the floor, the ankle may be brought into dorsiflexion against the resistance of the free weight (Fig. 19-21). Again, when this exercise can be performed for three sets of 10 repetitions each, the weight may be increased in 1- or 2-pound increments. A similar exercise may be performed on various cable or Universal machines, with simple modifications of a handle to a foot strap.

577

Section 1 FOOT AND ANKLE
Chapter 19 Rehabilitation of the
foot and ankle linkage system

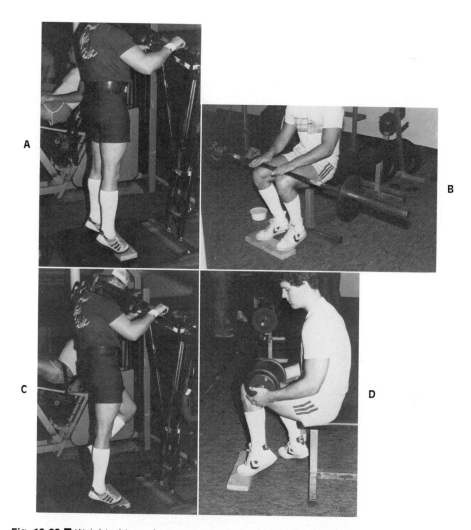

Fig. 19-20 ■ Weighted toe raises are performed with knees straight **(A)** and flexed **(B)**. Eccentric exercise can be done lifting weight with both legs and lowering it with only injured limb **(C)**, or using hands to help lift weight before lowering it with only injured limb **(D)**.

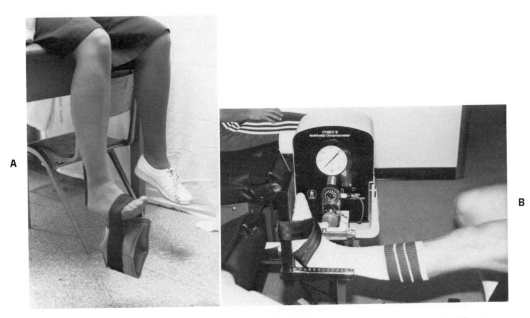

Fig. 19-21 ■ Both isotonic **(A)** and isokinetic **(B)** exercises are used to strengthen dorsiflexors of ankle.

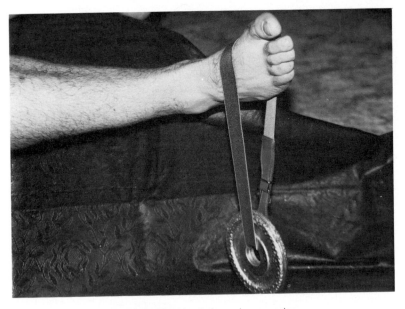

Fig. 19-22 ■ Isotonic inversion exercise.

very important for stabilizing the heel and preventing excessive motion of the subtalar joint in pronation and also for ensuring that the heel does not slide laterally off the sole. The side and rear walls should be as deep as possible without interfering with ankle joint motion.

We have found that most athletes tend to have tight heel cords with a limited amount of ankle joint dorisflexion. For this reason, the sole should be higher at the rearfoot than in the forefoot. This will help relax the Achilles tendon and decrease the incidence of chronic problems such as Achilles tendinitis. Lack of ankle dorsiflexion also increases the demand for pronation at the subtalar joint. Finally, the tendon and ankle areas should be padded to prevent cuts, blisters, or chafing.

Forefoot.

With respect to forefoot construction, shock absorbency is less important than in the rearfoot. However, a soft shock-absorbant material should exist between the outersole and the foot in the midsole areas. Drez felt that the studded outer sole ("waffle sole") provided more traction and shock absorption than the solid sole. He hypothesized this was because of its ability to reduce torsional stress.[11]

The shoe's upper should be strong enough to ensure that the foot will be held securely and that the sides of the toe box will not rip out. A round toe box of at least 1 to 1½ inches in height, as measured 1 inch from the outside of the top of the shoe, is important to prevent crowding of the toes. At toe-off the metatarsophalangeal joint dorsiflexes 25 to 30 degrees, and the sole of a running shoe must have enough intrinsic flexibility to allow for this or at least provide a rocker effect within the construction of the sole. A rigid sole that does not allow for this motion will produce increased stress over the gastrocnemius-soleus area.* To test for this, one can press the toe of the shoe

---

*Editor's note: This is a **linkage system** effect.

against a bathroom scale and note the force needed to produce flexion. Drez states this should be no more than 10 pounds.[11]

The flexibility of the forefoot sole in the cleated shoe differs from that in the running shoe. Because the repetitive gait cycle in running is not seen in sports such as football, the adherence to strict biomechanics differs. Torg felt that in selecting a cleated shoe, the sole should be rigid in the forefoot.[25] In the conventional football shoe, this is provided by the metal plates to which the posts are riveted. In the multipurpose cleated shoe, the manufacturer must reinforce the forepart of the sole.

Foot variation and shoewear

These then are general considerations. **It is of paramount importance when advising an athlete on shoe type to literally fit the shoe to the athlete and not vice versa.** In runners, this is absolutely critical. A runner with a tendency toward a **cavus** foot will generally have less motion within the joints of the foot and require more room on the top of the foot along the lacing area. This foot also has a tendency to break down the outside heel counter and the entire outside of the shoe as well as to flatten out the outside of the midsole and wear out the outside of the outersole. This foot type is also usually associated with a tighter than normal Achilles tendon, which forces the athlete to run more up on the forefoot or toes, resulting in excessive wear in the forward part of the sole under the ball of the foot (see Table 20-1). Because of the tightness, we also see excessive callus build-up under the entire ball of the foot, particularly under the area just behind the big toe.

Therefore in selecting a shoe for this foot type, we look for a strong heel counter, particularly on the outside, a relatively high heel to relieve stress on the Achilles tendon and balance out the front of the foot, and a midsole that is somewhat soft to dissipate the forces of heel contact, but not so soft as to flatten out

Table 20-1 ■ The cavus foot

Component	Effect
Less joint motion	Requires more room on top of the foot along the lacing area
	Breaks down outside heel counter and outersole
	Flattens outside of midsole
	Wears out outside of outersole
Tight heel cords	Excessive wear in the forepart of the sole under the ball of the foot
	Excessive callus build-up under the ball of the foot

Table 20-2 ■ Pes planus

Component	Effect
Excessive mobility	Excessive wear on inner side of sole
	Inner sole breakdown
Wide forefoot/ narrow heel	Difficult shoe fitting

with wear. A rubber with good memory is best for the midsole. The midsole should also be relatively substantial to withstand the stresses of a prominent forefoot and a forefoot striker. The outersole should be constructed of very tough, wear-resistant

---

CAVUS FOOT SHOEWEAR

Strong heel counter (particularly on outside)
Relatively high heel
Moderately soft midsole (rubber with good memory)
Wear-resistant outersole
Flexible forefoot (use the "10-pound rule")

---

rubber that can take considerable abrasive forces. Finally, the forefoot should be easily flexible under the ball of the foot, observing the "10-pound rule."

For athletes with **pes planus,** the shoe should be constructed slightly differently. Flatfeet are generally excessively mobile, and the foot has a tendency to move too much. In spite of this excessive mobility, however, the foot at heel strike is very often already flat and therefore does not dissipate the force of heel strike. Or, if the heel is not flat at heel strike, it flattens out too quickly and causes an excessive amount of stress along the inside of the foot and leg. In both cases, the foot is usually much wider than the high-arched foot, particularly in the front part of the

foot across the metatarsals. Not only is the forefoot wider but the heel is often narrow, making shoe fitting extremely difficult. To fit the front part of the foot, a wider shoe is needed, which leaves the heel loose. Often this requires a shoe that is either too small in the forefoot or too large in the heel (see Table 20-2).

A flatfoot is also generally straighter than most neutral or high-arched feet. Historically, North American shoes have been constructed on a model (last) that has a 6- to 8-degree inward flare. A cavus foot would have an even greater curve to it, in most cases. Some shoes on the market are constructed on a straight last, and generally these fit a flatfoot better.

Again, as in the shoe for the high-arched foot, we look for an elevated heel in the shoe for flatfoot. The difference, however, between a flatfoot with a tight Achilles tendon and a high-arched foot with a tight Achilles tendon is that the flatfoot has the ability to compensate for the tightness by excessively pronating or flattening the foot, whereas the high-arched foot does not. Most people with flatfeet also tend to hit at heel strike on the inside of their heel, which causes the inside of the sole to flatten out considerably faster than the outside of the sole. This results in a breakdown of the shoe toward the inside and leaves the foot in an unsupported position.

To address this problem of excessive wearing of the inner side of the sole with pronation, some manufacturers now use a higher-density rubber or some type of plug medially to limit the amount and rate of pronation or flattening of the foot. Again, it must be pointed out that the

---

SHOEWEAR FOR ATHLETES WITH PES PLANUS

High-density rubber with medial plug to limit
  pronation
Flexible at metatarsophalangeal joint area
Innersole arch support

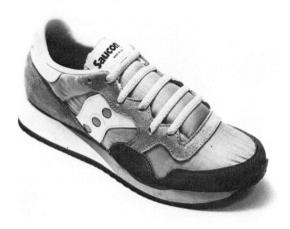

shoe should be easily flexible at the metatarsophalangeal joint area in the ball of
the foot. It is also wise for these people to
look for a shoe that comes with an innersole arch support for two reasons: (1)
such a shoe is usually a little deeper and
accommodates a custom-made orthotic
more easily if needed, and (2) the support
itself will often help limit some of the excessive flattening (Fig. 20-2).

Fig. 20-2 ■ Modern running shoe with firm heel
counter. Well-padded sole in hindfoot and
forefoot and slight flare at heel.

Summary of ideal shoewear design and construction

We can summarize the ideal characteristics of a running shoe, or a shoe used in
running sports, based on current concepts of the art and science of shoe design
and construction:

1. It is usually better to have a shoe
   with strong heel counters that fit
   well around the foot and that lock
   the shoe around the foot.
2. There should always be good flexibility in the forefoot where the toes
   bend.
3. It is preferable to have a fairly high
   heel, since most athletes have tight
   Achilles tendons.
4. The midsole should be fairly soft, but
   not too soft, and should not flatten
   out too easily.
5. The heel counter should be high
   enough to surround the foot and also
   allow for an orthotic device. It is
   therefore preferable to have a shoe
   that comes with an insole or orthotic
   sock lining, because these shoes are
   often designed with a higher counter
   to allow more room for the foot, and
   the counter can be removed if one is
   already wearing or expects to wear a
   custom orthotic.

6. The heel counter should be securely
   fastened to the sole so that the
   counter does not bend or come loose
   at this attachment.
7. Last but not least, one must be sure
   that the shoe has been quality constructed. Things to look for are the
   stitching along all the seams, the
   quality of rubber both in the midsole
   and outersole, the bonding between
   the heel counter and the sole, and
   the bonding between the outersole
   and midsole. Be sure that the
   counter of the shoe is perpendicular
   to the sole and that together the
   counter and sole are perpendicular
   to the ground. This should be viewed
   from the back of the shoe.

The material used in the construction
of the shoe is of equal concern. In the
construction of uppers, cowhide, nylon,
plastic, and canvas are the most commonly used materials. Of these, cowhide
and nylon dominate the market. Cowhide
tends to be the superior material overall
with respect to wear, breathability, and
fit. Nylon generally does quite well, but it
does not stretch well, and therefore fitting
becomes a problem in that the nylon will
not mold itself in time to the contours of

```
┌─────────────────────────────────────────┐
│      SHOE CONSTRUCTION MATERIALS         │
│ Cowhide   Excellent wear, breathability, │
│             and fit                      │
│ Nylon     Excellent wear                 │
│           Fitting may be a problem be-   │
│             cause of poor stretchability │
│           Easily launderable             │
│ Vinyl     Poor ventilation               │
└─────────────────────────────────────────┘
```

the foot as will cowhide. A benefit of nylon, however, is that it is easily launderable. Most frequently, manufacturers combine nylon and cowhide with very satisfactory results. In some shoes, plastic or vinyl is used in construction of the upper. The major disadvantage of this is that the plastic does not breathe, and ventilation of the foot may be a problem.

Recently, some running shoe manufacturers have begun making uppers of Gore-Tex. This fabric has the distinct advantage of allowing the foot to breathe while forming a relatively impermeable barrier to liquid water (as opposed to vapor). This enables the foot to stay dry on wet days and yet allows it to breathe. There are a limited number of shoes on the market constructed of Gore-Tex, but the use of this fabric for shoe construction is promising.

Shoetypes

Gridiron shoes

In contact sports such as gridiron football, the cleated foot may remain fixed to the ground at impact, and increase the susceptibility to injuries of the lower extremities, in particular. Clearly, a violent force, either direct or rotational, applied to the trunk will be transmitted down the legs. If the foot is fixed firmly to the ground, the force will be dissipated through the lower extremities, often through rupture of the periarticular structures about the knee and ankle. Not surprisingly then, the relationship between the football shoe and the risk of injury has been studied in some detail. The typical conventional cleated football shoe

has seven ¾-inch cleats, each with a diameter of ⅜ inch.

Hanley oval cleat. Dr. Daniel Hanley of Bowdoin College was the first to implicate the heel cleats as a major contributor to lower extremity football injuries.[13] This stemmed from his observation that a substantial number of the injuries he saw at Bowdoin occurred in the open field and appeared to be caused by an abnormal torsion force transmitted to the knee from a firmly planted foot with heel cleats dug deeply into the turf. He subsequently developed the Hanley cleat—an oval, low-profile cleat designed to provide traction without digging into the turf to the extent that conventional cleats did. Hirata conducted a survey of all team physicians in the Ivy League to determine the effectiveness of the Hanley cleat in decreasing injuries. His results suggested that the cleat had indeed decreased the rate and severity of football injuries.[14]

Disk cleat. Dr. Morle Rowe also studied the effect of cleat configuration on injuries in football. He replaced the conventional heel cleats with a specially made plastic disk. He then compared its effectiveness to the conventional soles in both high- and low-topped shoes. In a study of 1,325 New York City varsity high-school players, he found that the low-cut disc heel shoe was superior to other types tested in reducing injuries. The most striking result in his study was the high rate of injury recorded with the low cut, conventionally cleated shoe, which had a record of injury far greater than any other equipment combination.[20] He felt that the proper choice of footwear could save the average football team up to two knee and ankle injuries per year.

Soccer-type shoe. A byproduct of his study, later followed up by other investigators, is the use of soccer-type shoes to reduce foot fixation and therefore injury (Fig. 20-3). The sole of this shoe is molded, in contrast to conventional cleats, which are bolted on. There are 12 cleats rather than 6, and each cleat tip has a diameter

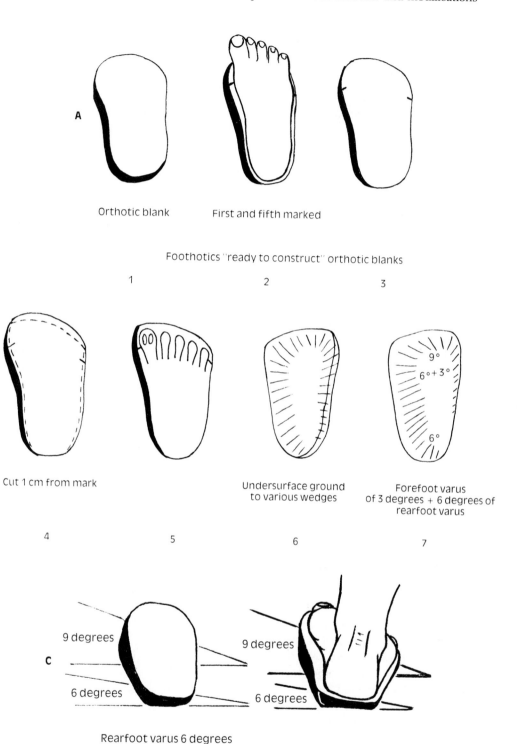

A

Orthotic blank   First and fifth marked

Foothotics "ready to construct" orthotic blanks

1   2   3

B

Cut 1 cm from mark   Undersurface ground   Forefoot varus
to various wedges   of 3 degrees + 6 degrees of
rearfoot varus

4   5   6   7

C

9 degrees   9 degrees

6 degrees   6 degrees

Rearfoot varus 6 degrees
Forefoot varus 3 degrees

8   9

Fig. 20-10 ■ A, Selection of orthotic blank and marking of metatarsal heads. **B,** Trimming and shaping of orthotic for patient with forefoot varus of 6 degrees. **C,** Resultant orthotic with 6 degrees rearfoot posting and 9 degrees forefoot posting.

ity in the material as with a rigid functional orthotic, and therefore the 9 degrees in the forefoot represents a sum of the rearfoot varus post of 5 degrees and the forefoot varus post of 4 degrees. The additional posting in the forefoot results from the additive thickness of material rather than the rigidity of the material, as is the case in a rigid orthotic (Fig. 20-10, B and C).

Donovan et al. have described the construction and use of another type of semisoft orthotic made primarily from Plastizote.[10] It is soft to semirigid in construct and therefore allows for good control and, in addition, provides a comfortable shock-absorbing cushion for the foot. They felt this made the device optimal for use in athletes. Its other advantages are that it is relatively easy to construct. There is no need for negative casting, and total construction time is approximately 30 minutes. Disadvantages of the device are that it is not as durable as the rigid type, with an average life of 6 to 18 months, and it is not applicable to all types of shoes, sometimes needing a somewhat deeper shoe. In addition, when using the device as a functional biomechanical device, it can be difficult to measure and construct the appropriate forefoot and rearfoot wedgings that are measured clinically.

The construction of the device is as described by Donovan. A precut piece of Aliplast* is placed over a precut piece of Plastizote* with rearfoot-forefoot Plastizote "posting strips" underneath both. All three pieces are then placed in a toaster oven set at 285° F (140° C) for 5 to 6 minutes until the materials are sufficiently soft.

With the patient's foot held in a neutral subtalar position, the patient stands on the Plastizote with his foot protected by two layers of Stockinette. Full weight bearing with equal forefoot and rearfoot pressure allows for adequate cupping around the heel. After 1 minute, the ma-

terials are set, the foot is removed, and the orthotic is ground out to a thickness of 1 to 2 mm laterally to fit easily in the shoe.

Semirigid orthotics

A more classic type of semirigid device is the one constructed with a flexible plastic such as polyethylene, polypropylene, or polyvinyl chloride. These provide a slightly less rigid platform than the acrylic orthotics, which will be described later. Semirigid orthotics will flex under unusual forces and are less likely to crack or break than the rigid acrylic orthotics. Semirigid orthotics include the University of California Biomechanics Laboratory (UCBL) devices, which are usually not wedged or posted, as well as orthotics described as "sports orthotics" made by various laboratories. The latter usually include forefoot or rearfoot posting or wedging. Semirigid orthotics require neutral-position casting, usually done in a non-weight-bearing position by manually loading the foot. We have found no specific advantages in semirigid orthotics over the semisoft functional orthotics. Some of the disadvantages of semirigid orthotics are (1) they are considerably more expensive because of the need for neutral-position negative casting, (2) the need to send them to an outside laboratory, which adds time to patient acquisition, and (3) the inability to make forefoot adjustments after the device is constructed. If the orthotic is causing irritation in the arch area, it cannot be easily lowered without sending it back to the laboratory. The break-in period for these orthotics is usually less than for a rigid orthotic, but much longer than for a semisoft functional orthotic.

Rigid orthotics

Rigid functional orthotics are the most expensive and most complicated to construct and provide the most rigid control of any of the types of orthotic devices. The initial step in the construction of a rigid

---

*Both by Alimed, Boston, MA.

orthotic is the construction of a cast of the foot in neutral position. It is very important to make sure that the foot is in the neutral position when constructing the cast. If there is doubt, the error should be toward pronation. This will result in an orthotic that provides slightly less correction, but this is much better tolerated by the patient than an overcorrected orthotic.

A negative mold of the cast is made, and then an acrylic plastic is heated and pressed over the mold. The orthotic is then posted or wedged appropriately. This creates the final product, a relatively rigid functional orthotic.

One of the disadvantages of the rigid orthotic is that the foot sometimes has a difficult time tolerating a rigid orthotic, and an adjustment period is needed because of the rigidity of the material. Blistering may occur over the longitudinal arch, and various adjustments may be required before the orthotic can be worn comfortably. This neccessitates multiple return visits to the physician before a successful fit is achieved, a somewhat time-consuming procedure.

Rigid orthotics can provide excellent rearfoot control when used in proper shoes. They can be used successfully by the distance runner. However, as runners begin to increase their speed and run more on their toes, as in shorter events,

---

FUNCTION OF ORTHOTICS

- Control foot motion
  Limit pronation, *or*
  Aid pronation to help foot function around
    neutral position
- Neutralize forefoot-to-rearfoot relationship

---

they usually need a softer and more flexible orthotic. It has been our general experience that any type of orthotic can work well if it is functional. A functional orthotic is one that controls the motion of the foot, either by limiting or aiding pronation, to help the foot function around

its neutral position. It specifically neutralizes the forefoot-to-rearfoot relationship.

A functional biomechanical orthotic is not synonymous with a rigid orthotic. Any type of material can be constructed into a functional biomechanical orthotic if the biomechanical principles outlined by Root, Mann, and Sgarlato are followed. The difference between a soft functional orthotic and a rigid functional orthotic is that in a rigid orthotic the forefoot to rearfoot relationship is established by the rigidity of the plastic material, whereas the soft functional orthotic maintains the forefoot-to-rearfoot relationship by the thickness of the wedges in the forefoot and rearfoot.

■ ■ ■

It is also our general experience that, once a need for orthotics has been established, a person should wear the orthotic not only for sports but for everyday use as well. This is particularly difficult, though not innsurmountable, for women. We have found that the preorthotic devices are particularly useful and offer a compromise, since they can be worn comfortably in pump-style shoes. They can also be increased in thickness as the need arises and as the patient tolerates them. There are several laboratories that also make orthotics that conform to dress shoes. It has been our general feeling that orthotics are a useful modality of treatment and for that reason should be readily available to patients at a reasonable cost. Finally, one must remember that any orthotic is only as good as the shoe that houses it. For that reason it is important to emphasize the need for a well-constructed shoe.

Some inserts are simply designed for the purpose of improving impact-absorbing qualities, and make no pretense to being an "arch support." There is a variety of commerical products available now that are simply designed to be inserted into the shoe and increase the "softness" of the footwear, and in so doing decrease the impact transmission to the lower extremity. The most effective of these at this time appears to be Sorbothane. Sorbothane is available as a heel insert and is particularly useful in such conditions as os calcis apophysitis or Achilles tendinitis. It is also available as a full-sole insert and can be useful to patients with a variety of overuse type injuries to the lower extremities. Research on this material has demonstrated that it can decrease the impact transmission to the lower extremity by 20% to 30%. The major drawback of this material is that it is quite heavy. While it can indeed be useful in training shoes for distance running, it probably should not be used by an elite runner in competition.

REFERENCES

1. Adkinson, J., and Garrick, J.G.: High school football injuries: a comparison of synthetic playing surfaces, Paper presented at the American College of Sports Medicine, Philadelphia, 1972.
2. Bates, J.B., Osternig, L.R., Mason, B., and James, L.S.: Foot orthotic devices to modify selected aspects of lower extremity mechanics, Am. J. Sports Med. 7:338, 1979.
3. Bramwell, S.T., Requa, R.K., and Garrick, J.G.: High school football injuries: a pilot comparison of playing surfaces, Med. Sci. Sports 4:160, 1972.
4. Cameron, B.M., and Davis, O.: The survival football shoe: a controlled study, J. Sports Med. 1:16, 1973.
5. Cavanagh, P.R., The running shoe book, Mountain View, Calif, 1981, World Publications.
6. Clark, J.E., Frederic, E.C., and Cooper, L.B.: Effects of shoe cushioning upon ground reaction forces in running, Int. J. Sports Med. 4:247, 1983.
7. Clarke, J.E., Frederic, E.C., and Hamill, C.L.: The effects of shoe design parameters on rearfoot control in running, Med. Sci. Sports Exerc. 15:376, 1983.
8. Clarke, J.E., Frederick, E.C., and Hamill, C.L.: The study of rearfoot movement in running. In Frederick, E.C., ed.: Sports shoes and playing surfaces, Champaign, Il., 1984, Human Kinetics Publishers, Inc.
9. Clement, D.B., and Taunton, J.E.: A guide to the prevention of running injuries, Aust. Fam. Physician 10:156, 1981.
10. Donovan, J., Scardina, R., Frykberg, R., Hill, C., and Lucchini, E.: Sports orthotic device, J. Am. Podiatry Assoc. 69:571, 1979.
11. Drez, D.: Running footwear, Am. J. Sports Med. 8:140, 1979.
12. Frederick, E.C., Clarke, J.E., and Hamill, C.L.: The effect of running: shoe design or attenuation. In Fredericks, E.C., ed.: Sports shoes and playing surfaces, Chicago, 1984, Human Kinetics Publishers, Inc., pp. 190-198.
13. Hanley, D.F.: Controllable external factors in lower extremity injuries, Paper presented at the Medical Society of the State of New York Symposium on Medical Aspects of Sports, 1969.
14. Hirata, I.: The Hanley cleat and the Ivy League: a progressive report, J. Am. Coll. Health Assoc. 17:369, 1969.
15. Krahenbuhl, G.S.: Speed of movement with varying footwear conditions on synthetic turf and natural grass, Res. Q. Am. Assoc. Health Phys. Educ. 45:28, 1974.
16. MacLellan, G.: Skeletal heel strike transients, measurements, implications and modifications by footwear. In Frederick, E.C., ed.: Sports shoes and playing surfaces, Champaign, Ill. 1984, Human Kinetics Publishers, Inc., pp. 76-86.
17. Mann, R.A.: Paper presented at American Academy of Orthopaedic Surgeons annual meeting, New Orleans, May 1980.
18. Micheli, L.J.: Overuse injuries in children's sports: the growth factor, Orthop. Clin. North Am. 14:337, 1983.
19. Nigg, B., Denoth, J., Kerr, B., Lueth, S., Smith, D., and Staroff, A.: Load sports shoes and playing surfaces. In Frederick, E.C., ed.: Sports shoes and playing surfaces, Champaign, Ill., 1984, Human Kinetics Publishers, Inc.
20. Rowe, M.: Varsity football knee and ankle injuries, N.Y. State J. Med. 69:3000, 1969.
21. Subotnick, S.I.: The abuses of orthotics in sports medicine, Phys. Sportsmed. 3:73, 1975.
22. Subotnick, S.I.: The flat foot, Phys. Sportsmed. 9:85, 1981.
23. Torg, J.S.: Athletic footwear and orthotic appliances, Clin. Sports Med. 1:157, 1982.
24. Torg, J.S., and Quendenfeld, J.C.: Effect of shoe type and cleat length on incidence and severity of knee injuries among Philadelphia high school football players, Res. Q. 42:203, 1971.
25. Torg, J.S., and Quendenfeld, J.C.: The shoe surface interface and its relationship to football knee injuries, Am. J. Sports Med. 2:261, 1974.

LEG

Injuries to the leg in athletes

Marc J. Friedman

Injuries to the leg are not uncommon among athletes. James et al. have documented the incidence of injuries to this area in their runners' clinic[51] (Table 21-1). The diagnosis of injuries in this region is difficult, but attention to anatomy and precise physical examination, coupled with appropriate adjunctive tests, will allow specific diagnosis and treatment.

Table 21-1 ■ Most common running injuries

Type	Prevalence (%)
Knee pain	29
Posterior tibial syndrome	13
Achilles tendinitis	11
Plantar fasciitis	7
Stress fractures	6
Iliotibial tract tendinitis	5

From James, S.L., Bates, B.T., Osterning, L.R.: Am. J. Sports Med. **6:**40, 1978.

The linkage concept plays an important role in the leg. Distal pathologic conditions, such as forefoot and heel imbalances, may manifest as leg pain. Proximal rotational variability can lead to problems in the leg. When evaluating leg pain, one must examine the entire linkage system to completely assess the biomechanical balance of the lower extremities.

■ ANATOMY
Osseous structures

The leg comprises the tibia and fibula, which are united both at the proximal and distal ends and in the middle by the interosseous membrane. The proximal tibiofibular joint is an articulation between the head of the fibula and the posterolateral aspect of the lateral tibial condyle.

The interosseous membrane passes downward and laterally from the interosseous crest of the tibia to that of the fibula. Superiorly, at the proximal level of the tibial tubercle, the anterior tibial artery enters the anterolateral compartment of the leg.

The tibiofibular syndesmosis represents a thickening of the interosseous membrane at the distal aspect of the leg above the ankle. This consists of the anterior and posterior tibiofibular ligaments and the transverse fibers, sometimes described as the inferior transverse ligament.

The body of the tibia is described as having three borders—anterior, medial, and interosseous—and three surfaces—medial, posterior, and lateral. The anterior border and medial surface are subcutaneous. The tibial tuberosity receives the patellar ligament proximally. The medial and lateral surfaces of the tibia show no anatomic grooves; however, the posterior surface is marked in its upper third by the line of the soleus muscle. The attachments, both origins and insertions of the muscles of the leg, are shown in Figs. 21-1 and 21-2.

The head of the fibula is subcutaneous; the peroneal nerve courses below the neck of the fibula and is thus particularly vulnerable to injury.

The body of the fibula has three borders—interosseous, anterior, and posterior—and three surfaces—medial, lateral, and posterior. The large posterior surface is marked by a medial crest.

Muscles of the leg
Posterior

The muscles of the calf are in two compartments within the deep fascia, separated from each other by a deep transverse fascia. The gastrocnemius, soleus, and plantaris muscles occupy the superficial compartment; the popliteus, flexor hallucis longus, flexor digitorum longus, and tibialis posterior occupy the deep compartment and arise in part from the covering fascia. The nerves and vessels reside first in the superficial compartment but penetrate the transverse septum to run in the deep compartment.

The gastrocnemius and soleus share a common tendon of insertion on the calcaneus and are called the triceps surae (Fig. 21-3). The plantaris also inserts on the calcaneus.

The **gastrocnemius** is most superficial. It consists of two heads that arise from the posterior aspect of the capsule of the knee and the posterior condyles of the femur. The medial head is larger. A bursa lies deep to each of these heads at its origin. The popliteal vessels run downward between the medial and lateral heads of the gastrocnemius. The lateral head may

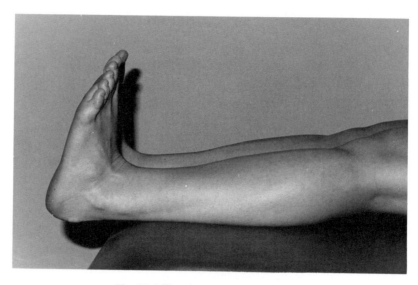

Fig. 21-6 ■ Active dorsiflexion exercise.

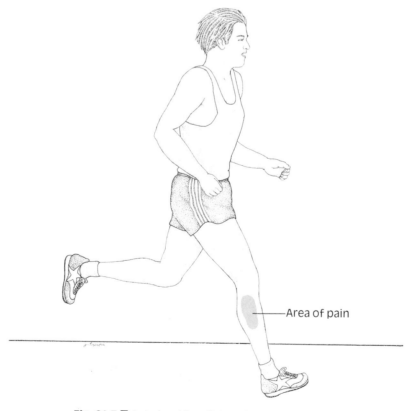

Fig. 21-7 ■ Anterior shin splints. Pain is lateral to tibia.

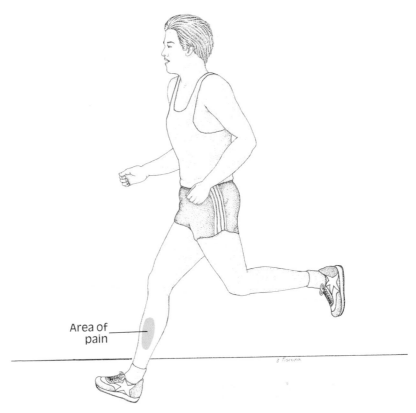

Fig. 21-8 ■ Posterior shin splints. Pain is medial to tibia.

over the posterior compartment (Fig. 21-8). The pain is usually described as aching and variable in intensity. Onset of symptoms is associated with the rhythmic, repetitive exercises of walking and running. Initially pain may occur only during exercise, but with continued stress the pain may be felt during regular daily activity.

When one examines the patient, pain may be elicited on either flexion or extension of the foot against resistance, depending on the involved muscles. Weakness of the involved muscles is generally found and can be determined by either manual muscle testing or Cybex evaluation. Toe walking may be painful for the patient with posterior shin splints. It may also be noted that there is diminished inversion of the heel in the affected leg as a result of pain in the tibialis posterior muscle. The time at which the athlete is examined is important, since the findings will vary depending on the length of time the symptoms have been present. For example, in runners the lesion may be initially well localized. Often the coach or trainer can make the diagnosis quite simply, since the symptoms are minimal and the signs quite specific. An orthopedist may not see the patient for several days, and by this time the signs and symptoms are advanced, making localization difficult.

Many limb alignment abnormalities contribute to shin splints. Mann and Hagy have shown that the muscles in each compartment act as a unit during running.[69] The anterior muscles become active at the time of toe-off, and activity continues through the entire swing phase and first 80% of the stance phase. In long-distance runners and joggers, the ground-to-shoe contact is made with the foot in a flatfoot or slightly flat-heel to flatfoot position. With the dorsiflexors firing, the tibia is accelerated over the fixed foot, apply-

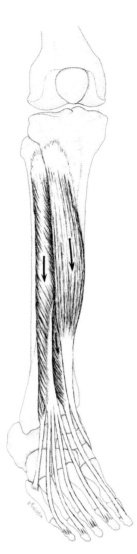

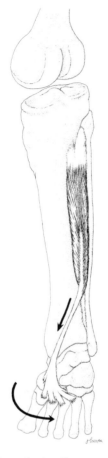

Fig. 21-9 ■ Pain and tenderness may occur in anterior compartment muscles *(arrows)* as a result of weakness or imbalance.

Fig. 21-10 ■ Excessive traction may occur on hyperpronated foot leading to pain in region of the tibialis posterior *(arrows)*.

ing a torque to move the body through space. Dorsiflexion probably cushions the impact of the body against the ground. Since anterior compartment activity contributes to shock absorption at foot strike, large loads are transmitted to these muscles. Hence running on hard surfaces or running in improper running shoes with either a hard heel or no cushion will lead to inflammation of the anterior compartment muscles as a result of overload.

An individual's ability to withstand load also depends on the strength of the mus-

cles. Hence weak anterior muscles will not be able to withstand excessive loads and tenderness may ensue as a direct result of muscle weakness (Fig. 21-9). According to Andrews, the activity of the tibialis anterior muscle during the stance phase prevents a "foot slap" in the runner who contacts the ground heel first. A varus foot or forefoot imbalance and malalignment can therefore cause overuse injury to the tibialis anterior.[4]

The posterior calf muscles are active for about the first 80% of the stance phase.[69] The activity begins in the last 25% of the swing phase. The muscle activity seems to control or modulate the rapid dorsiflexion activity. Brody states that during midstance the foot is pronated and the tibia internally rotated.[15] As the muscle is firing, the tendon may be abnormally stressed as a result of a hypermobile, pronated foot or increased heel eversion (Fig. 21-10). James has suggested that pronation of the foot may be a compensatory mechanism for various other alignment conditions, such as tibia vara, subtalar joint varus, forefoot supination, and heel cord tightness leading to functional equinovarus.[51] Weakness of the posterior muscles may contribute to inflammation.

Treatment

Shin splints, an overuse injury, therefore has many contributing causes. The basic problem is muscle overload. It

---

FACTORS CONTRIBUTING TO SHIN SPLINTS

Anterior
  Muscular
    Weak anterior muscles
  Equipment
    Poor running shoes (hard heel/minimal cushion)
  Training errors
    Hard running surface
    Inappropriate increase in mileage or speed
  Malalignment
    Varus foot
    Forefoot imbalance
Posterior
  Muscular
    Weak posterior muscles
    Tight heel cords with functional equinovarus
  Training errors
    Hard running surface
    Inappropriate increase in mileage or speed
  Malalignment
    Hypermobile, pronated foot
    Increased heel eversion
    Tibia vara
    Subtalar varus
    Forefoot supination

TREATMENT OF SHIN SPLINTS

Phase 1
  Rest
  Ice application ⎫ 10 to 15 minutes, 2 to 3
  Ice massage   ⎭   times a day

  Antiinflammatory medication (for severe shin splints)
  Cardiorespiratory exercises
  Well-leg exercise
Phase 2
  Progressive resistance exercise
  Ice therapy
  Stretching
  Cardiorespiratory exercises
  Well-leg exercise
Phase 3
  Review of equipment, anatomic factors
  Fabrication of appropriate orthoses
  Return to limited running
    Every other day
    Limited mileage/speed
    Appropriate surface (track, if possible)
    Level ground
    Continue stretching and strengthening exercises
Phase 4
  Return to sport or full running program
  Continue stretching and strengthening exercises

---

may result from muscle weakness, anatomic malalignment, or errors in training technique (inappropriate surface, poor-quality shoes, excessive mileage). Injury-producing stresses must be decreased and the inflamed musculotendinous tissue must be allowed to heal. A rest from the causative activity is the primary treatment.

The length of the rest period varies, depending on the severity of the inflammation. It may be as short as 1 or 2 days in very mild cases to a number of weeks in severe cases. In a study of 2777 first-year midshipmen at the United States Naval Academy, the average time lost from running programs as a result of shin splints was 8 days.[5]

During the acute phase of shin splints, the area of pain and tenderness should receive ice treatments for 10 to 15 minutes two to three times per day. Elevation and

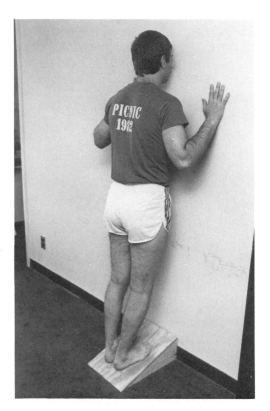

Fig. 21-11 ■ Calf stretching for anterior shin splints.

a brief course of antiinflammatory medication may be useful in the more severe cases. When pain and tenderness are diminished, the athlete is begun on an appropriate progressive resistance exercise program. For the athlete with anterior shin splints, strengthening of the tibialis anterior, extensor hallucis longus, and extensor digitorum communis muscles is prescribed.* This is combined with stretching of the antagonist muscle groups, predominantly the triceps surae (Fig. 21-11). Strengthening of the tibialis posterior, flexor hallucis longus, and flexor digitorum longus muscles is used for athletes with posterior shin splints.* Stretching of the heel cord is also prescribed for posterior shin splints. Exercise sessions are followed by ice therapy to the inflamed area.

_____
*For details, see Chapter 7.

During this treatment program, the athlete is encouraged to participate in sports that do not stress the affected muscles. This is very important when dealing with any recreational or professional athlete who wants very much to maintain his or her aerobic condition. In this regard, a runner with painful shin splints should be encouraged to bicycle (using the heel to push off), swim (without kicking or kickboard), or do circuit weight training. Total avoidance of sports activities is very poorly tolerated in these athletes and is undesirable for cardiovascular fitness.

Immobilization of the limb in a rigid type of cast or short leg orthosis that prevents ankle and foot motion is not recommended; this only leads to further muscle atrophy and prolongs the treatment period. Andrish et al. found that those midshipmen treated with cast immobilization had, on average, the longest loss of running time.[5]

Following amelioration of symptoms and documented strength and flexibility gains, the athlete's limb alignment, shoewear, and training program are thoroughly reviewed before running is resumed. An athlete with posterior shin splints and a hypermobile, pronated foot is given soft arch supports (Fig. 21-12) or a rigid orthotic device (Fig. 21-13). The orthosis prevents or reduces compensatory pronation; this is accomplished with a medial heel and forefoot wedge. A neutral orthotic is prescribed for patients with anterior shin splints and a varus alignment of the foot. All athletic shoes should have an appropriate firm, but not hard, well-cushioned heel. The athletes are instructed in limiting their speed and mileage initially. They should not run daily at first and must run on a track or other appropriate soft surface. Running on level ground is also suggested. A progressive resistance program and flexibility exercise are continued until the athlete reaches preinjury mileage, speed, and frequency and is asymptomatic. Of course, mainte-

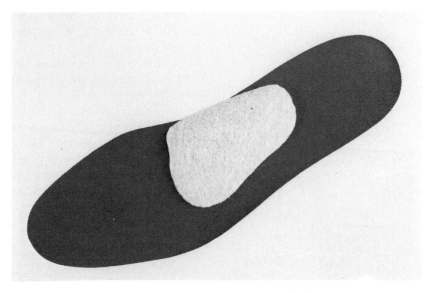

Fig. 21-12 ■ Spenco insert with arch support.

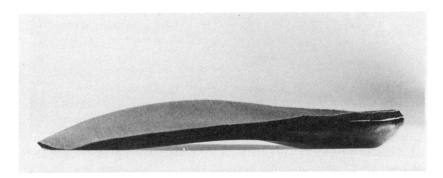

Fig. 21-13 ■ Hard plastic orthotic with Spenco cover.

nance flexibility programs are continued throughout the athlete's running career.

Medial tibial stress syndrome

The medial tibial stress syndrome is usually seen in runners. It has, however, been noted in athletes participating in tennis, volleyball, rope jumping, calisthenics, basketball, and long-jumping. The major complaint of these athletes has been pain in the posteromedial portion of the distal tibia after running or jumping (Fig. 21-14). Various causes have been proposed for the pain, including periostitis,[81] stress microfracture,[52] deep posterior compartment syndrome,[93] or stress fractures.[27]

Clinical findings

These athletes all complain of pain in the distal posteromedial aspect of the tibia. The pain starts after exercise and is generally relieved by rest. However, patients may not be relieved of pain by resting, and the characteristic pain can persist for hours or sometimes even days.[111,112] In Mubarak's group of 12 patients, the pain was exacerbated by weight bearing and relieved by rest. The description of the pain ranged from a dull aching discomfort to an intense, persistent pain aggravated by any physical activity.[81]

A localized area of tenderness over the posteromedial edge of the distal one third of the tibia is found. Occasionally there

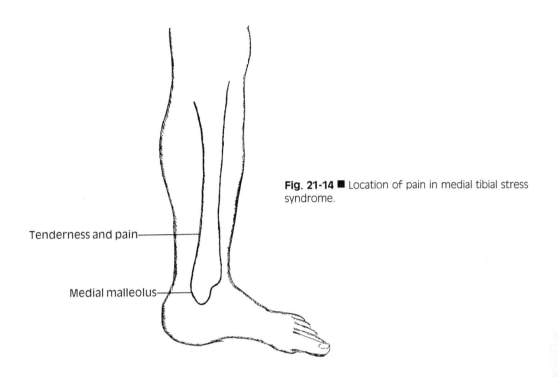

Fig. 21-14 ■ Location of pain in medial tibial stress syndrome.

Tenderness and pain

Medial malleolus

may be weakness and atrophy of the posterior compartment muscles. The neurologic and circulatory examination reveals normal findings. Excessive pronation of the feet may be found.[81] After exercise, the painful area becomes more symptomatic. Mubarak has described an injection test that consists of local injections of an anesthetic agent (xylocaine). In his patients, injections into the affected area relieved the pain and allowed the patients to exercise without discomfort.

Roentgenographic findings

Plain anteroposterior and lateral roentgenograms may be entirely normal. A small percentage of patients will have hypertrophy of the cortex or subperiosteal new bone formation in the painful region. Technetium pyrophosphate bone scanning may be useful for the patient with normal roentgenograms (Fig. 21-15). A pattern of diffuse increased uptake along the posteromedial portion of the tibia can occasionally be found. This pattern of diffuse, longitudinal uptake has by some authors been called a "stress reaction." This diffuse pattern is clearly different from

the localized, intense uptake found in a stress fracture.[24] Bone scans, like plain roentgenograms, can also be negative in this condition.

Compartment pressure testing

Much of the controversy over the cause of medial tibial stress syndrome has arisen as a result of the compartment pressure finding in these patients. Puranen presented a series of 22 patients who were clinically diagnosed as having medial tibial stress syndrome. He measured intracompartment pressures, using the wick catheter technique during exercise. Higher intramuscular pressures in the deep posterior muscle compartments were found in the patients with medial tibial stress syndrome than in the control subjects.[94]

Mubarak et al. used the wick catheter and slit catheter techniques to measure the deep posterior compartment pressures in 12 patients with this syndrome.[81] Measurements were taken at rest, during isokinetic exercise (dorsiflexion and plantar flexion), and after exercise. Slightly higher pressures were found during exer-

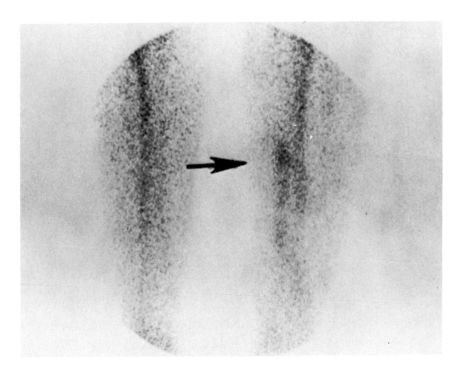

Fig. 21-15 ■ Bone scan demonstrating area of mild uptake (arrow) along posteromedial edge of distal one third of tibia in patient with medial tibial stress syndrome.
From Mubarak, S.J., and Hargens, A.R.: Compartment syndromes and Volkmann's contracture, Philadelphia, 1981, W.B. Saunders Co.

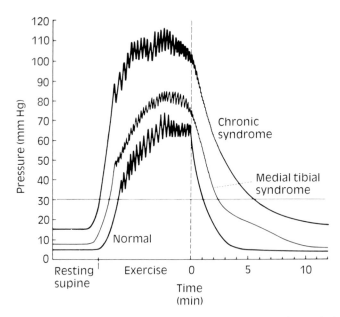

Fig. 21-16 ■ Illustrative compartment pressures recorded from wick catheter during exercise of a normal subject, a patient with medial tibial stress syndrome, and a patient with a chronic compartment syndrome. The pressures in normal subject and patient with chronic compartment syndrome were taken from anterior compartment, pressures in patient medial tibial stress syndrome from deep posterior compartment.
From Mubarak, S.J., Gould, R.N., Lee, Y.F., Schmidt, D.A., and Hargens, A.R.: Am. J. Sports Med. **10**:201, 1982.

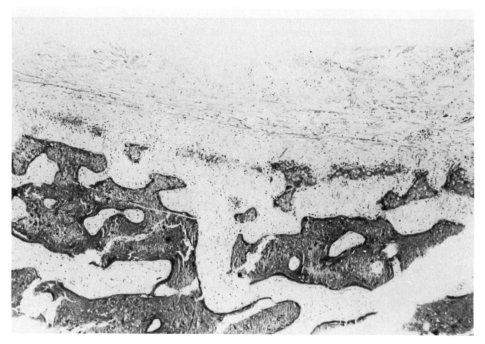

Fig. 21-17 ■ Undecalcified section obtained from edge of tibia in patient with medial tibial stress syndrome. Calluslike area (dark seams) outlining trabeculae indicate bone formation (original magnification 64 times, Goldner stain).
From Johnell, O. et al.: Clin. Orthop. **167**:180, 1982.

cise, but the values were considerably lower than the values found in patients with chronic compartment syndromes (Fig. 21-16). They concluded that the medial tibial stress syndrome did not represent a compartment syndrome.

Wallenstein studied several patients in a manner similar to Mubarak's. His patients with posteromedial tibial pain did not have increased intramuscular pressure in the deep posterior compartment even when in pain; he also concluded that medial tibial stress syndrome was not a chronic compartment syndrome.[110]

Muscle lactate studies

Wallenstein has studied percutaneous muscle biopsy specimens from patients with medial tibial stress syndrome and anterolateral lower leg pain. Patients with pain in the anterior tibial compartment were found to have an after exercise rise in lactate concentration that paralleled the rise in intramuscular pressure. The increase in lactate disappeared after fas-

ciotomy. Patients with medial tibial stress syndrome did not have any increase in muscle lactate concentration after exercise, although pain was present.[31,111] This study therefore also supports the concept that medial tibial stress syndrome is not a chronic compartment syndrome.

Pathology

Johnell et al. biopsied the tibia and associated areas of soft tissue during fasciotomies of 35 patients with medial tibial stress syndrome.[52] They found signs of increased metabolic activity (e.g., osteoblast activity, vascular ingrowth, or increased osteoid areas) in 22 of the 35 tibial samples (Fig. 21-17). Only one sample had an inflammatory lesion in the periosteum. None of the histologic findings consistent with increased metabolic activity were found in any of the 10 control biopsies. Since stress fractures imply increased localized metabolic activity, they concluded that stress microfracture causes medial tibial stress syndrome.

Mubarak studied biopsy material from the fascia obtained during posterior deep compartment fasciotomies for medial tibial stress syndrome and found inflammation and vasculitis.[81] However, as Mubarak pointed out, inflammation is a common finding in the region of a stress fracture.[27]

Treatment

Medial tibial stress syndrome probably results from stress microfracture secondary to repetitive load. Although roentgenograms and bone scans may be normal, the diagnosis can be made clinically by the characteristic pain and tenderness.

Since the cause is not a chronic compartment syndrome, treatment should be conservative. Rest is therefore the cornerstone of treatment for this condition. Athletic participation can resume when pain and tenderness subside. Modification of athletic participation is indicated to preserve aerobic capacity and general physical fitness. Certainly swimming or an appropriate circuit training program is valuable to maintain cardiovascular fitness during the healing process. Before resuming competition the athlete should begin an appropriate strengthening and stretching program. Emphasis should be on the development of strength in the posterior tibialis, flexor hallucis longus, and flexor digitorum longus muscles. Heel cord and tibial posterior stretching may also be of value during the rehabilitation process.

Stress fractures

Stress fractures were first described by the German military surgeon Briehaupt[14] in 1855 and were first discerned on roentgenograms by Stechow[105] in 1897. The entity may also be called a "fatigue fracture" or an "insufficiency fracture." Stress fractures are defined as partial or complete fracture of bone caused by an inability to withstand nonviolent stress that is applied in a rhythmic, repeated, subthreshold manner.[73] It is important to appreciate that stress fracture is an example of

bone remodeling rather than an acute fracture[74] (Fig. 21-18). Bone remodeling occurs in accordance with Wolff's law: Every change in the form and function of a bone is followed by certain definite changes in its internal architecture and secondary alterations in its external conformation. However, a bone's ability to remodel in response to the mechanical stress placed on it may be exceeded. The clinical manifestation of this situation is pain. Histologically, microfractures in the bone may be found initially. If the overload stress is continued, apparent stress fractures become obvious radiographically.

An "insufficiency" fracture is produced by normal physiologic stress applied to bone with *deficient* elastic resistance. The patient with an insufficiency fracture has decreased elastic resistance secondary to a wide variety of disorders resulting in decreased mechanical strength of bone. A "fatigue" fracture occurs when abnormal stress is applied to bone with *normal* elastic resistance. This occurs when the athlete simply overloads normal bone.[91,113]

It is interesting to note that stress fractures are primarily seen in humans, racehorses, and racing greyhounds, since these train for maximum performance in the presence of some pain[9,26] (Fig. 21-19).

Distribution of stress fractures

There are significant differences between the various types of athletic endeavor and types of stress fracture. Running sports affect the fibula and tibia; jumping sports affect the pelvis and femur; basketball affects the patella, calcaneus, femur, and pubis.

In military recruits, the incidence of metatarsal stress fractures in basic training appears to be approximately 40%. In contrast, metatarsal stress fractures in athletes compose only 20% of all stress fractures.[11,17,18,39] The fibula is the site of approximately 25% of the stress fractures in athletes, as opposed to only 2% in the military recruits. Overall, the fibula and

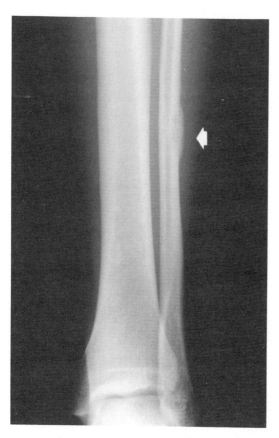

Fig. 21-22 ■ Distal fibular stress fracture.

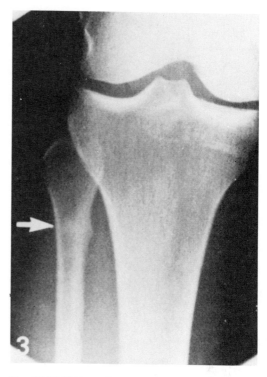

Fig. 21-23 ■ Stress fracture of proximal fibula in young jogger who developed pain after increasing her distance.
From Blair, W.F., and Hanley, S.R.: Stress fracture of the proximal fibula, Am. J. Sports Med. **8**:212, 1980.

Treatment

Treatment will vary, depending on the location of the fracture; it generally involves decreasing the stress applied to the bone.

Distal fibula. The most frequent stress fracture in runners involves the distal third of the fibula, 5 cm above the lateral malleolus[77] (Fig. 21-22). Lateral ankle pain is a common first indication a distal fibula stress fracture should be differentiated from peroneal tendinitis in the presence of chronic instability.[28] This is a "low-risk" stress fracture; other sports activities can easily be substituted while the fracture heals. Bicycling, walking rather than running, and swimming are all excellent substitutes for maintaining cardiorespiratory fitness while the stress fracture heals. It should be explained to the athlete that activity can be increased gradually, as long

as the pain does not recur. Any attempt at running after a fibular stress fracture is diagnosed should be strictly prohibited for a minimum of 3 weeks. During the period of healing, it is important to instruct the athlete carefully in appropriate heel cord, ankle stretching, and strengthening exercises to avoid ankle stiffness or weakness after the fracture has healed.

Some patients with distal fibular stress fractures have symptoms with simple full weight-bearing ambulation. In these rare cases, cast immobilization or partial weight-bearing ambulation may also be considered for two to three weeks until the inflammation resolves.

Proximal fibula. Rarely, a stress fracture may occur in the proximal fibula (Fig. 21-23). Blair and Hanley[12] reported a stress fracture in the neck of the fibula in a young jogger who tried to "run through" pain in the upper leg. Their review of the

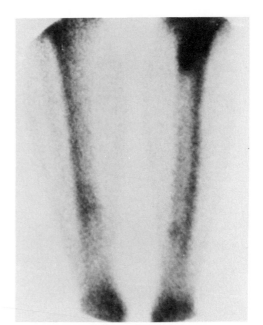

Fig. 21-24 ■ Bone scan demonstrating stress fracture of proximal tibia.

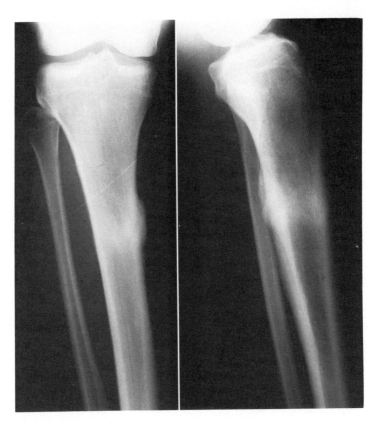

Fig. 21-25 ■ Marked periosteal bone formation associated with healing of tibial stress fracture in collegiate football player.
From the ISMAT Collection.

Fascial defects

Fascial defects may occur in the legs of patients with recurrent compartment syndromes. These are strictly a pressure phenomenon. When compartment pressures reach particularly high levels, one or more fascial defects may develop in the weakened areas of fascia. Herniation of muscle through the defect may occur (Fig. 21-33). Reneman[98] noted fascial defects over the anterior and/or lateral compartment in nearly 60% of his patients. He noted that the defects may be unilateral or bilateral, solitary or multiple, and present in both symptomatic and asymptomatic persons. Mubarak[82] has encountered the fascial defects much less frequently (30%). Mubarak noted that most fascial herniations are located in the lower third of the leg overlying the anterior intermuscular septum between the anterior and lateral compartment[82] (Fig. 21-34). At this point, a branch of the su-

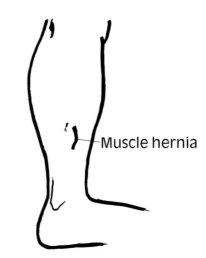

Fig. 21-33 ■ Fascial hernia in anterior compartment.

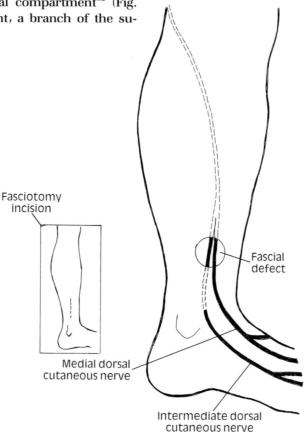

Fig. 21-34 ■ Fascial defect in lateral third of leg through which superficial peroneal nerve may exit.

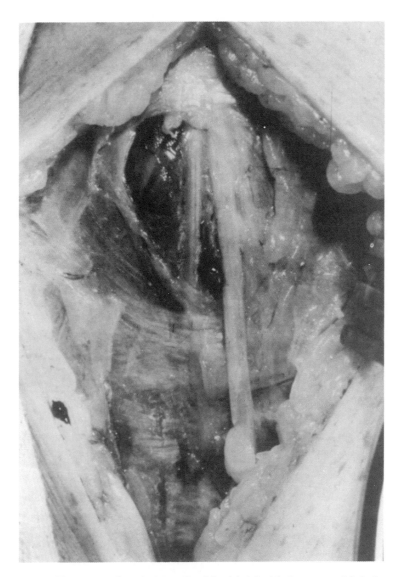

Fig. 21-35 ■ Intraoperative photograph of fascial defect in lower one third of patient's right leg. Medial dorsal cutaneous nerve is to right, exiting defect, and intermediate dorsal cutaneous nerve is to left.

From Mubarak, S., and Hargens, A.: Exertional compartment syndromes. In American Academy of Orthopaedic Surgeons, Symposium on the foot and leg in running sports, St. Louis, 1982, The C.V. Mosby Co.

perficial peroneal nerve exits the lateral compartment through a small opening in the fascia. An enlargement of this opening, with deficiency of the fascia in this region, may lead to muscle herniation and ischemia of the herniated muscle after exercise. Also muscle herniation may cause irritation of the superficial peroneal nerve or neuroma formation (Fig. 21-35).

Treatment

Treatment of muscle herniations secondary to fascial defects in the setting of increased intracompartmental pressure measurements are treated in a similar fashion to chronic exertional compartment syndromes. The involved compartment should be released with the release extending into the area of fascial hernia-

tion so that there is no remaining constriction of the muscle at the area of the
fascial defect. Care must be taken during
surgery to visualize the nerves in the area
of the fascial defect to protect them from
injury during surgery.

Popliteal artery entrapment syndrome

When a patient is initially seen with exercise-related leg pain and the distal
pulses are compromised or absent, one
should strongly consider the diagnosis of
popliteal artery entrapment syndrome. In
this condition, anatomic anomalies in the
popliteal fossa create intermittent occlusion of the popliteal artery. Several structures have been recognized as being responsible for this problem. In some cases,
the artery, traveling in its normal course,
is compressed by an aberrant insertion of
the gastrocnemius or plantaris muscle.[47]
Most of the reported cases have described
an anomalous relationship between the
popliteal artery and the gastrocnemius
muscle.[67,68] Lowe and Whelan have described a compression of the popliteal
artery caused by a fibrotic popliteus muscle rather than the gastrocnemius.[66] An
anomalous condition may arise where the
artery passes medially and below the medial head of the gastrocnemius muscle,
passing deep to the popliteus muscle
where it is compressed.[25]

Clinical findings

The majority of patients reported in the
literature are male, and more than 25%
are reported to have bilateral conditions.[21]
The patients often characterize the pain,
an intermittent claudication, in various
ways. Some describe it as a sensation of
cramping and tightness; others describe
increased fatigue forcing them to eventually stop walking and rest. In most, simply
resting for a few minutes while standing
is sufficient to relieve the pain. If there is
a need to sit down and elevate the extremity or if it takes more than a few minutes
for the pain to abate, then one should suspect a primary disease process rather

than chronic arterial insufficiency as the
cause of pain. As the condition progresses
and ischemia becomes more severe, pain
at rest may occur. The patient may rub
the foot or put it in a dependent position.
Cold or elevation of the foot increases
the pain. The physician should inquire
whether there has been vascular disease
involving the coronary or cerebral vessels,
whether the patient smokes, and the family history regarding diabetes. A reasonable index of arterial insufficiency is the
distance the patient can walk at a normal
stride before claudication occurs. A city
block is approximately 300 feet. If claudication distance is less than 600 feet, it indicates significant occlusion; a distance
over 1800 feet indicates only mild disease.

At times the location of pain allows an
estimation of the level of the occlusion.
Calf pain correlates to occlusion in the superficial femoral or in the popliteal artery. Pain in the anterior and lateral aspects of the legs or dorsum of the foot
suggests occlusion in the anterior tibial
artery.

On physical examination, distal pulses
are generally diminished and may be
completely absent. Some special maneuvers have been described to elicit a change
in pulse intensity as a result of popliteal
artery entrapment. These include active
plantar flexion or passive dorsiflexion of
the foot with the knee hyperextended.
However, since McDonald[75] has demonstrated that pulse reduction may also occur in normal individuals, these special
maneuvers may be of limited value.

When dealing with vascular causes of
leg pain, one must also consider venous
stasis. Venous pain usually is made worse
by standing and is relieved by elevation.
Pain is localized usually in the posterior
calf. It is also occasionally associated with
swelling of both the calf and the foot and
ankle.[55]

Treatment

The differential diagnosis of this condition should include early arteriosclerosis,

cystis adventitial disease, Buerger's disease, traumatic intimal tears, and other causes of external compression.

If the history and physical examination point toward the diagnosis of popliteal artery entrapment syndrome, an arteriogram is indicated. The natural history of this disease is characterized by progressive structural changes to the popliteal artery at the site of entrapment. With progressive hyperplasia of the intima and narrowing of the lumen, an arteriogram will demonstrate occlusion or abnormal flow characteristics through the area of compression.

Regardless of the type of anatomic anomaly, the treatment, following confirmation of the diagnosis by arteriography, is surgery. Since the artery may be significantly damaged, the surgeon must be prepared to resect the artery in the area of constriction and replace it with a saphenous vein graft. At the time of surgery, a Fogarty catheter should be used to remove any thrombotic material from the distal vessels, since diminished flow through these vessels may have created an environment for formation of thrombosis. Following surgery, the patient's pulses should return to normal and the symptoms subside.

Effort-induced venous thrombosis

A recently described condition of the lower extremity is effort-induced venous thrombosis. This condition should be included in the differential diagnosis of effort-associated leg pain.

Effort-induced thrombosis has been reported in joggers who are in their thirties and forties.[43] The athletes are otherwise healthy individuals without hematologic abnormalities. The onset occurs as a sharp pain in the posterior aspect of the leg. Characteristically the athlete does not seek medical attention and tries to run through the pain, believing its cause to be a muscular strain. However progressive calf swelling, pain when the leg is in a dependent position, and echymosis differ-

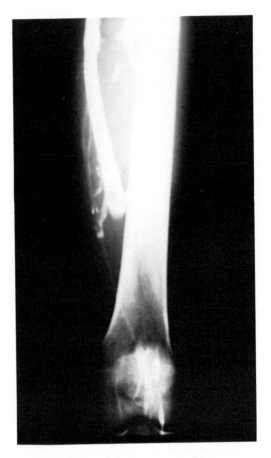

Fig. 21-36 ■ Deep vein thrombosis of leg demonstrated by venogram performed through dorsal vein of foot. Extensive nature of thrombosis is evident. Thrombosis occurred during sprinting. From Harrey, J.S.: Am. J. Sports Med. **6**:400, 1978.

entiate this condition from a simple strain. Elevation of the leg is found by the patient to be the only comfortable position.

On examination, the calf circumference is markedly increased and the calf is tender. The diagnosis is confirmed with venography (Fig. 21-36).

Treatment of deep vein thrombosis in these individuals is with anticoagulant medication and elevation of the limb. Initially heparin is used, then a course of coumadin is prescribed, as for any patient with deep vein thrombosis.

The importance of recognizing this condition is obvious. Effort-induced thrombosis in the upper extremity has been found to have a 12% incidence of pulmonary embolism.[29] Early recognition and treatment should avert this potentially serious complication.

The cause of effort-induced thrombosis is obscure. One theory contends that thrombosis follows repetitive or unusual muscular activity.[43] Another contributing factor may be hemoconcentration during exercise, leading to a hypercoagulable state.[2]

Tendinitis

Pathophysiology

Muscle can be injured by excessive compressive force, such as from a contusion. If extensive tensile force is applied, the muscles "overstretch," causing a strain. Overstretching the muscle or tendon usually occurs when the functional unit is overloaded in the eccentric muscle contraction phase.

Factors that predispose the musculotendinous unit to injury are inadequate conditioning, inadequate warm-up, fatigue, prior muscle injury, scarring, or overstretching. Prior steroid injections lead to weakening of the collagen in the tendon.[8,55] Immobilization, such as in a cast or splint, can also lead to significant weakening of the tendon.

The degree of injury can be classified according to the amount of disruption. Mild or first-degree strain results in a less than 5% disruption of the structural musculotendinous units. A moderate or second-degree strain consists of more significant but still incomplete disruption of the musculotendinous unit and involves a complete muscular tear. A severe or third-degree strain is a complete rupture of a muscle or tendon, leading to a ragged appearance. Avulsion at the origin or insertion of the tendon into bone is equivalent to a third-degree strain.

The individual's age and the relative strength of the musculotendinous unit determine the precise point of rupture. Failure occurs at the weakest point in the system. In children, the growth plate is usually the weakest point, and therefore avulsion fracture to the epiphyseal plate is most likely to occur. In middle age, there is increasing degeneration of collagen fibers within the tendon, and this often makes the tendons the weakest point. Rupture of the muscle itself is susceptible to tear in all age groups.

In comparing various treatment modalities, it becomes apparent that a specific definition must be given, since the condition "tendinitis" is broad, encompassing a variety of pathologic states. Clancy[23] has enlarged Puddu's original classification,[92] which is helpful in understanding the pathophysiology of tendon injury (see boxed list below).

CLASSIFICATION OF TENDON INJURIES

Tenosynovitis and tenovaginitis—an inflammation of only the paratenon, either lined by synovium or not

Tendinitis—an injury or symptomatic degeneration of the tendon, with a resultant inflammatory reaction of the surrounding paratenon

  Acute—symptoms present less than 2 weeks

  Subacute—symptoms present longer than 2 weeks but less than 6 weeks

  Chronic—symptoms present 6 weeks or longer

    Interstitial microscopic failure

    Central necrosis

    Frank partial rupture

    Acute complete rupture

Tendinosis—asymptomatic tendon degeneration due to either aging, accumulated microtrauma, or both

  Interstitial

  Partial rupture

  Acute rupture

From Clancy, W.: Tendinitis in runners. In D'Ambrosia, R.D., and Drez, D., eds.: Prevention and treatment of injuries to runners, Chicago, 1982, Charles Slack, Inc.

Tenosynovitis represents an inflammation of only the paratenon. **Tendinitis** represents an injury or systematic degeneration of the tendon, with a resultant inflammatory reaction of the surrounding paratenon. This in turn may be broken down into subdivisions, depending on the length of time the symptoms have been present. Acute tendinitis encompasses those conditions in which symptoms have been present for less than 2 weeks; subacute tendinitis involves symptoms that have been present for more than 2 weeks but less than 6 weeks; and chronic tendinitis is that in which symptoms are present for 6 weeks or longer. Chronic tendinitis can further be divided into interstitial microscopic failure, central necrosis, frank partial rupture, and acute complete rupture. This subdivision of chronic tendinitis is based on changes found at surgery by Clancy.[23]

Tendinosis is an asymptomatic tendon degeneration resulting either from aging or cumulative microtrauma or both. The findings of tendinosis were first described by Puddu et al.[92] and have also been noted by others.[7,23]

Pathologic changes consist of either mucoid, fatty hyaline degeneration, or calcification and bone metaplasia. These changes were initially noted when biopsies were taken of acute ruptures of the Achilles tendon in previously asymptomatic patients.[64] With time and continued loading, some patients may develop clinical symptoms and the condition would then be termed tendinitis.

Clinical findings

Achilles tendinitis. The Achilles tendon is formed by the fusion of fibers from the medial and lateral heads of the gastrocnemius and the soleus. Injury can occur at any point along the musculotendinous unit. In a growing child the site of injury can be the origin or insertion of the tendon into an apophysis.

Achilles tendinitis is the most commonly reported form of tendinitis. Clinically the onset of the pain occurs 3 to 4 hours after exercise. Patients often complain of pain when they climb stairs, although normal walking does not produce discomfort. The classic area of pain is 2 to

Table 21-3 ■ **Most prevalent etiological factors in 109 athletes with Achilles tendinitis**

Factor	Cases
Training errors	82
Sudden increase in mileage	13
Single severe session	11
Increase in intensity	6
Hill training	4
Return from layoff	4
Combination	44
Alignment factors	
Varus with functional pronation	61
Valgus pes cavus foot	6
Gastrocnemius/gastrocsoleus	
Insufficiency in strength and flexibility	41
Ineffective footwear	11

From Clement, D.B., Taunton, J.E., and Smart, G.W.: Am. J. Sports Med. **12:**179, 1984.

3 centimeters above the superior lip of the calcaneus.

On examination, some crepitation may be noted with active motion. In patients with chronic tendinitis, thickening and tenderness of the tendon is common.

Predisposing factors that are highly associated with Achilles tendinitis should be sought during the examination (Table 21-3). These include heel valgus, pronation, femoral anteversion, or a tight gastrocsoleus complex.

The athlete's training history must be carefully obtained. In runners, James et al. demonstrated that up to 75% of injuries result from training errors.[51] Insufficient warmup, inflexible shoes, abnormal foot strike secondary to abnormal hindfoot mobility, and inappropriate increase in mileage or a too rapid return from a layoff from running will also contribute to inflammation of the tendinous unit. It must be appreciated that the entire lower extremity functions as a unit and if the hamstrings are also tight, this will place an inordinate amount of tension on the gastrocsoleus complex.

Posterior tibial tendinitis. Posterior tibial tendinitis is generally characterized by pain in the tendinous portion of the posterior tibial tendon along the posterior, inferior edge of the medial malleolus. It is usually seen during the beginning of a training program and is often associated with running on hard surfaces. According to Clancy, foot pronation is the most common anatomic variation seen with this entity.[23] Pain may be elicited with inversion of the foot against resistance, holding the foot in a plantar flexed position. It is important to rule out stress fracture of the distal tibia in patients with pain localized in this area.

Extensor tendinitis. Extensor tenosynovitis results in crepitation of the extensor tendons anteriorly above the ankle with plantar flexion and dorsiflexion of the foot. This can result from the athlete's shoelaces being too tight.

Peroneal tendinitis. The peroneal area is an uncommon site for tendinitis. When the patient is initially seen with pain along the peroneal tendons distally, one must be careful to exclude stress fracture of the lateral malleolus. Pain can be elicited on eversion of the foot against resistance. Often a muscle imbalance can be demonstrated with Cybex testing in patients with peroneal tendinitis. Peroneal tendinitis is also seen with chronic lateral ankle instability.

Treatment

In patients with acute **tenosynovitis,** rest from the causative activity, contrast baths (cold and heat, ending with cold), and oral antiinflammatory medication generally produce fairly rapid recovery within 2 to 3 weeks. In some cases that do not resolve despite these measures, an analysis of the training measures should be undertaken.

In patients with acute **tendinitis,** a program of rest, contrast baths, and gentle stretching usually improves the condition within 2 to 3 weeks. Oral nonsteroidal antiinflammatory medication can usually make the patient more comfortable in the acute phase; however, it has not been shown to significantly decrease the period

the athlete requires before return to active sports participation. When the involved area is not tender to palpation, the athlete may gradually return to activity. In some cases, appropriate lifts may be built into the shoes to reduce the tensile stress applied to the affected muscle-tendon unit. For Achilles tendinitis, a ½-inch heel lift can be inserted into the running shoe. For peroneal tendinitis, an outer sole lift can be used. In patients with posterior tibialis tendinitis, a medial heel wedge is prescribed to limit pronation.

Following reduction of symptoms, the athlete concentrates on stretching to prevent further injury.* **The importance of stretching in these conditions cannot be overemphasized.**

When tendinitis has been present for up to 6 weeks (subacute), a minimum of 2 to 3 months will be necessary to resolve on the previously described regimen. Careful stretching of the Achilles with both the knee extended and flexed is shown in Fig. 21-37.

With the knee flexed, the medial and lateral heads of the gastrocsoleus, which is inserted above the knee joint, are released, thereby isolating the soleus muscle.

In patients with chronic tendinitis, the recovery period is again significantly prolonged. It is recommended that conservative therapy be employed for at least 3 to 6 months before recommending surgery; in most cases a minimum of six months is necessary. At times, a brief 4- to 6-week period of cast immobilization is indicated.

Surgery consists of incising the tendon sheath and examining the tendon by palpation. It is important to appreciate that the tendon may be entirely normal-appearing on first inspection; however, after a longitudinal incision is made into the body of the tendon in the area of tenderness, some obvious pathologic changes are usually noted. Once a significant area of defect is found, it is excised longitudi-

*For details see Chapter 7.

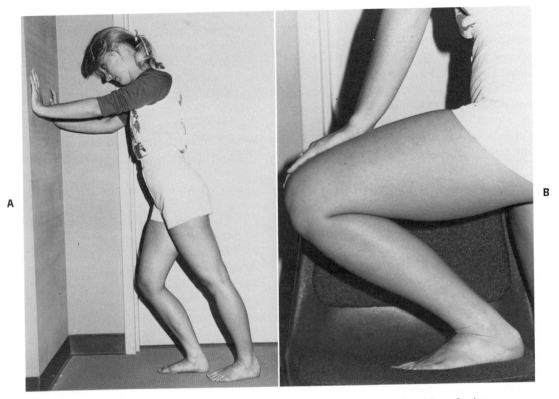

Fig. 21-37 ■ **A,** Heel cord stretching of gastrocnemius. **B,** Heel cord stretching of soleus.

nally. If the defect is not too large, the tendon is closed. In some cases the defect will be large, and either the plantaris tendon is used to reinforce the area or a musculotendinous gastrocnemius flap is turned down (Fig. 21-38). Postoperatively the patients are placed in a short-leg cast for 2 weeks, followed by gentle mobilization. At all times in the first 8 weeks of mobilization the patient must wear a heel lift to protect the repaired tendon. Patients with large defects requiring tenoplasty are initially immobilized for 6 to 8 weeks to allow healing.

Complete rupture of the Achilles tendon was first described by Paré in 1575 (Fig. 21-39). For diagnosing a complete Achilles tendon rupture, the Thompson test is the easiest and most consistent diagnostic method[108] (Fig. 21-40). No pressure is applied to the medial head of the gastroc in Fig. 21-40, *A*. Pressure on the

head of the gastroc produces plantar flexion of the foot *only* if the Achilles tendon is intact (Fig. 21-40, *B*).

Arner and Lindholm[7] presented 92 cases of subcutaneous Achilles tendon rupture, which was then complete in all cases. In most of the early Achilles tendon rupture articles (1955-1956) it was felt that partial tear of the Achilles tendon was extraordinarily rare. However, Gillstrom and Ljungqvist[40] reported on 90 patients operated on for partial rupture of the Achilles tendon during the period 1965 to 1974. Follow-up included clinical and roentgenographic examination and electromyography. The mean follow-up time was 5.2 years; and 82% of the patients were satisfied, 10% were unsure of the success of their result, and 8% were not satisfied. Of the competitive athletes, 76 returned to competitive sports after an average of 9.2 months, and 90% of the noncompetitors

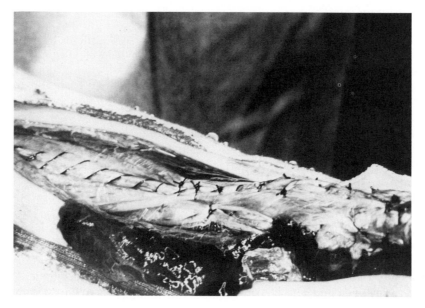

Fig. 21-38 ■ Achilles tendon defect repaired with gastrocnemius fascial reinforcement followed resection of degenerated tendon.

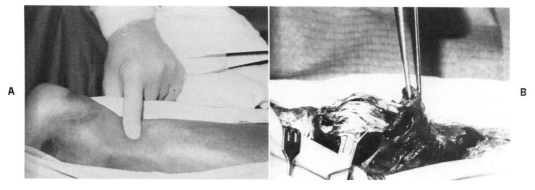

Fig. 21-39 ■ **A,** Defect in Achilles tendon clinically apparent with rupture. **B,** Surgical findings.

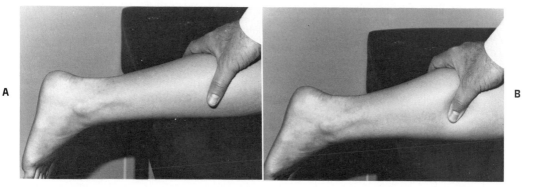

Fig. 21-40 ■ Thompson test. **A,** No pressure on gastrocnemius. **B,** Pressure on gastrocnemius and associated plantar flexion. If Achilles tendon is torn, plantar flexion does not accompany pressure.

resumed full physical activity after 8.7 months. Their results show that after operative treatment most of the patients could resume full physical activity.

In 1979 Ljungqvist and Persson[65] reported that electromyographic examination was useful to discern partial rupture of the Achilles tendon. They noted that decreased electrical activity on either the medial or lateral portion of the gastrocnemius muscle was present, depending on which was torn. In most of the cases of partial rupture, the H reflex was normal.

Quenuj and Stoianovitch[95] in 1929 advocated surgical repair based on cases from the literature. Lea and Smith[59] published results that documented nonsurgical treatment as giving good results.[59]

One of the major objections to nonsurgical treatment, however, has been the high incidence of rerupture. Most reports cite an incidence of approximately 10%.[59,62,87,95] Inglis et al.[46] had an incidence of 29% and Jacobs et al.[50] reported a rate of 22%. In these series, rerupture may have been caused by a shorter period of immobilization. Nistor[88] reviewed 25 papers comprising a total of 2647 ruptures in which surgical complications had been recorded. The major complications were deep infections, 1% (24 patients); fistulae, 3% (76 patients); necrosis of the tendon or skin, or both, 2% (52 patients); and rerupture, 2% (45 patients).

Only a few authors have used objective measurements to assess plantar flexion strength, which is another area of controversy regarding surgical versus nonsurgical repair. A Cybex dynamometer has been used in three studies. Sjostrom et al.[103] analyzed plantar flexion strength in nine surgically treated patients and compared it with changes in the type of muscle fibers. There was no correlation. Shields et al.[101] reported that the strength of plantar flexion averaged 85% of that on the uninjured side in 32 patients after operation. They found reduced strength on the uninjured side as compared to uninjured (control) tendons. Inglis et al.[46] compared the results of surgical and nonsurgical treatment in 30 surgically treated and 14 nonsurgical patients and found that the patients were weak on the injured side but that the reduction in strength was less in the group that was treated surgically. Nistor[88] reported a random series of 105 consecutive cases of closed acute rupture of the Achilles tendon. He found little difference in the results for two treatment groups between surgically treated and nonsurgical patients. The frequency of major complications was about the same in both groups of patients. There were two reruptures and two deep infections in patients that had operations as compared to five reruptures in conservatively treated patients.

Based on these data, we recommend surgical repair of complete rupture of the Achilles tendon in high-performance athletes. Repair should also be undertaken in those recreational athletes who participate in ballistic sports (e.g., tennis, basketball, racquetball, volleyball).

Postoperatively the athlete's cast is changed several times during the period of immobilization. At each cast change, the tension on the gastrocsoleus complex is maintained to retard the profound muscle hypotrophy noted when muscles are immobilized without tension. Indeed, Haggmark and Eriksson[42] have shown that cast immobilization for 6 weeks after Achilles tendon repair leads to a 23% decrease in the cross-sectional area of the calf muscles and selective type I fiber atrophy of the soleus muscle.[42]

Tennis leg

The term "tennis leg" refers to a partial tear of the medial head of the gastrocnemius; it was first described in 1884.[44] Although called tennis leg, this clinical condition can occur in any sport that includes side-to-side motion.

Clinical findings

The typical history consists of sudden calf pain as if the calf had received a direct blow while making a sharp cutting

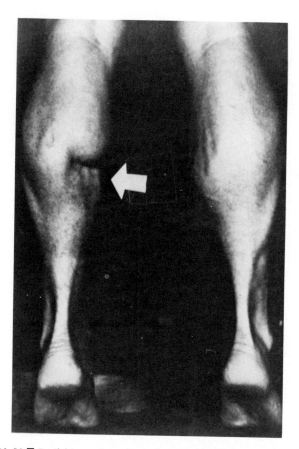

Fig. 21-41 ■ Partial tear of medial head of gastrocnemius—"tennis leg."
From Zarins, B., and Ciullo, J.V.: Clin. Sports Med. **2**:167, 1983.

movement. Usually the knee is extended and the ankle dorsiflexed. The injury generally causes the player to stop playing and, depending on the severity, to seek medical attention. At that time there may be significant echymosis and swelling about the medial calf. At times a palpable defect in the medial gastrocnemius fascia is noted (Fig. 21-41). Dorsiflexion of the foot is painful and often restricted.

Arner and Lindholm[6] described 20 injuries with this mechanism and diagnostic pattern. They performed surgery on five patients, all of whom were described as having a transverse rupture at the junction between the medial gastrocnemius and its tendinous expansion. During surgery, exploration of the plantaris tendon in this particular series revealed that the plantaris tendon is always intact.

Treatment

The primary treatment should be to reduce the pain and swelling. Ice, compression, elevation with partial or complete non-weight-bearing ambulation should be instituted for 2 or 3 days. After this, contrast baths may be given with gentle stretching, depending on the degree of the symptoms. It is important to perform gentle, gradual stretching so as to align the healing scar tissue in the torn gastrocnemius.

A ½-inch heel lift can be used briefly to aid ambulation. No ballistic activity is allowed until motion, strength, and power have been totally restored. For some patients a ½-inch heel lift is built into the athletic shoes to take the stress off the gastrocsoleus complex. Following resumption of sports, a careful preexercise

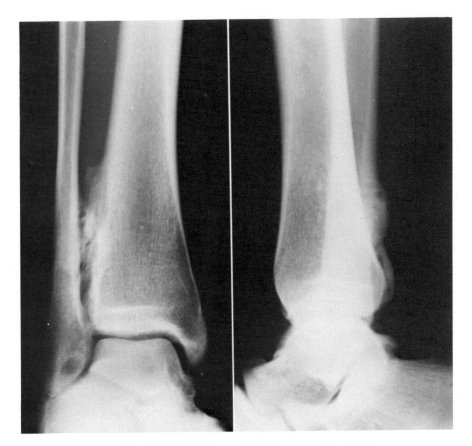

Fig. 21-42 ■ Distal tibiofibular synostosis in a young football player.
From the ISMAT Collection.

stretching routine involving the hamstring and gastrocsoleus complex is carried out.

Millar[79] reported a series of 720 patients over a 12-year period who were treated conservatively. In Millar's series, 61 of the patients were relieved in 1 week, 26% in 2 weeks, 8% in 3 weeks, and 5% took longer than 3 weeks.

Our personal experience indicates that it can take 2 to 3 months to recover from a significant partial tear of the medial head of the gastrocnemius. However, the overall prognosis is excellent for return to function following appropriate conservative therapy.

Tibiofibular synostosis

Ossification of the interosseous membrane may develop from a single severe injury or from recurrent, less severe episodes of trauma. In a single severe injury, tearing of the anterior and posterior tibiofibular ligaments and lower third of their interosseous membrane occurs, with splitting of the fibula away from the tibia. The talus usually tilts, as in an inversion, internal rotation ankle sprain. This appears to be associated with avulsion of these structures in varying degrees from their periosteal insertion. Bone develops from either side as a flat exostosis or across the interosseous membrane, causing a synostosis (Fig. 21-42). Synostosis may also occur proximally along the interosseous membrane (Fig. 21-43).

The formation of bone is unrelated to normal growth or normal physiology. The exact mechanism is unknown. The athlete

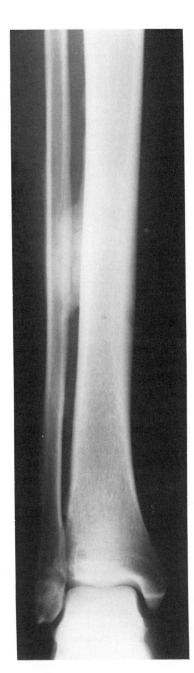

Fig. 21-43 ■ Proximal tibiofibular synostosis occurring after interosseus membrane sprain in a professional football player.
From the ISMAT Collection.

may complain of a spasmlike feeling in the leg. The ankles may feel unstable and movements are slow, especially with cutting movements. Limitation of motion may be noted on examination.

If the initial injury is treated effectively by ice and compression, a lesion may not develop. The synostosis has most often occurred after recurrent inversion ankle sprains. If activity is diminished, surgery can usually be avoided. Whiteside et al.'s experience[114] with this condition led them to believe that partial ossification of the distal tibiofibular syndesmosis is compatible with normal ankle function and that even total synostosis may be relatively asymptomatic.

However, if the disability is so severe that it prevents the individual from participating in sports, surgery is indicated.[76] Surgery consists of synostectomy. Surgery must be delayed until the bone is mature. At this time the bone scan should be "cold" and the alkaline phosphatase return to normal. Recurrence after surgery may be common; some authors[99] feel that repeated surgery may be necessary to free the distal fibula.

REFERENCES

1. Abrahams, M.: Mechanical behavior of tendons in vitro, Med. Biol. Eng. **5:**433, 1967.
2. Ali, M.S., Kutty, S.M., and Corea, J.R.: Deep vein thrombosis in a jogger. Am. J. Sports Med. **12:**169, 1984.
3. American Medical Association Subcommittee on Classification of Sports Injuries: Standard nomenclature of athletic injuries, Chicago, 1966, AMA.
4. Andrews, J.R.: Overuse syndromes of the lower extremity, Clin. Sports Med. **2:**137, 1983.
5. Andrish, J.T., Bergfeld, J.H., and Walheim, J.: A Prospective study on the management of shin splints. J. Bone Joint Surg. **56A:**1697, 1974.
6. Arner, O., and Lindholm, A.: "What is tennis leg?" Acta Chir. Scand. **116:**73, 1958.
7. Arner, O., Lindholm, A., and Orell, S.R.: Histological changes in subcutaneous rupture of the Achilles tendon: a study of 74 cases, Acta Chir. Scand. **116:**484, 1958.
8. Bar, R.D., et al.: Electrodiagnosis in the entrapment of the intermediate dorsal cutaneous branch of the superficial peroneal nerve, Orthop. Rev. **2:**105, 1982.

9. Bateman, J.K.: Broken hock in the greyhound: repair methods and the plastic scaphoid, Vet. Rec. **70:**621, 1958.

10. Bauman, J.V., et al.: Intramuscular pressure during walking: an experimental study using the wick catheter, Clin. Orthop. **145:**292, 1979.

11. Bingham, J.A.: Stress fractures of the femoral neck, Lancet **2:**13, 1945.

12. Blair, W.F., and Hanley, S.R.: Stress fracture of the proximal fibula, Am. J. Sports Med. **8:**212, 1980.

13. Brahms, M.A., Fumich, R.M., and Ippolito, V.D.: Atypical stress fracture of the tibia in a professional athlete, Am. J. Sports Med. **8:**131, 1980.

14. Briehaupt, M.D.:Zur Pathologie des menschlichen Fusses, Med. Zeitung **24:**169, 1955.

15. Brody, D.A.: Running injuries; Clinical symposium, Summit, N.J., 1980, vol. 32, no. 4, CIBA Pharmaceutical Co.

16. Brooker, A.R., and Pewzenshki, C.: Tissue pressure to evaluate compartmental syndrome, J. Trauma **19:**689, 1979.

17. Brubaker, C.E., and James, S.L.: Injuries to runners, J. Sports Med. **2:**189, 1974.

18. Burrows, H.J.: Fatigue infraction of the middle tibia in ballet dancers, J. Bone Joint Surg. **38B:**83, 1956.

19. Cahill, B.R.: Stress fracture of the proximal tibial epiphysis: a case report, Am. J. Sports Med. **5:**186, 1977.

20. Carton, R.W., Dainauskas, J., and Clark, J.W.: Elastic properties of single elastic fibers, J. of Appl. Physiol. **17:**547, 1962.

21. Cassells, S.W., Fellows, B., and Axe, M.J.: Another young athlete with intermittent claudication, Am. J. Sports Med. **11:**180, 1983.

22. Ciullo, J.V., and Zarins, B.: Biomechanics of the musculotendinous unit: relation to athletic performance and injury, Clin. Sports Med. **2:**71, 1983.

23. Clancy, W.G.: Tendinitis and plantar fasciitis in runners, and prevention and treatment of running injuries. Reprinted in Orthopedics **6:** 1983.

24. D'Ambrosia, R.D., et al.: Interstitial pressure measurements in the anterior and posterior compartments in athletes with shin splints, Am. J. Sports Med. **5:**127, 1977.

25. Delaney, T.A., and Gonzalez, L.L.: Occlusion of the popliteal artery due to muscular entrapment, Surgery **69:**97, 1971.

26. Devas, M.B.: Shin splints or stress fractures in the metacarpal bones in horses and shin soreness or stress fractures of the tibia in man. J. Bone Joint Surg. 49B:310, 1967.

27. Devas, M.B.: Stress fracture of the tibia in athletes or shin soreness, J. Bone Joint Surg. **40B:**227, 1958.

28. Devas, M.B., and Sweetman, R.: Stress fractures of the fibula, J. Bone Joint Surg. **53A:**507, 1971.

29. Dunphy, H.E., and Lawrence, W.W.: Effort thrombosis. In Surgical Diagnosis and Treatment, Los Altos, Calif., 1977, Lange Medical Publishers.

30. Elliott, D.H.: The mechanical properties of tendon in relation to muscular strength, Ann. Phys. Med. **9:**127, 1967.

31. Eriksson, E., and Walinstein, R.: Can research into muscle morphology and muscle metabolism improve orthopedic treatment? Presented at the Associated Meeting Western Orthopedic, Las Vegas, Nevada, October 16, 1979.

32. Ernst, C.B., and Kaufer, H.: Fibulectomy-fasciotomy: an important adjunct in the management of lower extremity arterial trauma, J. Trauma **11:**365, 1971.

33. Frankel, V.H., and Nordin, M.: Basic biomechanics of the skeletal systems, Philadelphia, 1980, Lea & Febiger.

34. Garfin, S.R., Mubarek, S.J., and Owens, C.A.: Exertional anterolateral compartment syndrome, J. Bone Joint Surg. **59A:**404, 1977.

35. Garrick, J.G.: Early diagnosis of stress fractures and their precursors. Presented at New Orleans Academy of Orthopedic Surgeons, February 2, 1976.

36. Gay, S.J., and Hunt, T.E.: Reuniting of skeletal muscle after transection, Anat. Rec. **120:**853, 1954.

37. Gershuni, D.H., et al.: Ultrasound evaluation of the anterior musculofascial compartment of the leg following exercise, Clin. Orthop. **167:**185, 1982.

38. Geslien, G.E., et al.: Early detection of stress fractures using 99M Tc-polyphosphate, Radiology **121:**683, 1976.

39. Gilbert, R.S., and Johnson, H.S.: Stress fractures in military recruits—a review of 12 years' experience, Milit. Med. **131:**716, 1966.

40. Gillström, P., and Ljungqvist, R.: Long-term results after operation for subcutaneous partial rupture of the Achilles tendon, Acta Chir. Scand. (suppl.) **482:**78, 1978.

41. Greaney, R.B., et al.; Distribution and natural History of stress fractures in U.S. Marine recruits, Radiology **146:**349, 1983.

42. Haggmark, T., and Eriksson, E.: Hypotrophy of the soleus muscle in man after Achilles tendon rupture, Am. J. Sports Med. **7:**121, 1979.

43. Harvey, J.S.: Effort thrombosis in the lower extremity in a jogger, Am. J. Sports Med. **6:**400, 1978.

44. Hood, W.P.: Lancet 2 (Quoted annotation in British Medical Journal 1969–July 28, 1980).

45. Horn, C.E.: Acute ischemia of the anterior tibial muscle and the long extensor muscles of the toes, J. Bone Joint Surg. **27A:**615, 1945.

46. Inglis, A.E., Scott, W.N., and Sculco, T.P.: Ruptures of the tendoachilles: an objective assessment of surgical and non-surgical treatment, J. Bone Joint Surg. **58A:**990, 1976.

47. Insua, J.A., Young, J.R., and Humphries, A.W.: Popliteal artery entrapment syndrome, Arch. Surg. **101:**771, 1970.

48. Jackson, D., and Bailey, D.: Shin splints in the young athlete: a non-specific diagnosis, Phys. Sports. Med. **3**(3):45, 1975.

49. Jackson, D.W., and Strizak, A.M.: Stress fractures in runners, excluding the foot, In Mack, R., ed.: AAOS Symposium on the foot and leg in Running sports, St. Louis, 1980, The C.V. Mosby Co.

50. Jacobs, D., et al.: Comparison of conservative and operative treatment of Achilles tendon rupture, Am. J. Sports Med. **6:**107, 1978.

51. James, S.L., Bates, B.T., and Osterning, L.R.: Injuries to runners, Am. J. Sports Med. **6:**40, 1978.

52. Johnell, O., Rausing, A., Wandeberg, B., and Westlin, N.: Morphological bone changes in shin splints, Clin. Orthop. **167:**180, 1982.

53. Kelly, R.P., and Whitesides, T.E.: Transfibular route for fasciotomy of the leg, J. Bone Joint Surg. **49A:**1020, 1967.

54. Kennedy, J.C., and Roth, J.H.: Major tibial compartment syndromes following minor athletic trauma, Am. J. Sports Med. **7:**201, 1979.

55. Kennedy, J.C., and Willis, R.B.: The effects of local steroid injections on tendons: a biomechanical and microscopic correlative study, Am. J. Sports Med. **4:**11, 1976.

56. Kiiskinen, A., and Heikkinen, E.: Effect of prolonged physical training on the development of connective tissues in growing mice. Proceedings of the Second International Symposium on Exercise and Biochemistry, Abstract, p. 25, 1973.

57. Kimball, P.R., and Savastano, A.A.: Fatigue fractures of the proximal tibia, Clin. Orthop. **70:**170, 1970.

58. Kirby, N.G.: Exercise ischemia in the fascial compartment of soleus, J. Bone Joint Surg. **52B:**738, 1970.

59. Lea, R.V., and Smith, L.: Non-surgical treatment of tendoachilles rupture, J. Bone Joint Surg. **54A:**1398, 1972.

60. Leach, R.E., and Corbett, M.: Anterior tibial compartment syndrome in soccer players, Am. J. Sports Med. **7:**258, 1979.

61. Leach, R.E., Hammond, G., and Stryker, W.S.: Anterior tibial compartment syndrome: acute and chronic, J. Bone Joint Surg. **49A:**451, 1967.

62. Lildoholdt, T. and Munch-Jorgensen, T.: Conservative treatment of Achilles tendon rupture: a follow-up study of 14 cases, Acta Orthop. Scand. **47:**454, 1976.

63. Logan, J.G., Rorabeck, C.H., and Castle, G.S.P.: The measurement of dynamic compartment pressure during exercise, Am. J. Sports Med. **11:**220, 1983.

64. Ljungqvist, R.: Subcutaneous partial rupture of the Achilles tendon, Acta Orthop. Scand. (suppl.) **113:**1, 1968.

65. Ljungqvist, R., and Persson, A.: Electrophysiological observations in cases of partial and total rupture of the Achilles tendon, J. Electroenceph. Klen. Neurophysiol. **31:**239, 1971.

66. Lowe, J.X., and Whelan, T.J.: Popliteal artery entrapment syndrome, Am. J. Surg. **109:**620, 1965.

67. Lysens, R.J., et al.: Intermittent claudication in young athletes: popliteal artery entrapment syndrome Am. J. Sports Med. **11:**177, 1983.

68. Madigan, R.P., and McCampbell, B.R.: Thrombosis of the popliteal artery in a jogger, J. Bone Joint Surg. **64A:**1490, 1981.

69. Mann, R.A., and Hagy, J.: Biomechanics of walking, running and sprinting, Am. J. Sports Med. **8:**345, 1980.

70. Martens, M.A., et al.: Chronic leg pain in athletes due to a recurrent compartment syndrome, Am. J. Sports Med. **12:**148, 1984.

71. Matsen, F.A., et al.: Monitoring of intramuscular pressure, Surgery **79:**702, 1976.

72. Mavor, G.E.: The anterior tibial syndrome, J. Bone Joint Surg. **38B:**513, 1956.

73. McBride, A.M.: Stress fractures in athletes, J. Am. Sports Med. **3:**212, 1976.

74. McBride, A.M.: Stress fractures in runners. In D'Ambria, R.D., and Drez, D., ed.: Prevention and treatment of running injuries, Thorofare, N.J., 1982, Charles Slack, Inc.

75. McDonald, P.T., et al.: Popliteal artery entrapment syndrome: clinical, noninvasive and angiographic diagnosis, Am. J. Surg. **139:**318, 1980.

76. McMasters, J.H., and Scranton, P.E.: Tibiofibular synostosis, Clin. Orthop. **3:**172, 1975.

77. McPhee, H., and Franklin, C.M.: "March fracture" of the fibula in athletes, JAMA **131:**574, 1946.

78. Mercia, M., Brennan, R.E., and Edigan, J.: Computed tomography of stress fractures, Skeletal Radiol. **8:**193, 1982.

79. Millar, A.P.: Strains of the posterior calf musculature ("tennis leg"), Am. J. Sports Med. **7:**172, 1979.

80. Moss, A.A., Gamsu, G., and Gannant, H.K.; Computed tomography of the body, Philadelphia, 1983, W.B. Saunders Co.

81. Mubarak, S.J., et al.: The medial tibial stress syndrome: a cause of shin splints, Am. J. Sports Med. **10:**201, 1982.

82. Mubarak, S., and Hargens, S.: Exertional compartment syndromes. In Mack, R., ed.: AAOS Symposium on the foot and leg in running sports, St. Louis, 1982, The C.V. Mosby Co.

83. Mubarak, S.J., et al.: The wick catheter technique for measurement of intramuscular pressure: a new research and clinical tool, J. Bone Joint Surg. **58A:**1016, 1976.

84. Mubarak, S.J., and Owens, C.A.: Double incision fasciotomy of the leg for decompression and

compartment syndromes, J. Bone Joint Surg. **59A**:184, 1977.

85. Mubarak, S.J., Owen, C.A., Garfin, S., and Hargens, S.J.: Acute exertional superficial posterior compartment syndrome, Am. J. Sports Med. **6**:287, 1978.

86. Meurman, K.O.A., and Elfving, S.; Stress fractures in soldiers: a multifocal bone disorder, Radiology **134**:483, 1980.

87. Nistor, L.: Conservative treatment of fresh subcutaneous rupture of the Achilles tendon, Acta Orthop. Scand. **47**:459, 1976.

88. Nistor, L.: Surgical and non-surgical treatment of Achilles tendon ruptures, J. Bone Joint Surg. **63A**:394, 1981.

89. Noyes, F.R.: Functional properties of knee ligaments and alterations induced by immobilization, Clin. Orthop. **123**:210, 1977.

90. Orava, S., Puranen, J., and Ala-Ketola, L.: Stress fractures caused by physical exercise, Acta Orthop. Scand. **49**:19, 1978.

91. Pentecost, R.L., et al.: Fatigue insufficency in pathologic fractures, JAMA **187**:1001, 1964.

92. Puddu, G., Ippolito, E., and Postacchini, F.: Classification of Achilles tendon disease, Am. J. Sports Med. **4**:145, 1976.

93. Puranen, J.: The medial tibial syndrome, J. Bone Joint Surg. **56B**:712, 1974.

94. Puranen, J., Alavaikko, A.: Intracompartmental pressure increased on exertion in patients with chronic compartment syndrome in the leg, J. Bone Joint Surg. **63A**:1304, 1981.

95. Quenuj, R.S., and Stoianovitch, L.: Ruptures to tendon d'Achille. Rev. Chir. **67**:647, 1929.

96. Quorfordt, P., et al.: Intramuscular pressure, muscle blood flow, and skeletal muscle metabolism in chronic anterior tibial compartment syndrome. Clin. Orthop. **179**:284, 1983.

97. Reneman, R.S.: The anterior and lateral compartment syndromes of the leg, The Hague, 1968, Mouton Publishers.

98. Reneman, R.S.: The anterior and lateral compartmental syndrome of the leg due to intensive use of the muscles. Clin. Orthop. **113**:69, 1975.

99. Rorabeck, C.H., Bourn, R.B., and Fowler, P.J.: Tibiofibular synostosis and recurrent ankle sprains in high performance athletes, Am. J. Sports Med. **6**:204, 1978.

100. Roub, L.W., et al.: Bone stress: a radionuclide imaging perspective, Radiology **132**:431, 1979.

101. Shields, C.L., et al.: The Cybex II evaluation of surgical repair to Achilles tendon ruptures, Am. J. Sports Med. y:369, 978.

102. Siddiqui, A.R.: Bone scans for early detection of stress fractures, N. Engl. J. Med. **298**:1033, 1978.

103. Sjostrom, M., et al.: Achilles tendon injury plantar flexion strength and structure of the soleus muscle after surgical repair, Acta Chir. Scand. **144**:219, 1978.

104. Somer, K., and Meurman, K.O.A.: Computed tomography of stress fractures, J. Comput. Assist. Tomogr. **6**:109, 1982.

105. Stechow, A.W.: Fussoedem und Roentgenstrahlen, Dtsch. Mil-Aerztl Zeitg. **26**:465, 1897.

106. Strait, J.L.: Early diagnosis of stress fractures by bone scintography. Presented at Dallas American Academy of Orthopedic Surgeons, February 27, 1978.

107. Symeonides, P.P.: High stress fracture of the fibula, J. Bone Joint Surg. **42B**:508, 1960.

108. Thompson, T.C., and Doherty, J.H.: Spontaneous rupture of the tendon of Achilles: a new clinical diagnostic test, J. Trauma **2**:126, 1962.

109. Vogt, P.R.: Ischemic muscular necrosis following marching. Unpublished paper, Oregon State Medical Society Meeting, September 4, 1943, cited by C.E. Horn, 1945.

110. Wallenstein, R.: Results of fasciotomy in patients with medial tibial stress syndrome or chronic anterior compartment syndrome, J. Bone Joint Surg. **65A**:1252, 1983.

111. Wallenstein, R. and Eriksson, E.: Is medial lower leg pain (shin splint) a chronic compartment syndrome? In Mack, R.P., ed.: AAOS symposium on the foot and leg in running injuries. C.V. Mosby St Louis, 1982.

112. Wallenstein, R., and Karlsson, J.: Histochemical and metabolic changes in lower leg muscle in exercised-induced pain, Int. J. Sports Med. **5**:31, 1984.

113. Weaver, J., and Francisco, C.: Pseudofractures, J. Bone Joint Surg. **22A**:610, 1940.

114. Whiteside, L.A., Reynolds, F.C., and Ellasser, J.C.: Tibiofibular synostosis and recurrent ankle sprains in high performance athletes, Am. J. Sports Med. **6**:204, 1978.

115. Whitesides, T.E., et al.: Tissue pressure measurements as a determinant for the need of fasciotomy, Clin. Orthop. **113**:43, 1975.

116. Wilcox, J.R., Moniot, A.L., and Green, J.P.: Bone scan in the evaluation of exercise-related stress injuries, Radiology **123**:699, 1977.

117. Wright, S.: Applied physiology, ed. 10, London, 1961, Oxford University Press.

ADDITIONAL READINGS

Bates, B.T., et al.: Foot orthotic devices to modify selected aspects of lower extremity mechanics, Am. J. Sports Med. **7**:338, 1979.

Clement, D.B., Taunton, J.E., and Smart, G.W.: Achilles tendinitis and peritendinitis: etiology and treatment, Am. J. Sports Med. **12**:179, 1984.

Carter, A.B., Richards, R.L., and Zachary, R.B.: The anterior tibial syndrome, Lancet **2**:928, 1949.

Clement, D.B.: Tibial stress syndrome in athletes, Am. J. Sports Med. **2**:81, 1974.

Clancy, W.G., Neidhart, D., and Brand, R.L.: Achilles tendinitis in runners—a report of five cases, Am. J. Sports Med. **4**:46, 1976.

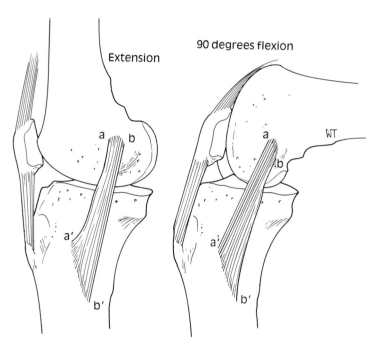

Fig. 22-7 ■ Effect of joint motion on superficial MCL. During flexion, knee tightens *A-A'* and conversely, during extension, *B-B'* tightens.

stressing of the knee following an incision in the superficial MCL alone was 4 to 5 mm, with the maximum at 30 to 40 degrees of flexion. Subsequently, incising the deep MCL led to a small statistically insignificant increase in valgus opening.[33] If the deep MCL, oblique portion of the MCL, and posterior capsule were incised initially, no significant increment in valgus opening was seen. However, following resection of the only remaining medial structure, the superficial MCL, 5 to 7 mm of opening were seen, with the maximum at 30 degrees.[33]

FUNCTIONS OF THE SUPERFICIAL MCL

- Primary restraint against valgus stress
- Prevention of external rotation of tibia on the femur
- Secondary restraint against anterior tibial translation (with absent ACL)

A second function of the medial structures is to prevent external rotation of the tibia on the femur. Following sectioning of the deep MCL, a minimal increase in external rotation of the tibia was noted. Incising the oblique fibers of the MCL and posterior capsule as well had only a minimal affect. When the superficial MCL was also cut, a near doubling effect of external tibial rotation with the knee at 0 degrees of flexion was seen. This effect was magnified if the knee was flexed, resulting in a tripling of external rotation from 6 to 18 degrees at 90 degrees of flexion.

If the sequence was reversed, most of the increment in external rotation was seen by sectioning only the superficial MCL.[33]

A third function of the superficial MCL is as a secondary restraint against anterior tibial translation if the ACL was absent. We have noted that sectioning all of the structures of the medial side of the knee, including the superficial MCL, oblique fibers, deep MCL, and capsule will not increase anterior tibial translation if the ACL is intact.[31] Conversely, if the ACL is incised first, then sectioning the superficial MCL will significantly increase the anterior tibial translation. However, no such effect is seen by sectioning the oblique fibers of the MCL, posterior capsule, or deep MCL.

Thus it is concluded that the superficial MCL is the prime static support against a valgus stress. It is an important restraint against external tibial rotation and a secondary restraint against anterior tibial translation if the ACL is absent. The oblique portion of the MCL and the deep MCL appear to play no role in preventing anterior tibial translation with or without an intact ACL. If the ACL is intact, they contribute minimally to valgus resistance and only after the superficial MCL is incised. It would appear likely that they would help to resist further valgus opening if both the ACL and superficial MCL were injured.

■ LATERAL ASPECT OF THE KNEE

Injuries to the lateral side of the knee, while relatively uncommon, have a complex anatomy that requires a sound understanding to enable the surgeon to restore these tissues to their proper anatomic alignment.

Surgical anatomy

In reviewing the lateral side of the knee it is useful once again to think in terms of a three-layer concept. As discussed by Seebacher et al., layer one consists of the fascia lata with its thickening, the iliotibial band tract[30] (Fig. 22-8, A, and 22-9). This layer extends posteriorly to include the biceps tendon and the posterior expansion, which lies over the peroneal nerve. Anteriorly it extends to the patella and includes the layer of the prepatellar bursa. (see Figs. 22-8, A, and 22-9)

Anteriorly, layer two is formed by the patellar retinaculum, which is adherent to layer one at the edge of the patella. Posteriorly (Fig. 22-8, B), layer two is incomplete, with extensions to the lateral intermuscular septum, fabella, lateral meniscus, and tibia. Proximally, the patellofemoral ligament includes components to

the lateral intermuscular septum and others to the fabella (see Fig. 22-8, B). More distally, the fibers insert on the meniscus, forming the meniscopatellar ligament. These fibers thus run from the patella to the lateral meniscus with extensions to Gerdy's tubercle. Layers one and two are adherent not only at the edge of the patella; some fibers from the patellofemoral ligament join the iliotibial band (layer one) just distal to the lateral intermuscular system.

Layer three forms the lateral part of the joint capsule, attaching directly to the femur proximally and tibia distally, to form an attachment to the meniscus that extends to the tibia as the coronary ligament (see Fig. 22-9). Anteriorly, this layer is separate and deep to layer two. Just posterior to the iliotibial band, layer three divides into two layers, separated by the inferior genicular artery (Figs. 22-9 and 22-10). The superficial portion of layer three encompasses the lateral collateral ligament (LCL) and terminates at the fabellofibular ligament. The deeper portion of layer three is the more recently developed portion of the capsule evolutionarily, having formed as the fibula receded from its articulation with the femur.[30] The deeper portion of layer three passes along the edge of the lateral meniscus (Fig. 22-11), forming the coronary ligament. A hiatus within this layer allows for passage of the popliteus tendon. The deeper lamina of layer three ends at the arcuate ligament, which crosses the popliteus muscle running from the styloid process of the fibula to join the posterior oblique ligament on the femur.

Three anatomic variations of the arcuate and fabellofibular ligaments are

ANATOMIC VARIATIONS OF THE ARCUATE AND FABELLOFIBULAR LIGAMENTS	
Arcuate ligament alone	13%
Fabellofibular ligament alone	20%
Both present	67%

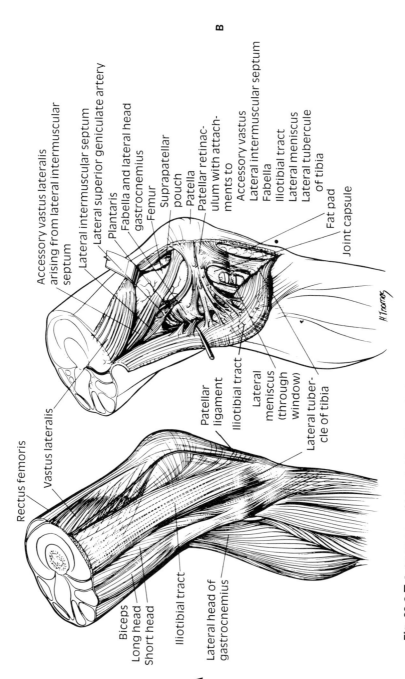

Fig. 22-8 ■ **A,** Layer one of lateral side of knee, including iliotibial tract and biceps. **B,** Layer two, including patellar retinaculum and patellofemoral and patellomeniscal ligaments.

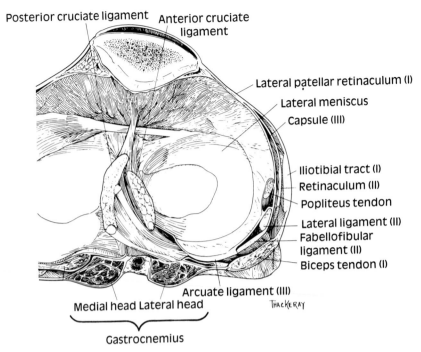

Posterior cruciate ligament   Anterior cruciate
ligament

Lateral patellar retinaculum (I)

Lateral meniscus

Capsule (III)

Iliotibial tract (I)
Retinaculum (II)
Popliteus tendon
Lateral ligament (II)
Fabellofibular
ligament (II)
Biceps tendon (I)

Arcuate ligament (III)

THACKERAY

Medial head   Lateral head

Gastrocnemius

Fig. 22-9 ■ Cross-section demonstrating layered approach to lateral side of knee.

noted in this region. In 13% of specimens, the arcuate ligament alone was seen reinforcing the capsule posteriorly. In 20%, only the fabellofibular ligament was seen, while in 67%, both structures were present. These variations could be predicted by the presence or absence of a fabella. When the fabella is large or robust, a large

---

**RELATIONSHIP OF ARCUATE AND
FABELLOFIBULAR LIGAMENTS
TO FABELLA**

Large fabella → Robust fabellofibular ligament

Absent fabella → Large arcuate ligament

---

fabellofibular ligament is seen, but if it is absent, the arcuate ligament predominates.[30] In fact, Last pointed out that there is a such a complexity of fiber arrangement at this site that careful dissection can make almost any pattern desired.[20] However, it appears that there are two limbs of the arcuate ligament, a medial

and a denser lateral ligament. Both come from the fibular styloid process, with the medial branch arching over the popliteus tendon to join the oblique ligament and the lateral extending to the femur and popliteus tendon. The popliteus muscle arises from the posterior tibial surface and has two insertion sites (Fig. 22-12). Generally, a large portion of the muscle inserts directly into the posterior portion of the lateral meniscus to insert on the femur deep and anterior to the LCL.

Last has noted that the popliteus muscle insertion acts to hold the lateral meniscus posteriorly as knee flexion occurs.[20] In crossing the lateral meniscus the tendinous portion of the popliteus muscle creates an opening in the deep lamina of layer three, but it is still extraarticular, because it is covered by synovium. The region over the meniscus is generally free, but in some specimens Last has noted an attachment of the popliteus tendon to the meniscus.

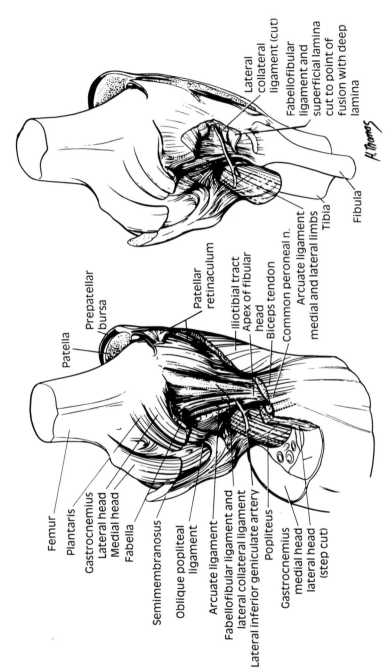

Fig. 22-10 ■ Dissection demonstrating layer three. Posteriorly, this layer divides into superficial and deep lamina separated by inferior genicular artery.

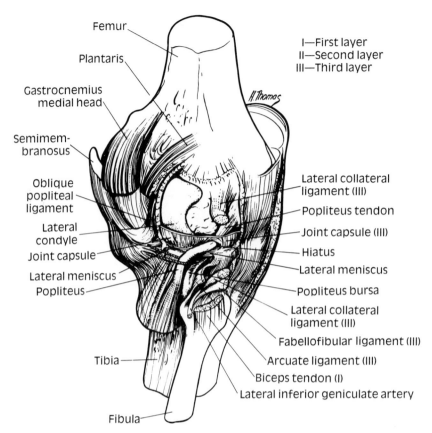

Femur

Plantaris

Gastrocnemius
medial head

Semimem-
branosus

Oblique
popliteal
ligament

Lateral
condyle

Joint capsule

Lateral meniscus
Popliteus

Tibia

Fibula

I—First layer
II—Second layer
III—Third layer

H. Thomas

Lateral collateral
ligament (III)

Popliteus tendon

Joint capsule (III)

Hiatus

Lateral meniscus

Popliteus bursa

Lateral collateral
ligament (III)

Fabellofibular ligament (III)

Arcuate ligament (III)

Biceps tendon (I)

Lateral inferior geniculate artery

Fig. 22-11 ■ Posterolateral view demonstrating popliteus tendon and muscle with its insertion into lateral meniscus.

POSTERIOR ATTACHMENTS OF LATERAL MENISCUS
Slip from popliteus
Ligaments of Wrisberg and Humphrey (variable)

MENISCOFEMORAL LIGAMENTS
Ligament of Wrisberg—Posterior to PCL
Ligament of Humphrey—Anterior to PCL

Two additional ligaments play a role in the function of the lateral meniscus as described by Last. These are the ligaments of Wrisberg and Humphrey. These ligaments pass from the posterior horn of the lateral meniscus to the medial femoral condyle. The ligament of Wrisberg lies posterior to the posterior cruciate ligament (PCL), and the ligament of Humphrey lies anterior (see Fig. 22-12, *B*). These ligaments are not uniformly pres-ent, being noted by Heller and Langman in only 35% of their specimens.[14] The ligament of Humphrey can be quite large and create problems in diagnosing damage to the PCL when viewed anteriorly. Last felt that these ligaments exist to hold the posterior arch of the lateral meniscus in a constant relationship to the femur, thus preventing injury in flexion and external rotation of the femur.[20]

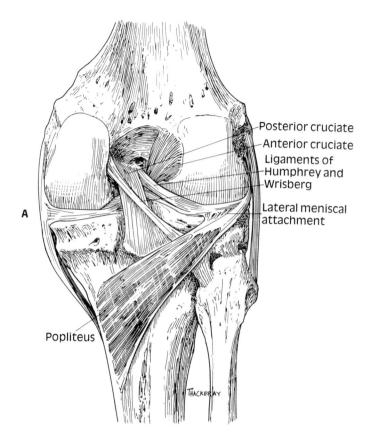

Posterior cruciate

Anterior cruciate

Ligaments of Humphrey and Wrisberg

Lateral meniscal attachment

A

Popliteus

THACKERAY

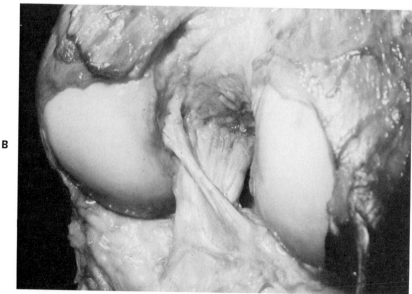

B

Fig. 22-12 ■ **A,** Posterior view of knee demonstrating popliteus muscle origin. **B,** Anatomic dissection depicting PCL and ligament of Wrisberg.
B from the ISMAT Collection.

Table 22-1 ■ Static constraints of the posterolateral aspect of the knee

	LCL*	Deep†	LCL and deep	PCL*	PCL and deep and LCL
Varus rotation	Maximum of 3.6 degrees at 30 degrees of flexion	No effect	↑ of 8.9 degrees at 30 degrees of flexion	No effect	↑ of 15.6 degrees at 60 degrees of flexion
External rotation	No effect	↑ of 5.8 degrees at 90 degrees of flexion	↑ of 14 degrees at 30 degrees of flexion	No effect	Extension—no change 90 degrees of flexion—of 9.5 degrees
Posterior tibial translation	No effect	No effect	↑ of 3-4 mm at 30 degrees of flexion	↑ Maximal at 60-90 degrees of flexion	At 30 degrees note 3.5 times excursion over isolated PCL

From Gollehon, D.L., Warren, R.F., and Torzilli, P.A.: The role of the posterior lateral and cruciate ligaments in human knee stability, J. Bone Joint Surg. (In press.)
*LCL, Lateral collateral ligament; PCL, Posterior cruciate ligament.
†Popliteus tendon and arcuate ligament.

Functional anatomy

The anatomy of the posterolateral corner of the knee appears to play a combined role in varus, anterior and posterior translation of the tibia on the femur, and internal and external rotation (Table 22-1).

In our selective cutting experiments we have not seen any increase in anterior tibial translation as long as the ACL is intact, regardless of which tissues are incised laterally. In contrast, we have found that posterior tibial translation will occur after incising the LCL and popliteus tendon complex despite an intact PCL.[11] This increment is small (3 to 5 mm) but significant. More importantly, we have noted marked increments in rotation externally after incising the LCL and popliteus. Incising either the LCL or popliteus alone did not provide enough of an increment to be statistically significant, but the combined cuts were highly significant, averaging 15 to 20 degrees. Incising the PCL alone did not increase forced external tibial rotation, but cutting the PCL after the LCL and popliteus tendon resulted in a further increment.

Incising the ACL alone has not significantly increased either internal or external rotation, but this changes dramatically if the LCL and popliteus are incised first. In this situation, large increments in both external and internal tibial rotation are seen.[24]

In reference to varus opening, we have found only small increments by incising the LCL. These have increased considerably if the popliteus was also incised.

It would appear that the LCL and popliteus act in concert in preventing varus opening, external tibial rotation, and posterior displacement. This effect will vary with the degree of knee flexion.

The popliteus muscle-tendon unit appears to be able to function both as a muscle and as a ligament. The key to this is the tibial attachment site, which is quite broad. If tension is placed in a distal direction on the muscle fibers, considerable motion is seen. In contrast, if the tendon is grasped proximally and a proximal force exerted, very little motion is seen, even if the entire joint attachments are incised. This would suggest that the popliteus muscle-tendon unit performs as a ligament in a proximal direction, but in a distal direction it functions as a muscle, creating internal tibial rotation.

muscle unit in the body. The quadriceps is essentially a uniarticular muscle unit; only the rectus femoris spans two joints, with its origin from direct and indirect heads located just anterior to the hip joint. The remainder of the quadriceps, the vastus lateralis, vastus intermedius, and vastus medialis, take origin from essentially the anterior one half of the femur. The rectus femoris makes up only about 15% of the cross-sectional area of the quadriceps femoris,[35] and this muscles' function as a hip flexor is minimal and secondary. The primary function of the quadriceps during gait is to prevent collapse of the flexing knee from heel strike to midstance. Indeed, its electromyographic activity ceases when the body's center of gravity passes anterior to the axis of the knee joint. The common point of attachment for the four muscles is the patella, the largest sesamoid bone in the body. The fibers of attachment of the rectus femoris continue over the anterior surface of the patella and become confluent with the patellar ligament. The pinnation angles (attachment angles) of the vastus lateralis are slight, 5 to 10 degrees, in a lateral direction. The fibers of the vastus intermedius are almost straight, as are the bulk of the fibers from the vastus medialis. Only the terminal portion of the vastus medialis, the so-called vastus medialis obliquus, diverges from this pattern: it has a variably increasing pinnation, approximately 50 to 60 degrees, as it inserts into the medial portion of the patella. Anatomically, the vastus medialis obliquus is *not* a separate muscle,[35] but rather a continuous extension of the vastus medialis. The same is true when muscle activity is measured electromyographically, as shown by Perry.[27] The four heads function as a unit, without a selective increase in activity in the vastus medialis obliquus during terminal extension.

The patella is integral to the function of the quadriceps mechanism. Technically a sesamoid bone, the patella is located in the tendon of the quadriceps muscle. Its anterior surface has the shape of a rounded triangle with the apex inferior and the primary tendinous-ligamentous attachments at the superior and inferior poles. The blood supply to the patella has been described by Scapinelli,[28] and it enters primarily through orifices located in the middle of the anterior surface. The posterior surface of the patella is oval in shape, and the articular cartilage on its surface is the thickest in the human body. The articular surface is divided into facets, the largest being the lateral facet. The longitudinal ridge separates the lateral from the medial facet. A second ridge subdivides the medial half into medial and odd facets. Additional soft tissue attachments are the medial and lateral patellar retinacula, extensions of the quadriceps tendon. Medially, this retinaculum is confluent with the fused layers one and two of the medial side of the knee. Laterally, discrete thickening, such as the epicondylopatellar or lateral patellofemoral ligament of Kaplan, can be identified.

The distal end of the femur articulates with the patella by means of the femoral trochlea, which is made up of a lateral and medial facet. The lateral is the larger, being both longer and taller an average of 5 mm, according to Cassalls. The trochlea blends with fibrocartilage into the supratrochlear fat pad, which has a synovial covering. Medially, a ridge has been described by Outerbridge at the entrance to the trochlea groove, with the postulate that it contributes to the etiology of medial facet chondromalacia.[26]

There have been numerous descriptions of both clinical and roentgenographic determinants of patellar position with respect to the femur and the rest of the leg (Fig. 22-17). One of the more common is the Q angle, a clinical measure, which is the angle subtended by connecting the central point on the patella with the anterior superior iliac spine above and the tibial tubercle below. Normal values average 15 degrees plus or minus 3, according to Insall et al.[16] The lateral tracking vector, or valgus vector, is a clinical measure of lateral movement of the pa-

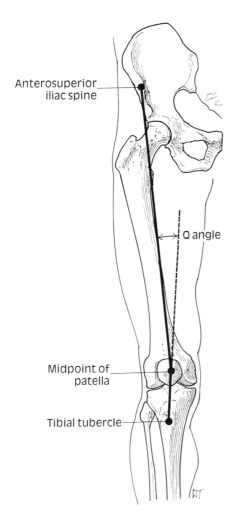

Anterosuperior
iliac spine

Q angle

Midpoint of
patella

Tibial tubercle

Fig. 22-17 ■ Diagrammatic representation of quadriceps, or Q angle.

tella. Performed with the knee in full extension, it is a measure of the sudden lateral shift of the patella associated with quadriceps contraction.

Roentgenographically, the common measures of patellar position are the Merchant angle,[25] the lateral patellofemoral angle, and the patellofemoral index of Laurin.*[7] Normal Merchant angles are −6 degrees (medial) with a standard deviation of 11 degrees. The Laurin angle should open laterally in the normal patient. Pa-

tella alta, as defined by Insall and Salvati,[17] is a measure of patellar tendon length and patellar height as determined on the lateral roentgenograms. Normal values are up to a ratio of 1:2.

■ PATELLOFEMORAL CONTACT

Goodfellow,[12] using a contrast method, has demonstrated that initial patellofemoral contact occurs at approximately 20 degrees of knee flexion along the inferior margin of the patella in a narrow, broad, continuous band across both the medial and lateral facets. As flexion of the knee proceeds, the contact area moves superiorly on the patella from the ridge between the odd and medial facets to the lateral facet (Fig. 22-18). The odd facet fails to make contact until about 135 degrees of knee flexion, and here it comes into contact with the lateral margin of the medial femoral condyle. Up to about 90 degrees of knee flexion, only the articular surface of the patella is in contact with the trochlea; past 90 degrees, the broad quadriceps tendon begins to make contact with the trochlear groove. Patellofemoral contact areas[9] increase up to about 90 degrees of the knee flexion. However, load is increasing at the same time and at a greater degree, so that force-per-unit area is also increasing through flexion. It is of note that these increasing loads occur in models in which knee flexion is resisted. When viewed with regard to the extending knee, there is a decrease in patellofemoral contact area at the same time there is an increase in load. Lieb and Perry[22] have shown that almost twice the quadriceps force is needed for the terminal 15 degrees of extension for the arc of motion from 90 degrees to −15 degrees.

Viewed clinically, the patellar tracking is a gentle C, open laterally.[15] In the terminal 20 degrees of extension, stability is affected only by the soft tissues. Once the patella has entered the trochlea, bony contact and compressive forces add functional stability to the joint.

---

*See Chapter 26 for details of techniques.

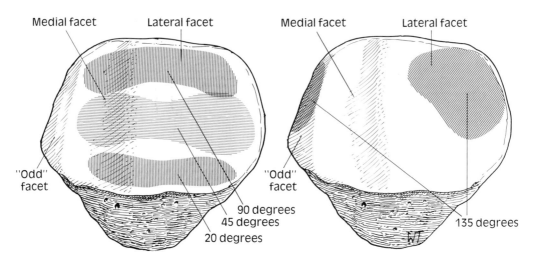

Fig. 22-18 ■ Patellar contact areas with increasing knee flexion. There is superior migration of the contact area of patella.

■ ANATOMY OF THE CRUCIATE LIGAMENTS
Anterior cruciate Ligament (ACL)

The ACL is attached to a fossa on the posterior aspect of the medial surface of the lateral femoral condyle. The femoral attachment is in the form of a segment of a circle, with its anterior border straight and its posterior border convex. Its long axis is tiled slightly forward from the vertical, and the posterior convexity is parallel to the posterior articular margin of the lateral femoral condyle[2,10] (Fig. 22-19).

The tibial attachment of the ACL is a fossa in front of and lateral to the anterior tibial spine. At this attachment the ACL passes beneath the transverse meniscal ligament, and a few fascicles of the ACL may blend with the anterior attachment of the lateral meniscus. In some instances, fascicles from the posterior aspect of the tibial attachment of the ACL may extend to and blend with the posterior attachment of the lateral meniscus. The tibial attachment of the ACL is somewhat wider and stronger than the femoral attachment[2,10] (Fig. 22-20).

The ACL courses anteriorly, medially, and distally across the joint as it passes from the femur to the tibia. As it does, it twists on itself in a slight outward (lateral) spiral. This is because of the orientation of its bony attachments. The orientation of the femoral attachment of the ACL, with regard to joint position (flexion-extension), is also responsible for the relative tension of the ligament throughout the range of motion.[10]

The ACL is attached to the femur and tibia not as a singular cord but rather as a collection of individual fascicles that fan out over a broad, flattened area[2,10,19,34] (Fig. 22-21). These fascicles have been summarily divided into two groups: the anteromedial band (AMB), those fascicles originating at the proximal aspect of the femoral attachment and inserting at the anteromedial aspect of the tibial attachment; and the posterolateral bulk (PLB), the remaining bulk of fascicles, which are inserted at the posterolateral aspect of the tibial attachment. When the knee is extended, the PLB is taut, while the AMB is moderately lax. However, as the knee is flexed, the femoral attachment of the ACL assumes a more horizontal orientation, causing the AMB to tighten and the PLB to loosen[2,10] (Fig. 22-22).

While this designation provides a general idea as to the dynamics of the ACL through the range of motion, it is an over-

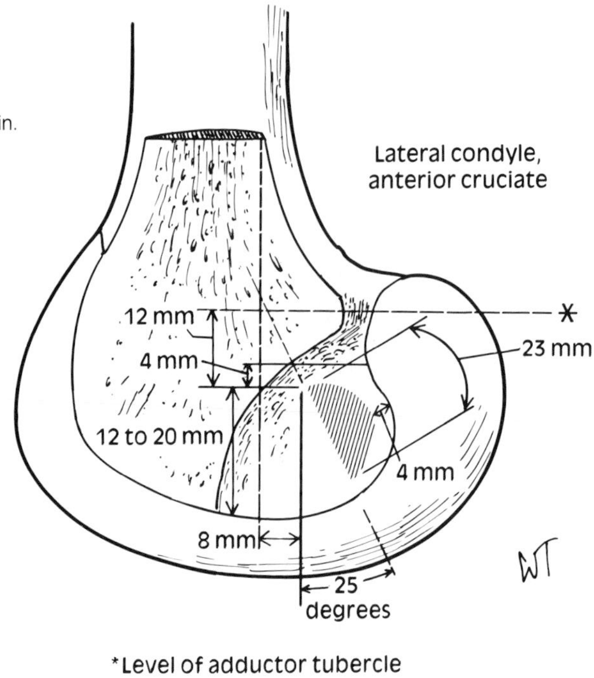

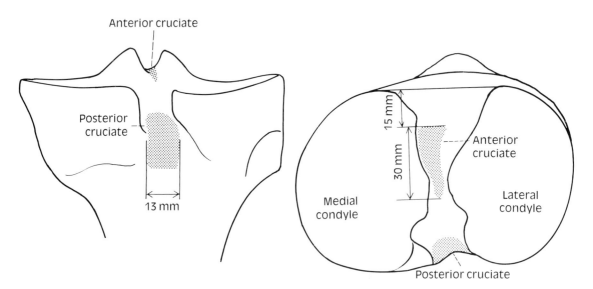

Fig. 22-19 ■ Drawing of medial surface of right lateral femoral condyle, showing average measurements and body relations of femoral attachment of ACL.
From Girgis, F.G., Marshall, J.L., and Monajem, A.R.S.: Clin. Orthop. **106**:216, 1975.

Lateral condyle, anterior cruciate

12 mm

4 mm

12 to 20 mm

8 mm

23 mm

4 mm

25 degrees

✳

*Level of adductor tubercle

Anterior cruciate

Posterior cruciate

13 mm

15 mm

30 mm

Anterior cruciate

Lateral condyle

Medial condyle

Posterior cruciate

Fig. 22-20 ■ Drawing of tibial plateau showing average measurements and relations of tibial attachment of anterior and posterior cruciate ligaments.
From Girgis, F.G., Marshall, J.L., and Monajem, A.R.S.: Clin. Orthop. **106**:216, 1975.

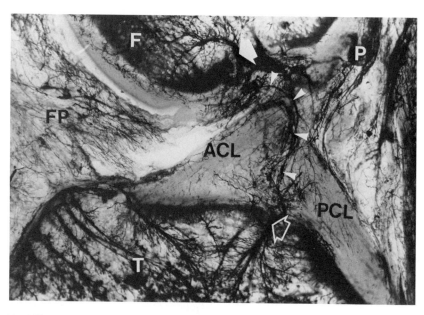

Fig. 22-30 ■ A 5 mm thick sagittal section of human knee joint (Spalteholz technique) showing vascularity of cruciate ligaments. Branches of middle genicular artery supply cruciate ligaments (small white arrows) as well as distal femoral epiphysis (large closed white arrow) and proximal tibial epiphysis (large open white arrow). *F,* femur, *T,* tibia; *FP,* infrapatellar fat pad; *P,* popliteal artery; *ACL,* anterior cruciate ligament; *PCL,* posterior cruciate ligament.

of the ligament and the fact that these fascicles tighten and loosen through the range of motion.

Blood supply to the cruciate ligaments

The blood supply to the ACL and PCL arises from the ligamentous branches of the middle genicular artery as well as some terminal branches of the inferior genicular arteries.[2,23,29]

The cruciate ligaments are covered by a synovial fold that originates at the posterior inlet of the intercondylar notch and extends to the anterior tibial insertion of the ligament, where it joins the synovial tissue of the joint capsule distal to the infrapatellar fat pad. This synovial membrane, which forms an envelope about the ligaments, is richly endowed with vessels that originate predominantly from the ligamentous branches of the middle genicular artery (Fig. 22-30). A few smaller terminal branches of the lateral and medial inferior genicular arteries also contribute some vessels to this synovial plexus

through its connection with the infrapatellar fat pad. The synovial vessels arborize to form a weblike network of periligamentous vessels, which ensheath the entire ligament (Fig. 22-31). These periligamentous vessels then give rise to smaller connecting branches, which penetrate the ligament transversely and anastamose with a network of endoligamentous vessels (Fig. 22-32). These vessels, along with their supporting connective tissues, are oriented in a longitudinal direction and lie parallel to the collagen bundles within the ligament.[2,23]

The blood supply to the ACL and PCL is predominantly of soft tissue origin. While the middle genicular artery gives off additional branches to the distal femoral epiphysis and proximal tibial epiphysis, the ligamentous-osseous junctions of the cruciate ligaments do not contribute significantly to the vascular scheme of the ligaments themselves[2,23] (Fig. 22-33).

Although the PCL is in intimate contact

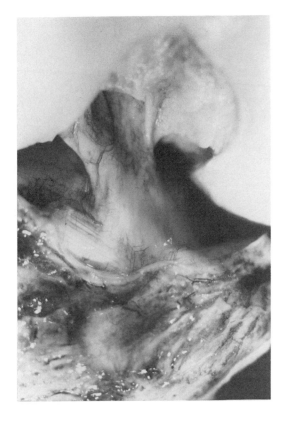

Fig. 22-31 ■ Human knee specimen injected with
India ink to show weblike network of
periligamentous vessels that ensheathes ACL.
From Arnoczky, S.P.: Orthop. Clin. North Am. **16:** 15, 1985.

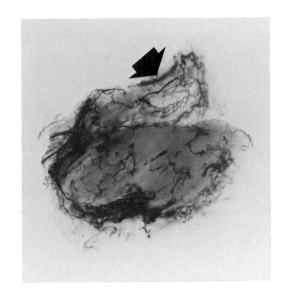

Fig. 22-32 ■ Cross-section of human ACL
(Spalteholz technique) demonstrating
periligamentous as well as endoligamentous
vasculature. Fold of synovial membrane (arrow)
can be seen supplying vessels to synovial covering
of the ligament.
Arnoczky, S.P.: Clin. Orthop. **172:**19, 1983.

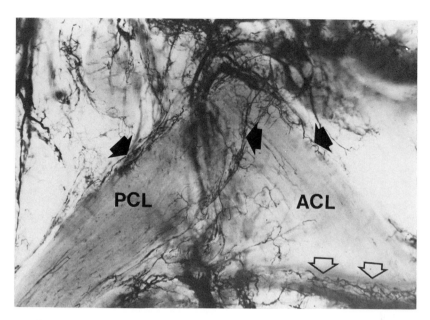

Fig. 22-33 ■ A 5 mm thick sagittal section of human knee joint (Spalteholz technique) showing periligamentous vasculature (black closed arrows) of anterior cruciate ligament *(ACL)* and posterior cruciate ligament *(PCL)*. Note that ligamentous osseous attachment of ligament (black open arrows) does not provide any vessels to vascular scheme of ligament.
Arnoczky, S.P.: Clin. Orthop. **16**:15, 1985.

with the ligamentous branches of the middle genicular artery and the vascular synovial tissue of the posterior joint capsule, there is no evidence to suggest that the PCL has a better vascular supply than the ACL.

Nerve supply to the cruciate ligaments

The cruciate ligaments receive nerve fibers from branches of the tibial nerve. These fibers penetrate the joint capsule posteriorly and course along with the synovial and periligamentous vessels surrounding the ligament. Smaller nerve fibers have also been observed throughout the substance of the ligament.[19] While the majority of fibers are associated with the endoligamentous vasculature and appear to have a vasomotor function, some fibers have been observed to lie alone among the fascicles of the ligament. It has been suggested that these fibers may serve some type of proprioceptive or sensory function.[19]

■ MENISCI
Anatomy of the menisci

The menisci are C-shaped discs of fibrocartilage interposed between the condyles of the femur and tibia. Properly regarded as functional extensions of the tibia, the menisci serve to deepen the surfaces of the articular fossae of the head of the tibia for reception of the condyles of the femur. The peripheral border of each meniscus is thick, convex, and attached to the inside capsule of the joint; the opposite border tapers to a thin, free edge.[13] The proximal surfaces of the menisci are concave and in contact with the condyles of the femur; their distal surfaces are flat and rest on the head of the tibia (Fig. 22-34).

The medial meniscus is somewhat semicircular in form. It is approximately 3.5 cm in length and considerably wider posteriorly than it is anteriorly[6,13] (Figs. 22-35 and 22-36). The anterior horn of the medial meniscus is attached to the tibial

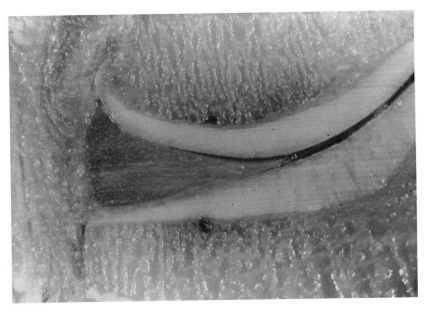

Fig. 22-34 ■ Frontal section of medial compartment of knee illustrating articulation of meniscus with condyles of femur and tibia.

plateau in the area of the anterior intercondylar fossa in front of the ACL. The posterior fibers of the anterior horn attachment merge with the transverse ligament, which connects the anterior horns of the medial and lateral menisci[13] (see Fig. 22-35). The posterior horn of the medial meniscus is firmly attached to the posterior intercondylar fossa of the tibia between the attachments of the lateral meniscus and the PCL. The periphery of the medial meniscus is attached to the joint capsule throughout its length. The tibial portion of this capsular attachment is often referred to as the coronary ligament.[13] At its midpoint, the medial meniscus is more firmly attached to the femur and tibia through a condensation in the joint capsule known as the deep medial ligament.[13]

The lateral meniscus is almost circular and covers a larger portion of the tibial articular surface than the medial meniscus; it is approximately the same width from front to back (see Figs. 22-35 and 22-36). The anterior horn of the lateral meniscus is attached to the tibia in front of the in-

tercondylar eminence and behind the attachment of the ACL, with which it partially blends. The posterior horn of the lateral meniscus is attached behind the intercondylar eminence of the tibia in front of the posterior end of the medial meniscus (see Fig. 22-36). While there is no attachment of the lateral meniscus to the LCL, there is a loose peripheral attachment to the joint capsule.

Several ligaments run from the posterior horn of the lateral meniscus to the medial femoral condyle, either just in front of or behind the origin of the PCL.[6] These are the ligaments of Humphrey (the anterior meniscofemoral ligament) and Wrisberg (the posterior meniscofemoral ligament).[6]

Blood supply to the menisci

The vascular supply to the medial and lateral menisci of the knee originates predominantly from the lateral and medial geniculate arteries (both inferior and superior). Branches from these vessels give rise to a perimeniscal capillary plexus within the synovial and capsular tissues of

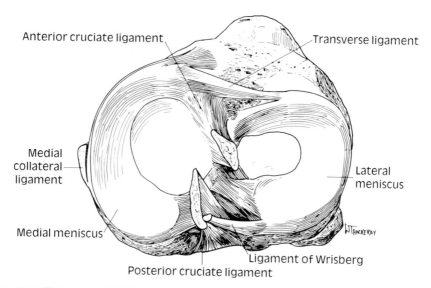

Fig. 22-35 ■ Drawing of tibial plateau showing shape and attachments of medial and lateral menisci.

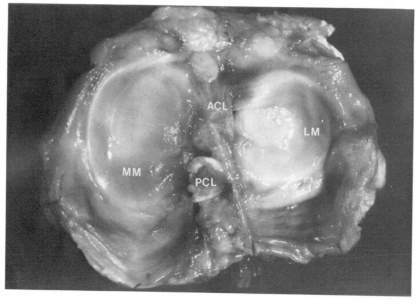

Fig. 22-36 ■ Photograph of tibial plateau illustrating position and shape of medial and lateral menisci.

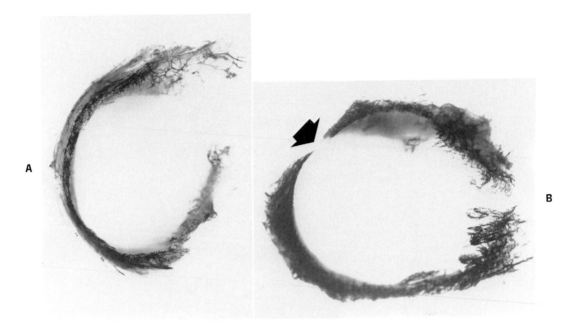

Fig. 22-37 ■ Superior aspect of medial **(A)** and lateral **(B)** menisci following vascular perfusion with India ink and tissue clearing using modified Spalteholz technique. Note vascularity at periphery of menisci as well as at anterior and posterior horn attachments. Absence of peripheral vasculature at posterolateral corner of lateral meniscus (arrow) represents area of passage of popliteal tendon.
From Arnoczky, S.P., and Warren, R.F.: Am. J. Sports Med. **10:**90, 1982.

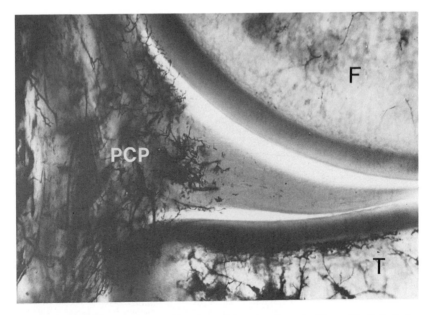

Fig. 22-38 ■ A 5 mm thick frontal section of medial compartment of knee (Spalteholz times three). Branching radial vessels from perimeniscal capillary plexus *(PCP)* can be seen penetrating peripheral border of medial meniscus. *F,* femur; *T,* tibia.
From Arnoczky, S.P., and Warren, R.F.: Am. J. Sports Med. **10:**90, 1982.

the knee joint. This plexus is an arborizing network of vessels that supplies the peripheral border of the meniscus throughout its attachment to the joint capsule[3] (Fig. 22-37). These perimeniscal vessels are oriented in a predominantly circumferential pattern, with radial branches directed toward the center of the joint (Fig. 22-38). Anatomic studies have shown that the degree of vascular penetration is 10% to 30% of the width of the medial meniscus and 10% to 25% of the width of the lateral meniscus.

The middle genicular artery, along with a few terminal branches of the medial and lateral genicular arteries, also supplies vessels to the menisci through the vascular synovial covering of the anterior and posterior horn attachments. These synovial vessels penetrate the horn attachments and give rise to endoligamentous vessels that enter the meniscal horns for a short distance and end in terminal capillary loops (Fig. 22-39). A small reflection of vascular synovial tissue is also present throughout the peripheral attachments of the medial and lateral menisci on both the femoral and tibial articular surfaces. (An exception is the posterolateral portion of the lateral meniscus adjacent to the area of the popliteal tendon.) This "synovial fringe" extends for a short distance (1 to 3 mm) over the articular surfaces of the menisci and contains small, terminally looped vessels. While this vascular synovial tissue adheres intimately to the articular surfaces of the menisci, it does not contribute vessels into the meniscal tissue.[3]

■ BLOOD SUPPLY TO THE KNEE

The blood supply to the knee is derived from branches of the following major arteries: the descending genicular artery, the medial and lateral superior genicular arteries, the medial and lateral inferior genicular arteries, the middle genicular artery, and the anterior and posterior tibial recurrent arteries[1,7,13,18,29] (Figs. 22-40 to 22-44).

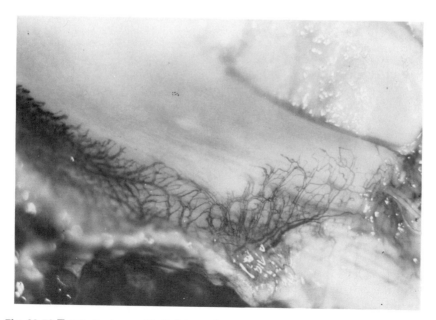

Fig. 22-39 ■ Anterior horn of India ink–perfused medial meniscus showing extension of vascular synovial fringe into synovial covering of anterior horn attachment.
From Arnoczky, S.P., and Warren, R.F.: Am. J. Sports Med. **10**:90, 1982.

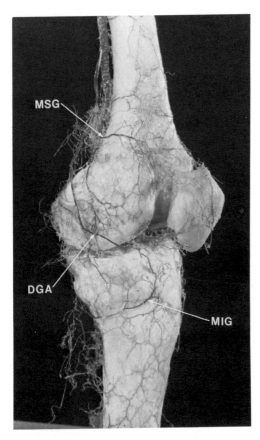

Fig. 22-40 ■ Anteromedial view of vascular cast specimen of knee showing location and branches of medial superior genicular artery *(MSG)*, descending genicular artery *(DGA)*, and medial inferior genicular artery *(MIG)*.

From Kaderly, R., Butler, D.L., and Noyes, F.R.: Trans. Orthop. Res. Soc. **8:**382, 1983.

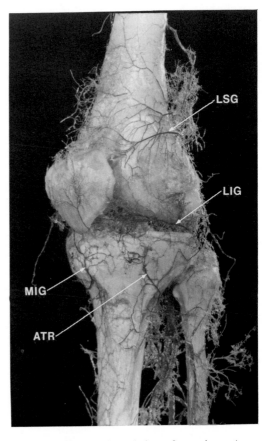

Fig. 22-41 ■ Anterolateral view of vascular cast specimen of knee showing location and branches of lateral superior genicular artery *(LSG)*, lateral inferior genicular artery *(LIG)*, medial inferior genicular artery *(MIG)*, and anterior tibial recurrent artery *(ATR)*.

From Kaderly, R., Butler, D.L., and Noyes, F.R.: Trans. Orthop. Res. Soc. **8:**382, 1983.

The **descending genicular artery** arises from the femoral artery just before it passes through the opening in the tendon of the adductor magnus and immediately divides into a saphenous and an articular branch. The saphenous branch accompanies the saphenous nerve to the medial side of the knee, passing between the sartorius and gracilis and anastomosing with the medial inferior genicular artery. The articular branch descends within the substance of the vastus medialis and anastomoses with the medial superior genicular artery. A branch from this vessel crosses proximal to the patella and forms an anastomotic arch within the lateral superior genicular artery.[13,29]

The **medial and lateral superior genicular arteries** arise on each side of the popliteal artery and wind around the femur immediately proximal to its condyles to the front of the knee. The medial superior genicular artery courses anterior to the semimembranosus and semitendinosus and proximal to the tendon of the biceps femoris.[13,29]

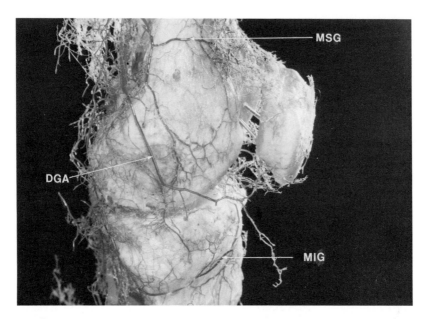

Fig. 22-42 ■ Medial view of vascular cast specimen of knee showing location and branches of medial superior genicular artery *(MSG)*, descending genicular artery *(DGA)*, and medial inferior genicular artery *(MIG)*.
From Kaderly, R., Butler, D.L., and Noyes, F.R.: Trans. Orthop. Res. Soc. **8**:382, 1983.

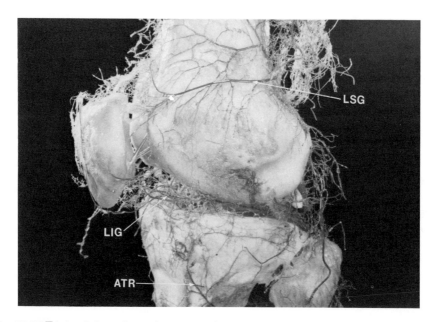

Fig. 22-43 ■ Lateral view of vascular cast specimen of knee showing location and branches of lateral superior genicular artery *(LSG)*, lateral inferior genicular artery *(LIG)*, and anterior tibial recurrent artery *(ATR)*.
From Kaderly, R., Butler, D.L., and Noyes, F.R.: Trans. Orthop. Res. Soc. **8**:382, 1983..

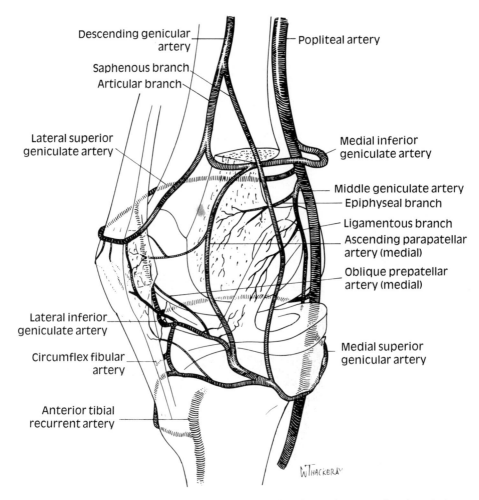

Descending genicular artery

Saphenous branch

Articular branch

Popliteal artery

Lateral superior geniculate artery

Medial inferior geniculate artery

Middle geniculate artery
Epiphyseal branch

Ligamentous branch

Ascending parapatellar artery (medial)

Oblique prepatellar artery (medial)

Lateral inferior geniculate artery

Circumflex fibular artery

Medial superior genicular artery

Anterior tibial recurrent artery

W THACKERAY

Fig. 22-44 ■ Schematic drawing of knee illustrating location and course of major arteries supplying joint.
From Arnoczky, S.P.: Orthop. Clin. North Am. **16**:15, 1985.

The **medial and lateral inferior genicular arteries** also arise from each side of the popliteal artery. These vessels originate just below the level of the joint space and pass under the gastrocnemius toward the front of the knee joint. The medial inferior genicular artery passes below the medial condyle of the tibia and deep to the medial (tibial) collateral ligament (MCL). The lateral inferior genicular artery passes proximal to the fibular head and deep to the lateral (fibular) collateral ligament (LCL) at the level of the joint line.[13,29]

The **middle genicular artery** arises from the popliteal artery and runs forward to penetrate the posterior joint capsule in the intercondylar notch. This vessel gives off branches that supply the distal femoral epiphysis, the cruciate ligaments, the synovial membrane, and joint capsule, as well as the proximal tibial epiphysis.[1,4,29]

The **anterior and posterior tibial recurrent arteries** arise from the anterior tibial artery and supply the anterior aspect of the knee joint. The anterior tibial recurrent artery ascends in the tibialis anterior muscle and assists in the formation of the patellar plexus by anastomosing with the medial and lateral inferior genicular arteries.[13,29]

REFERENCES

1. Arnoczky, S.P.: Blood supply to the anterior cruciate ligament and supporting structures, Orthop. Clin. North Am. **16**:15, 1985.
2. Arnoczky, S.P.: Anatomy of the anterior cruciate ligament, Clin. Orthop. **172**:19, 1983.
3. Arnoczky, S.P., and Warren, R.F.: Microvasculature of the human meniscus, Am. J. Sports Med. **10**:90, 1982.
4. Bousquet, M.G.: The traumatic rupture of the cruciate ligaments of the knee, Master's thesis, Lyons, France, 1969.
5. Branitgan, O.C., and Voshell, A.F.: The mechanics of the ligaments and menisci of the knee joint, J. Bone Joint Surg. **23**:44, 1941.
6. Bullough, P.G., Vosburgh, F., Arnoczky, S.P., and Levy, I.M.: The menisci of the knee. In Insall, J.D., ed.: Surgery of the knee, Edinburgh, 1984, Churchill Livingstone, pp. 135-146.
7. Crock, H.V.: The blood supply of the lower limb bones in man, Edinburgh, 1967, E.S. Livingstone.
8. Daseler, E.D., and Anson, B.J.: The plantarius muscle: an anatomical study of 750 specimens, J. Bone Joint Surg. **25**:822, 1943.
9. Ficat, P., and Hungerford, D.S.: Disorders of the patello femoral joint, Baltimore, Williams & Wilkins Co.
10. Girgis, F.G., Marshall, J.L., and Monajem, A.R.S.: The cruciate ligaments of the knee joint: anatomical, functional, and experimental analysis, Clin. Orthop. **106**:216, 1975.
11. Gollehon, D.L., Warren, R.F., and Torzilli, P.A.: The role of posterolateral and cruciate ligamentous structures in knee stability, J. Bone Joint Surg. (In press.)
12. Goodfellow, J., Hungerford, D.S., and Zindel, M.: Patello femoral joint mechanics and pathology. 1. Functional anatomy of the patello femoral joint, J. Bone Joint Surg. **58B**: 287, 1976.
13. Goss, M.: Gray's anatomy, ed. 29 Philadelphia, 1973, Lea & Febiger.
14. Heller, L., and Langman, J.: The menisco femoral ligaments of the human knee, J. Bone Joint Surg. **46B**:307, 1964.
15. Hungerford, D.S., and Barry, M.: Biomechanics of the patellofemoral joint, Clin. Orthop. **144**:9, 1979.
16. Insall, J., Falvo, K.A., and Wise, D.W.: Chondromalacia patellae: a prospective study, J. Bone Joint Surg. **58A**: 1, 1976.
17. Insall, J., and Salvati, E.: Patella position in the normal knee joint, Diagn. Radiol. **101**:101, 1971.
18. Kaderly, R., Butler, D.L., and Noyes, F.R.: A new vascular anatomic technique: vascular casts of human and cynamologous monkey knee joints, Trans. Orthop. Res. Soc. **8**:382, 1983.
19. Kennedy, J.C., Weinberg, H.W., and Wilson, A.S.: The anatomy and functioin of the anterior cruciate ligament as determined by clinical and morphological studies, J. Bone Joint Surg. **56A**: 223, 1974.
20. Last, R.J.: The popliteus muscle and the lateral meniscus, J. Bone Joint Surg. **32B**:93, 1950.
21. Laurin, C.A., Dussault, R., and Levesque, H.P.: The tangential x-ray investigation of the patellofemoral joint, Clin. Orthop. **144**:16, 1979.
22. Lieb, F.J., and Perry, J.: Quadriceps function: an anatomical and mechanical study using amputated limbs, J. Bone Joint Surg. **50A**:1535, 1968.
23. Marshall, J.L., Arnoczky, S.P., Rubin, R.M., and Wickiewicz, T.L.: Microvasculature of the cruciate ligaments, Phys. Sportsmed. **7**(3):87, 1979.
24. Marshall, J.L., Girgis, F.G., and Zelko, R.R.: The biceps femoris tendon and its functional significance, J. Bone Joint Surg. **54A**:1444, 1972.
25. Merchant, A.C., Mercer, R.L., Jacobsen, R.H., and Cool, C.R.: Roentgenograhpic analysis of patellofemoral congruence, J. Bone Joint Surg. **56A**:1391, 1974.
26. Outerbridge, R.E.: The etiology of chondromalacia patellae, J. Bone Joint Surg. **43B**:752, 1961.
27. Perry, J.: The mechanics of walking, Phys. Ther. **47**:778, 1966.
28. Scapinelli, R: Blood supply to the human patella, J. Bone Joint Surg. **49B**:563, 1967.
29. Scapinelli, R.: Studies on the vasculature of the human knee joint, Acta. Anat. **70**;305, 1968.
30. Seebacher, J.R., Inglis, A.E., Marshall, J.L., and Warren, R.F.: The structure of the posterolateral aspect of the knee, J. Bone Joint Surg. **64A**:536, 1982.
31. Sullivan, D.J., Levy, Sheskier, S. Torzilli, P.A., and Warren, R.F.: Medial restraints to anterior-posterior motion of the knee, J. Bone Joint Surg. **6A**:930, 1984.
32. Warren, L.F., and Marshall, J.L.: The supporting structures and layers on the medial side of the knee, J. Bone Joint Surg. **61A**:56, 1979.
33. Warren, L.F., Marshall, J.L., and Girgis, F.: The prime static stabilizer of the medial side of the knee, J. Bone Joint Surg. **56A**:665, 1974.
34. Welsh, R.P.: Knee joint structure and function, Clin. Orthop. **147**:7, 1980.
35. Wickiewicz, T.L., Roy, R.R., Powell, P.P., and Edgerton, V.R.: Muscle architecture of the human lower limb, Clin. Orthop. **179**:275, 1983.

ADDITIONAL READINGS

Alm, A., and Stromberg, B.: Vascular anatomy of the patellar and cruciate ligaments, Acta Chir. Scand. (Suppl.) **445**:25, 1974.

Arnoczky, S.P.: The blood supply of the meniscus and its role in healing and repair. In Finerman, G., ed.: Symposium on sports medicine: the knee, St. Louis, 1985, The C.V. Mosby Co.

Arnoczky, S.P., Rubin, R.M., and Marshall, J.L.: The microvasculature of the cruciate ligaments and its response to injury, J. Bone Joint Surg. **61A:**1221, 1979.

Basmajian, J.V., and Lovejoy, J.E.: Functions of the popliteus muscle in man, J. Bone Joint Surg. **53A:**557, 1971.

Brantigan, O., and Voshell, A.: The tibial collateral ligament: its function, its bursae and its relation to the medial meniscus, J. Bone Joint Surg. **25:**121, 1943.

Brantigan, O.C., and Voshell, A.F.: Ligaments of the knee joint: the relationship of the ligament of Humphrey to the ligament of Wrisberg, J. Bone Joint Surg. **28:**66, 1946.

Danzig, L.A., Newell, J.D., Guerra, J. and Resnick, D.: Osseus landmarks of the normal knee, Clin. Orthop. **156:**200, 1981.

Fulkerson, J.P., and Gossling, H.R.: Anatomy of the knee joint lateral retinaculum, Clin. Orthop. **153:**188, 1980.

Girgis, F., Marshall, J., and Monajeim, A.: The cruciate ligaments of the knee joint, Clin. Orthop. **106:**216, 1975.

Hey Groves, E.: The crucial ligaments of the knee joint: their function, rupture and operative treatment of the same, Br. J. Surg. **7:**505, 1920.

James, S.L.: Surgical anatomy of the knee. In Schulitz, K.P., Krahl, H. and Stein, W.H., eds.: Late reconstructions of the injured ligaments of the knee, Berlin, 1978, Springer-Verlag.

Kaplan, E.B.: The iliotibial tract: clinical and morphological significance, J. Bone Joint Surg. **40A:**817, 1958.

Kaplan, E.B.: The fabellofibular and short lateral ligaments of the knee joint, J. Bone Joint Surg. **43A:**169, 1961.

Kaplan, E.B.: Some aspects of functional anatomy of the human knee joint, Clin. Orthop. **23:**18, 1962.

Kennedy, J., Weinberg, H., and Wilson, A.: The anatomy and function of the anterior cruciate ligament, J. Bone Joint Surg. **56A:**223, 1974.

Last, R.J.: Some anatomical details of the knee joint, J. Bone Joint Surg. **30B:**683-688, 1948.

Müller, W.: Functional anatomy related to rotatory stability of the knee joint. In Chapchal, G., ed.: Injuries of the ligaments and their repair, Stuttgart, Georg Thieme Verlag, 1977, pp. 39-46.

Reider, B., Marshall, J.L., Koslin, B., Elmsford, B.R., and Girgis, F.G.: The anterior aspect of the knee joint, J. Bone Joint Surg. **63A:** 351, 1981.

Schultz, R.A., Miller, D.C., Kerr, C.S., et al.: Mechanoreceptors in human cruciate ligaments: a histologic study, J. Bone Joint Surg. **66A:**1072, 1984.

Voshell, A.F.: Anatomy of the knee joint. In Raney, R.B., ed.: American Academy of Orthopaedic Surgeons Instructional cause lectures, vol. 13, St. Louis, 1956, The C.V. Mosby Co., p. 247.

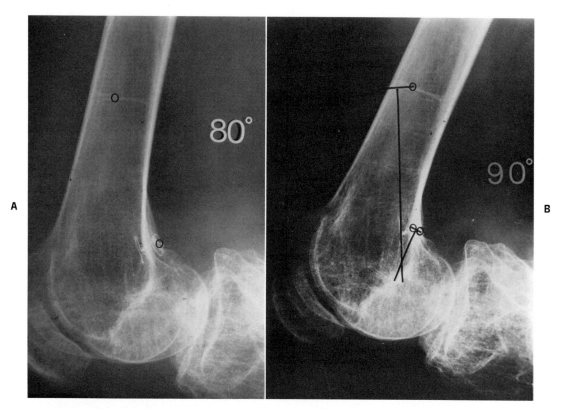

Fig. 23-4 ■ Locating instant center. **A,** Two easy-to-identify points on femur are designated on roentgenogram of knee flexed to 80 degrees. **B,** Roentgenogram is then compared with another in which knee is flexed to 90 degrees and on which same two points have been marked. Images of tibia are superimposed, and lines are drawn to connect each set of points. Perpendicular bisectors of these two lines then are drawn. Point at which they intersect locates instant center of tibiofemoral joint for motion between 80 and 90 degrees of flexion.
Courtesy Ian Goldie, M.D.

way through the entire range of flexion and extension in the knee can be plotted. The instant center pathway for the tibiofemoral joint in a normal knee is semicircular (Fig. 23-5).

Since the instant center pathway has been established, the surface joint motion can then be described. In each pair of superimposed roentgenograms the contact point between the tibiofemoral surfaces is marked and then a line is drawn to connect the contact point with the instant center. A second line, drawn at a right angle to the first, describes the direction of displacement (direction of change in the position) of the contact points. The second line (the direction of displacement line) will, in a normal knee, be tangential

to the tibial surface throughout each interval of motion from full extension to complete flexion. This tangentiality demonstrates that the femur is sliding on the tibial condyles (Fig. 23-6). In 1971, Frankel et al.[20] identified the instant center pathway and described the tibiofemoral surface motion in 25 normal knees—in intervals ranging from 90 degrees of flexion to full extension.[20] They found that tangential sliding existed in all cases.

Displaced instant centers

In the same study, Frankel et al. also plotted the instant center pathway for the tibiofemoral joint in 30 knees that had internal derangements.[20] In all 30 cases the instant center was displaced from its nor-

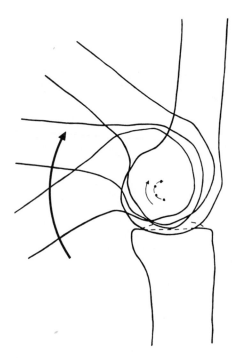

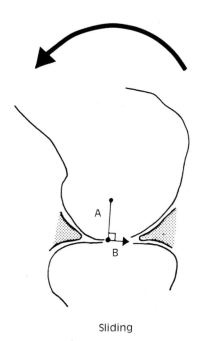

Sliding

Fig. 23-5 ■ Semicircular instant center pathway for tibiofemoral joint of 19-year-old man with normal knee.
Adapted from Frankel, V.H., and Nordin, M.: Basic biomechanics of the skeletal system, Philadelphia, 1980, Lea & Febiger.

Fig. 23-6 ■ In normal knee, line drawn from instant center of tibiofemoral joint to tibiofemoral contact point (line *A*) forms right angle with line tangential to tibial surface (line *B*). Arrow indicates direction of displacement of contact points. Line B is tangential to tibial surface, indicating that femur slides on tibial condyles during measured interval of motion.
From Frankel, V.H. and Nordin, M.: Basic biomechanics of the skeletal system, Philadelphia, 1980, Lea & Febiger.

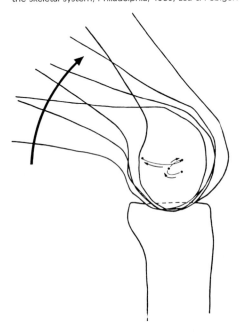

Fig. 23-7 ■ Abnormal instant center pathway for 35-year-old man with bucket-handle tear. Note that instant center jumps at full extension of knee.
Adapted from Frankel, V.H., Burstein, A.H., and Brooks, D.B.: J. Bone Joint Surg. **53A:** 945, 1971.

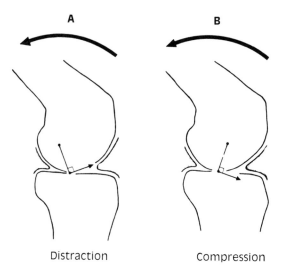

Distraction   Compression

Fig. 23-8 ■ Surface motion in two tibiofemoral joints with displaced instant centers. In both joints, line that is at right angle drawn between instant center and tibiofemoral contact point describes direction of displacement of contact points. **A,** Arrow in joint indicates that tibiofemoral joint willl be distracted with further flexion. **B,** Arrow in joint indicates that tibiofemoral joint will become compressed with further flexion. From Frankel, V.H. and Nordin, M.: Basic biomechanics of the skeletal system, Philadelphia, 1980, Lea & Febiger.

mal position during some portion of the joint motion analyzed. The abnormal instant center pathway of the knee of one subject—a 35-year-old man with a bucket-handle derangement—indicates that the instant center radically jumps at full extension of the knee (Fig. 23-7).

Extending and flexing a knee about a displaced instant center is like trying to close a door with a bent hinge. It will not fit smoothly into the door jamb. Likewise, in knees with displaced instant centers the tibiofemoral joint surfaces do not slide tangentially; instead they become either seriously distracted or compressed (Fig. 23-8).

A knee that is continually forced to move about a displaced instant center will gradually compensate for this derangement by stretching the ligaments and other supporting structures of the joint or by exerting abnormally directed and possibly high forces on the joint's articular surfaces. To continue the door hinge analogy, this would be similar to tearing the screws loose from the bent hinge, or damaging the door itself.[19]

Tamea and Henning[65] in 1981 used the instant center technique to study the effect of the pivot shift maneuver. Once the instant center for a given range of motion is determined, the surface velocity vector

of the weight-bearing part of the joint can be determined. Eight knees with suspected tears of the anterior cruciate ligament (anterior drawer sign positive, positive Lachman test, positive pivot shift) were compared to a control group of normal knees by using the instant center technique combined with the pivot shift maneuver. The control group showed a normal pattern of instant center progression. The surface velocity vectors were tangential to joint line surfaces. The group with anterior cruciate ligament tears showed a marked deviation from the normal pattern, analyzed in three separate phases. The sublux phase was present from 0 to 20 degrees of flexion and showed a displacement of the instant centers of rotation located anteriorly and near the joint line. The surface velocity vectors were not tangential to the joint surface at the point of joint contact.

The shift phase ranged from 20 to 40 degrees of flexion and showed a sudden marked displacement of the centrode to a posterior and more proximal position on the femur. The surface velocity vectors became tangential to the joint surface during this phase.

The reduced phase ranged from 40 degrees to about 90 degrees of flexion. The instant centers and the surface velocity vectors were identical to those of the control group through the remaining range of motion. Surgical or conservative treatment that does not result in a restoration of normal joint mechanics and an obliteration of the pivot shift cannot be expected to prevent long-term distractive internal derangements of the knee joint.[65]

It should be pointed out that the instant center technique is adapted to study primarily the knee motion in the sagittal plane and to analyze flexion and extension. Uncontrolled rotation of the tibia could result in an error in the interpretation of the roentgenogram.[2,17,67]

In 1983 Gerber and Matter[24] used the instant center technique to study the kinematics of acute ruptures of the anterior cruciate ligament before and after repair. They found that the abnormal instant center pathway noticed preoperatively could not be normalized by primary repair except in one case. Although the rated results of the patients were good or excellent, the objective evaluation showed that normal stability when compared to the other undamaged knee was achieved rarely.

The use of the instant center technique in the assessment of knee joint function seems to offer an objective method of evaluation to the investigator. The critical point in this technique is to avoid the rotation of the tibia, achieved by a standardized manner of investigation in which rotation is controlled. The stress examinations as used by Tamea and Henning offer an additional technique, but rotation still must be controlled.[65] The rotation in the knee occurs in the transverse plane, and abnormal rotation should be studied in the transverse plane to yield a more three-dimensional picture of knee function.[2]

Screw-home mechanism and internal derangements

Internal derangements of the tibiofemoral joint may also interfere with the screw-home mechanism, which is the combined action of knee extension and external rotation of the tibia (Fig. 23-9). The tibiofemoral joint has a figure-8, or helicoid, action; it is not a pure hinge joint. This helicoid action of the tibia about the femur during flexion and extension result from the anatomic specifications of the medial femoral condyle: it is approximately 1.7 cm longer than the lateral femoral condyle. Therefore, as the tibia slides on the femur from full flexion to full extension it also descends and ascends the contours and curves of the medial femoral condyle while, at the same time, it rotates externally. As the tibia returns to a position of full flexion, the entire helicoid motion is reversed. The complex screw-home mechanism provides the knee with a high degree of stability in any position. This would be unattainable if the tibiofemoral were a pure hinge joint.

Helfet test for external tibial rotation

Because the instant center technique cannot be used to analyze motion in the transverse plane, the Helfet test is used to determine whether external rotation of the tibia occurs during knee extension, which in turn indicates whether the screw mechanism is functioning properly.[29]

This clinical test is performed on a patient who is sitting, leg hanging freely, with 90 degrees of knee and hip flexion. The medial and lateral borders of the patella are outlined; the tibial tuberosity and the midline of the patella are marked. The alignment of the tibial tuberosity with the patella is checked. In a normal knee with 90 degrees of flexion, the tibial tuberosity lines up with the medial half of the patella (Fig. 23-10, *A*). Then the knee is fully extended and the shifting of the tibial tuberosity is identified. Normally the tibial tuberosity will move laterally during extension, and it will line up with the lateral half of the patella when full extension is reached (Fig. 23-10, *B*).

In a normal knee the rotational motion may be as great as half the width of the

66. Trent, P., Walker, P.S., and Wolf, B.: Ligament length patterns, strength and rotational axes of the knee joint, Clin. Orthop. **117:**263, 1976.

67. Walker, P.S.: Human joints and their artificial replacements, Springfield, Ill., 1977, Charles C Thomas.

68. Walker, P.S., and Erkman, M.J.: The role of the menisci in force transmission across the knee, Clin. Orthop. **109:**184, 1975.

69. Wang, J.B., and Marshall, J.: THe popliteus tendon as a static stabilizer of the knee, Paper presented at the 23rd Annual Meeting of the Orthopaedic Research Society, Las Vegas, February 1-3, 1977.

70. Wang, J., Rubin, R., and Marshall, J.: A mechanism of isolated anterior cruciate ligament rupture, J. Bone Joint Surg. **57A:**411, 1975.

71. Warren, L.F., Marshall, J.L., and Girgis, F.: The prime static stabilizer of the medial side of the knee, J. Bone Joint Surg. **56A:**665, 1974.

72. Watkins, M.P., Harris, B.A., Wender, S., Zarins, B., and Rowe, C.R.: Effect of patellectomy on the function of the quadriceps and hamstrings, J. Bone Joint Surg. **65A:**390, 1983.

73. Zarins, B., Rowe, C.R., Harris, B.A., and Watkins, M.P.: Rotational motion of the knee, Am. J. Sports Med. **11:**152, 1983.

chapter 24

Biomechanical analysis of knee stability

Peter A. Torzilli

Biomechanically, the knee is one of the most complex joints in the human body. There are several reasons for this complexity. First, knee motion is a truly general motion. No one fixed axis exists about which relative motion occurs, in contrast to such other constrained joints as the hip and elbow. The tibia is free to move in any direction relative to the femur. Second, the knee's complex kinematic motion is controlled by a unique set of soft tissue structures, namely, the cruciate and collateral ligaments and the menisci. Acting together with the muscles, these structures control and limit the permissible excursions experienced by the knee during function. Finally, the knee experiences joint reaction forces of many times body weight. These large forces not only compress the joint but also cause large shear forces, which must be restrained by the surrounding soft tissues.

Even though the knee is subjected to large joint forces, the intact knee is readily capable of providing stability and range of motion during normal activities. However, soft tissue injuries can change the mechanical performance of the knee, resulting in an unstable joint, a decrease in function, and possibly joint destruction. These injuries can occur during normal sports activities, to both the occasional athlete and professional, and as a result of trauma. A difficult task facing the examining physician is the diagnostic determination of the specific type of injury that has occurred to the knee. Just as important is the recognition and understanding of the biomechanical consequences of the injury.

This chapter deals with the biomechanical (objective) evaluation of the patient with an injured knee. To begin, we must define the terminology of motion and apply it to describe knee motion. With this background, we can discuss the abnormalities occurring in the injured knee. It is hoped that this chapter will further knowledge of the changes occurring after injury and aid in the clinical evaluation of the injured patient. In addition, I believe this chapter will aid in communicating this information to others.

■ TERMINOLOGY AND DESCRIPTION OF KNEE MOTION

The terms and methods for describing the motion of the knee are as varied as the people doing the describing.* In the past, this has caused some confusion. To avoid this, I will use the two concepts of **translation** and **rotation,** as described in textbooks on engineering mechanics.[15]

---

*References 17, 18, 25, 29, 34, 39, 44, 45, and 58.

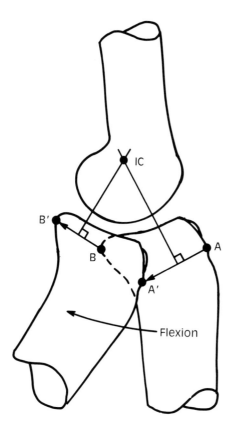

Fig. 24-7 ■ The instant center of rotation is located at intersection of perpendicular bisectors of lines connecting two displaced points on the tibia as knee flexes. Here points A and B move to A' and B', respectively.

ion position to another is identified (Fig. 24-7). The instant center is determined by locating the intersection of the perpendicular bisectors of the line connecting the displacement of each respective point. The path of the instant centers is determined by repeating this construction for each successive position of knee flexion.

I have treated knee flexion-extension as occurring about a single axis, that is, the mediolateral axis. In planar motion, the instant center appears as a point, the axis of rotation being perpendicular to the plane. However, we must realize that other motions will occur as the knee flexes. When these motions occur simultaneously with flexion-extension, the axis of rotation will no longer be perpendicular to the sagittal plane but will continually change its **direction and position**

with each successive position. While I will only consider planar motion in this section, the effect of tibial rotation should not be ignored.[3,11,47] A further discussion of this important mechanism is included in the next section.

It should also be remembered that, in studying the kinematics of motion between two bodies, either of the bodies can be chosen as the reference or fixed body about which the other moves. I have chosen the femur as the reference. However, similar results would be obtained if I used the tibia as the reference.

As previously mentioned, the velocity at any point on the tibia is in the direction perpendicular to a line drawn from the instant center to the particular point. This is especially important when referenced to the point of joint contact between the condylar surfaces. In general, five types of motion can occur at the point of contact. **Rolling** occurs when the instant center and the point of contact are coincident (Fig. 24-8, *A*). This is similar to a wheel rolling on the ground. Each point along the perimeter of the wheel contacts an equally spaced point on the ground. **Sliding** of the joint surfaces occurs when the velocity is tangential to the joint surfaces at the point of contact (Fig. 24-8, *B*). Minimal frictional loss occurs during sliding because of the smooth condylar surfaces and the excellent lubricating properties of the articular cartilage.[51] Sliding is the normal mechanism of motion in all diarthrodial joints. This condition always occurs when the instant center lies along a line that is perpendicular to the joint surface at the point of contact. As the distance from the instant center to the point of contact increases, the relative motion changes from pure rotation to pure translation (Fig. 24-8, *C*). If the distance becomes exceedingly great, the arc of motion of all points about the instant center (at infinity) approximates a straight line.

Whenever the instant center does not coincide with the point of joint contact on the articular surface, sliding will occur. In addition, sliding will still occur if the in-

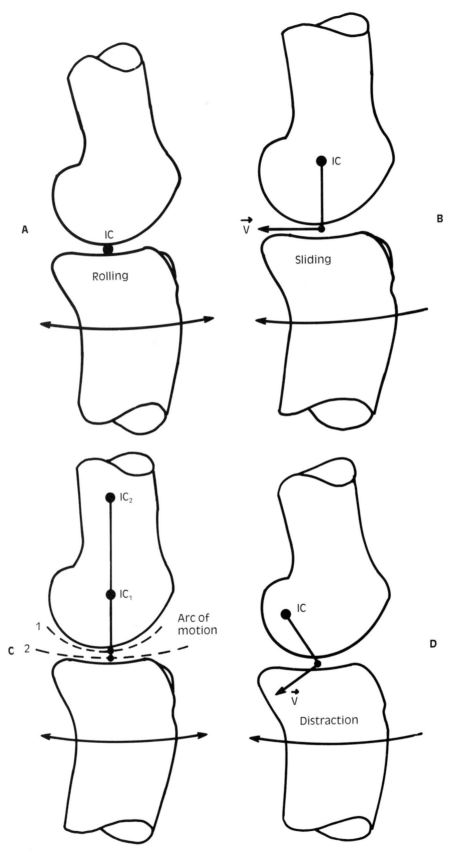

Fig. 24-8 ■ For legend see opposite page.

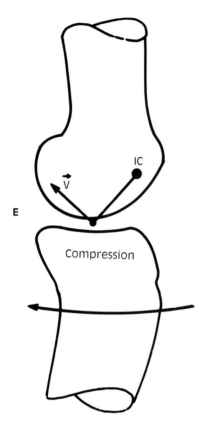

Fig. 24-8 ■ Rolling occurs when instant center coincides with point of joint contact. **B,** Sliding occurs when direction of velocity at the point of joint contact is tangential to articular surfaces. **C,** As instant center moves distal to point of joint contact, motion tends toward pure translation. **D,** If velocity of tibia at point of joint contact is directed away from femur, motion is one of joint distraction. **E,** On the other hand, if tibial velocity is directed into femur at point of contact, joint compression will result.

stant center does not lie on a line perpendicular to the articular surface at the point of joint contact, but the direction of the surface velocities will not be tangential to the articular surfaces. **Distraction** (separation) or **compression** of the articular surfaces will occur whenever the surface velocity is directed away from or into the opposing joint surface, respectively (Figs. 24-8, *D* and *E*). In general, both distraction and compression are abnormal. Joint compression is probably the more serious of the two, because it causes plowing of the articular cartilage and ex-

ceedingly high shear stresses. This type of motion usually leads to abnormal articular wear and can result in the formation of osteophytes to further alter the kinematics.

Normal knee flexion-extension is shown schematically in Fig. 24-9.* Motion proceeds from full extension to full flexion. Initially, the knee rolls during the first 10 to 15 degrees of flexion. The instant center of rotation is located at the point of contact on the articular surfaces. For flexion angles greater than approximately 10 to 15 degrees, the instant center moves proximally, and the tibia slides against the femur. As the knee approaches full flexion, the instant center will be suddenly displaced as the tibia impinges upon the femur because of the restraining effects of the ligaments and menisci. The velocity vector at the point of contact on the articular surface will be directed toward the femoral surface, indicating impingement of the tibia and joint compression.

If the direction of knee motion is reversed from full flexion to full extension, a similar path of instant centers will result. At hyperextension, the instant center will again be displaced as the joint is restrained from further motion.

Alterations in normal knee kinematics have been demonstrated in the injured or internally deranged knee.[1,3,10] Injured knees with a meniscal lesion demonstrate an abnormally positioned instant center at one or more positions of knee flexion. An example is shown in Fig. 24-10 of a knee with a displaced bucket-handle tear of the medial meniscus. The abnormally displaced instant center produced a nontangential velocity vector at the point of joint contact as the knee went into extension. This resulted in the joint surfaces being compressed and the joint locking. Cartilage corrosion and wear and osteophyte formation can also produce abnormal knee kinematics (Fig. 24-11). Again, joint compression and locking are usually

---

*References 3, 6, 10, 11, 31, 33, 46, and 56.

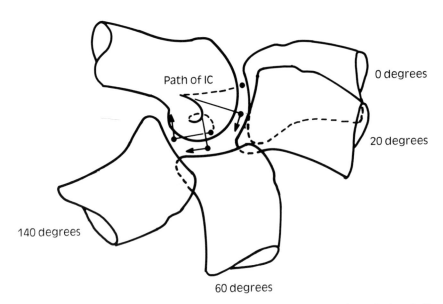

Fig. 24-9 ■ Schematic representation of path of instant centers during knee flexion. Rolling occurs during first few degrees of flexion. Thereafter articular surfaces slide smoothly. At full flexion, soft tissue constraints produced joint compression to stop motion. In extension, motion is reversed.

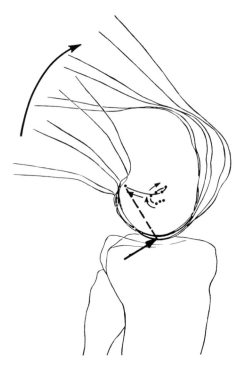

Fig. 24-10 ■ A 35-year-old man with displaced bucket-handle tear of medial meniscus. Instant center pathway is indicated. Note that instant center for 30 degrees of knee flexion is displaced posteriorly so that rotation about this point forces the joint surfaces together, producing blocking to extension.

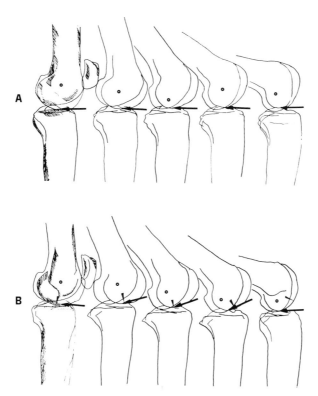

Fig. 24-11 ■ Surface velocities of both knees of a 48-year-old man who had had many episodes of locking of his left knee and mild persistent knee symptoms since an injury at age 18. Arthrotomy revealed torn and retracted anterior horn of medial meniscus, which was adherent to fat pad, and large area of wear on anterior aspect of medial femoral condyle with associated marginal osteophytes. **A,** Kinematic study of normal right knee. **B,** In symptomatic left knee, surface velocities are abnormal at from 10 to 50 degrees but not at 0 to 5 degrees and at 50 to 80 degrees of flexion, where tangential (sliding) motion was found despite obvious wear of the articular surface in contact area for these two positions.

From Frankel, V.H., Burstein, A.H., and Brooks, D.B.: J. Bone Joint Surg. **53A:**945, 1971.

found. In the contralateral, uninjured knee, normal sliding is present with the velocity vectors tangential to the articular surface at the point of joint contact.

No evidence has been found of abnormal kinematics in knees with absent anterior or posterior cruciate ligaments.[1,3] No change could be found in the location of the instant center of motion between intact knees and these without cruciate ligaments. Data indicate that the cruciate ligaments have a minor role in controlling passive knee motion during flexion and extension. Only near full extension or full flexion is their role believed to be significant. The anterior cruciate ligament is found to function near full extension and the posterior cruciate ligament to function only near full flexion.[3] The results indicate that the condylar geometry largely controls the normal rolling and sliding motion of the knee. However, whether this is true during dynamic situations, especially during gait, in which joint compressive forces are several times body weight, has yet to be determined.

■ IN VITRO BIOMECHANICAL KNEE STABILITY

Several in vitro studies exist that evaluate the contributions of the ligamentous and meniscal structures in controlling

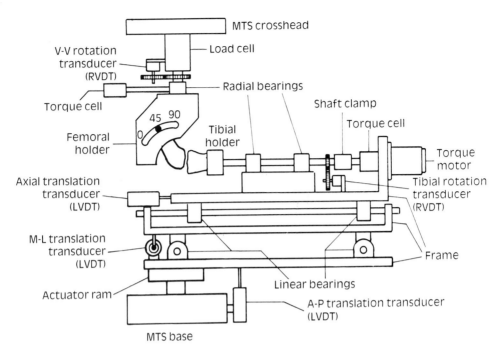

Fig. 24-12 ■ Schematic diagram of mechanical device to test in vitro knee motion. Entire test device is mounted on an MTS Materials Test System. An anteroposterior tibial force is applied through test machine base, an internal-external tibial rotation with torque motor, and a varus-valgus rotation with torque cell. For each fixed flexion position, 5 degrees of knee motion are measured using translation and rotation transducers shown here.

Adapted from Sullivan, D., Levy, I.M., Sheskier, S., Torzilli, P.A., and Warren, R.F.: J. Bone Joint Surg. **66A**:930, 1984.

knee motion.* These studies usually use a mechanical device or machine to apply a known load or torque to a cadaveric knee and measure the resulting translations and rotations. The machine attempts to simulate, as closely as possible, the knee stress test performed by the physician during the clinical examination. The objectives of these in vitro biomechanical tests are to evaluate the motion of the intact knee and then determine alterations in normal motion following removal or section of different ligamentous and meniscal structures.

A 5 DOF mechanical knee stress apparatus is shown in Fig. 24-12. The device allows anterior and posterior tibial translation, medial and lateral tibial translation, axial (proximal and distal) tibial translation, internal and external tibial rotation,

and varus and valgus tibial (femoral) rotation. The flexion angle is held fixed between 0 and 90 degrees. The apparatus is mounted on an MTS Materials Test System, which is capable of applying an anterior and posterior tibial force. In addition, an internal and external tibial torque can be applied by the attached torque motor and a varus and valgus torque applied manually through the femoral torque cell. The attached translation (LVDT) and rotation (RVDT) transducers continually record the 5 degrees of knee motion as the load and torque are applied.

The type of knee forces applied by the apparatus illustrated in Fig. 24-12 attempts to simulate the in vivo situation. Similar devices have been used by various investigators.[13,36,40,42,50] Other investigators have used knee test apparatus with less than 5 DOF.* While these types of appa-

---

*References 4, 7, 8, 12, 13, 16, 32, 36, 38, 40, 42, 50, 55, 56, and 58.

*References 7, 12, 32, 38, 55, and 56.

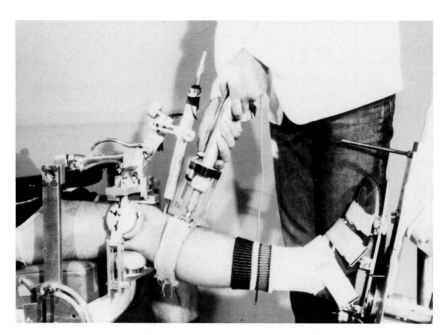

Fig. 24-26 ■ Anteroposterior test at 20 degrees of flexion using instrumented test device of Markolf et al. Subject is reclining to relax hamstrings while ankle is strapped securely to rigidly fixed foot rest. Approximately 10 kg of force is applied manually through instrumented handle attached to V-shaped padded plate strapped to anterior surface of tibia. Spring-loaded plunger maintains contact with tibial tubercle and measures any anteroposterior translation of tubercle.
Courtesy Keith L. Markolf.

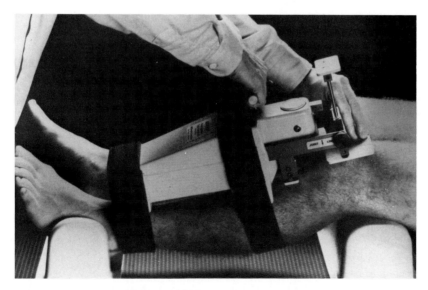

Fig. 24-27 ■ The KT-1000 Knee Ligament Arthrometer (Medmetrics Corporation, Inc., San Diego, CA) attached to lower limb. Anterior and posterior force is applied to tibia through attached handle. Amount of anterior and posterior tibial translation is measured by displacement of pads resting on patellar and tibial tubercle.
Courtesy L. Malcolm, Ph. D., San Diego, Calif.

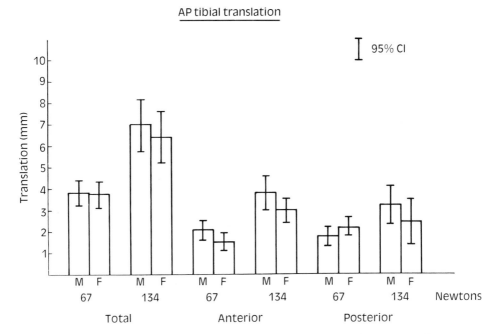

Fig. 24-28 ■ Anterior, posterior, and total tibial translation resulting from a 67- and 134-newton force (a 50 and 100 N joint line force, respectively) applied to the midtibia in 18 male (M) and 11 female (F) normal subjects.

motion resulting from an anterior and posterior tibial force in a group of 29 normal subjects. All tests were performed at 90 degrees of knee flexion. The results for tibial translation are shown in Fig. 24-28. No differences were found in the amount of total, anterior, or posterior translation between men and women or in the amount of anterior translation as compared to the amount of posterior translation. An important criterion for patient evaluation is the difference between the neutral or unloaded position of contralateral knees. In the injured patient, if the amount of anterior and posterior translation in each knee cannot be determined from the same neutral position, the results may be inaccurate. No *statistical* difference was found in the neutral position between contralateral sides in the normal subject group; however, certain individuals had very large differences in the neutral position between contralateral knees. This malalignment of the contralateral neutral position must be accounted for if

an accurate comparison is to be made between the uninjured and injured knee.

One of the major concerns in comparing contralateral knees is the variability in measurements between the contralateral sides. No *statistical* difference is found in normal knee motion between contralateral sides.[35,37,53] However, on an individual-to-individual comparison, it is found that large differences can exist between contralateral sides[37,53] (Fig. 24-29). Differences were as high as 5 mm.[53] With a 67-newton tibial load the mean *absolute* difference in total translation between contralateral knees measured 1.35 ± 1.31 mm, with 54% having less than 1 mm difference and 77% having less than 2 mm difference. On the other hand, at a higher, 134-newton load, the mean difference was 2.55 ± 1.21 mm, with only 10% being less than 1 mm and 45% being less than 2 mm. The greater load produced a statistically higher difference than for the lower load, p<0.01. This suggests that when using a biomechanical device, a smaller tib-

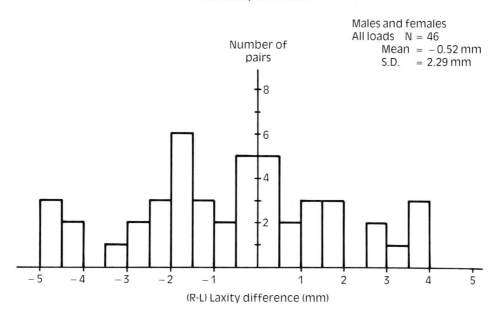

Fig. 24-29 ■ Difference in total translation between contralateral knees resulting from 67- and 134-newton load in 18 male and 11 female subjects.
From Torzilli, P.A., Greenberg, R.L. and Insall, J.N.: J. Bone Joint Surg. **63A**:960, 1981.

ial force should be used to lower the possible error in comparing contralateral sides.

In the normal group of subjects tested,[53] there was no significant amount of coupled femoral abduction-adduction or femoral rotation resulting from an anterior and posterior tibial force. The rotations measured less than a few degrees and demonstrated no consistent pattern. These in vivo results are similar to in vitro results, suggesting that the measurement of the coupled femoral rotations is probably not an important parameter for diagnostic purposes.

Contrary to femoral rotations, the tibia exhibited a preferred rotational direction, similar to in vitro results (Fig. 24-30). In 98% of the knees, an anterior force produced an internal tibial rotation, and in 82% of the knees, a posterior force produced an external rotation. As described earlier, the coupled rotation was believed to be caused by the moment exerted by the tensed anterior and posterior cruciate

ligaments about the axis for tibial rotation (see Figs. 24-16 and 24-19). This characteristic of knee motion may be very important in developing a method for diagnostic testing. In evaluating the injured patient, the magnitude of the measured parameter, in this case the amount of coupled tibial rotation, may not be as important as the characteristic of that parameter, the direction of tibial rotation. This is especially true when comparing the injured knee to the contralateral knee and a normal data base. Unfortunately, the presently available mechanical devices can only measure 1 DOF and thus are inadequate to reproduce this important finding. However, it is the concept of a change in the characteristic of knee motion in the injured patient, rather than the absolute measurement itself, that may well prove to be the best diagnositic procedure for evaluating ligamentous and meniscal injuries.

While measurement of normal knee motion is fairly well documented, data for

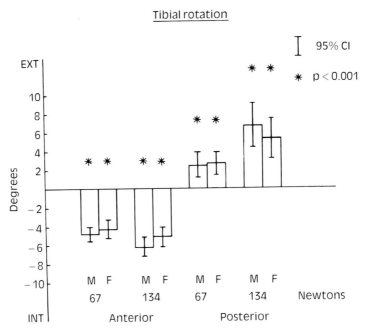

Fig. 24-30 ■ Application of an anterior force resulted in internal rotation of tibia, while application of posterior force resulted in external tibial rotation.

the injured knee and criteria for assessing isolated damage are still lacking, or at best insufficient. In Kennedy and Fowler's study[24] of 11 injured patients tested at 90 degrees of flexion, anterior translation ranged from 7 to 20 mm. However, of these only 8 had surgical verification of "a damaged or lax anterior cruciate ligament." An anterior translation of 5 millimeters was chosen as the upper limit for normal motion when later assessing knee injury.[24,25] In a study of 30 injuries involving the cruciate ligaments, Jacobson[19] subjectively evaluated each patient by classifying them as having abnormally elevated translations if (1) the movement was greater than the upper 97.5% confidence limit of the normal subjects, that is, for an anterior, posterior, or total translation greater than 7.4, 5.4 or 11.7 mm, respectively; or (2) there was a difference between the injured and uninjured side of greater than 3 mm. Injury predictive scores (probability of a true positive and true negative test) were higher for his mechanical test than for clinical examination

or evaluation with the patient under general anesthesia. After an initial data analysis, he later stated that a better injury predictive score could be obtained by using a difference of 4 mm between the injured and uninjured knees.[21] In 25 postmeniscectomy patients, Bargar et al.[2] measured total anteroposterior translation at 0, 20, and 90 degrees of flexion. Only at 20 degrees of flexion in knees with an absent medial meniscus and anterior cruciate ligament was the translation greater than both the contralateral normal side and a group of previously sampled normal subjects.[37] Otherwise, meniscectomy with or without an anterior cruciate ligament resulted in no significantly different results from normal individuals. In a similar study of 41 patients with absence of the anterior cruciate ligament (two with isolated injuries and the other 39 with associated meniscal and/or collateral ligament lesions), Kochan et al.[28] reported that the injured knee had a greater total anteroposterior translation when compared to the contralateral normal knee at 0, 20, and 90 degrees of flexion. However, examination of their data reveals that at 90 degrees of flexion the injured knee was equal to a previously sampled normal group of subjects,[37] and the uninjured side had less total translation.

Although several biomechanical measurements have been performed on injured knees, limited objective criteria have been established for evaluation of the injured patient. Many of the previous studies included patients with mixed multiple ligamentous damage,* who had undergone prior operative procedures,[14,20,24] and who, in some cases, had uncertain surgical verification of ligamentous injury.[25] Torzilli et al.[52] attempted to establish criteria by comparing groups of patients having similar ligamentous and/or meniscal injuries, including whether there had been any prior surgery. Thirty seven patients with unilateral knee injuries were evaluated. Prior surgery was performed on 10 patients at least 1 year before the stress test and included medial meniscectomy, patellar shaving, and loose body removal. All stress tests were performed at 90 degrees of flexion using a resultant anterior and posterior 50-newton force at the joint line (a 67-newton force was applied at midtibia). Shown in Figs. 24-31 to 24-33, respectively, is the amount of total, anterior, and posterior translation measured in the injured and uninjured knee of patients with (1) an isolated tear of the medial meniscus, (2) an isolated rupture of the anterior cruciate ligament, and (3) an isolated rupture of the anterior cruciate ligament and previous removal of the medial meniscus.

In patients with an isolated tear of the medial meniscus, there was no difference between contralateral knees for total, anterior, or posterior translation. In addition, there was no difference in either knee when compared to a previously tested normal group of subjects.[53]

*References 14, 20, 22, 24, 25, 27, and 28.

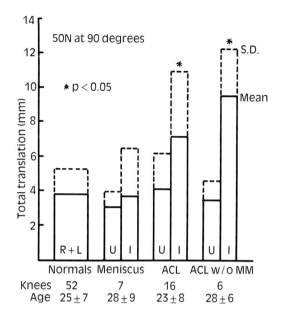

Fig. 24-31 ■ Total translation resulting from 50-newton joint line force at 90 degrees of knee flexion in normal group of subjects and group of patients with torn medial meniscus, ruptured anterior cruciate ligament, or ruptured anterior cruciate ligament with previous removal of the medial meniscus. *R*, right; *L*, left; *U*, uninjured side; *I*, injured side.

CASE #1: Two years ago this 32-year-old male twisted his left knee while dancing. There was some pain and swelling at that time, which gradually subsided. He again twisted his left knee 2 months ago while playing tennis. Recently, while he was squatting, the knee suddenly "locked," and he has had difficulty extending it. Physical examination revealed a positive tibial rotation test for the medial meniscus. Passively, the injured knee lacked the last few degrees of full extension and full flexion as compared to the opposite knee. Clinical stress testing indicated intact medial collateral and anterior cruciate ligaments. Patellar signs were negative. An arthrogram indicated a bucket-handle tear of the medial meniscus. Mechanical stress test analysis with a 50-newton joint load revealed the difference in neutral positions was 1 mm (injured side posteriorly translated). Shifting the injured knee with respect to the uninjured knee resulted in the following translations (in millimeters):

	Injured	**Uninjured**
Total	3.2	3.2
Anterior	1.1	1.0
Posterior	2.1	2.2

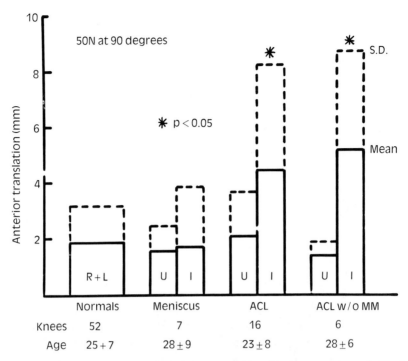

Fig. 24-32 ■ Amount of anterior translation measured for subject groups shown in Fig. 24-31.

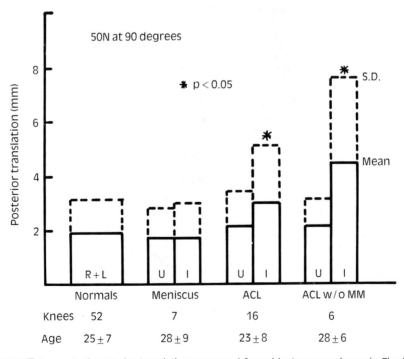

Fig. 24-33 ■ Amount of posterior translation measured for subject groups shown in Fig. 24-31.

Both knees were within the normal limits (95% confidence interval) of the normal group, as compared contralaterally and unilaterally. Surgical findings revealed a bucket-handle tear of the left medial meniscus.

Patients with an isolated tear of the anterior cruciate ligament had a significant increase in total, anterior, and posterior translation on the injured side as compared to the contralateral normal knee and when compared to the normal subject group (see Figs. 24-31 to 33). The uninjured knee demonstrated no abnormal translation. There was a small but not significant increase in translation in patients with a ruptured anterior cruciate ligament and previous surgical removal of the medial meniscus as compared to patients with an isolated rupture of the anterior cruciate ligament. Again, the contralateral uninjured knee was similar to the normal

subject group. Finally, there was no difference between patients with a rupture of the anterior cruciate ligament who had previous surgery not believed to affect knee stability and patients having either an isolated anterior cruciate ligament or a ruptured anterior cruciate ligament with previous medial meniscectomy (Fig. 24-34). In the 25 patients with a ruptured anterior cruciate ligament there was a significant increase in both anterior and posterior translation (see Fig. 24-34). This unusual finding of increased posterior translation may indicate a possible secondary mode of damage following anterior cruciate rupture. However, this could not be verified at the time of surgery.

CASE #2: Three months ago this 29-year-old female suffered a "giving way" of her right knee while running. Since then she has had recurrent episodes of swelling and has been

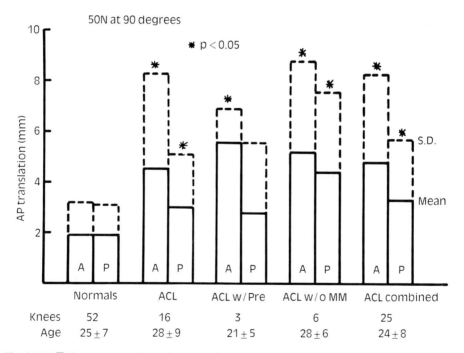

Fig. 24-34 ■ The amount of anterior (A) and posterior (P) translation resulting from 50-newton joint line force at 90 degrees of knee flexion. Data are for a normal group of subjects and on injured knee in patients with ruptured anterior cruciate ligament (ACL), ruptured anterior cruciate ligament and previous knee surgery not related to knee stability (ACL w/Pre), ruptured anterior cruciate ligament with prior removal of the medial meniscus (ACL w/o MM), and combined data for all three groups with rupture of anterior cruciate ligament.

unable to flex the knee completely. An arthrogram showed intact medial and lateral menisci with a possible anterior cruciate tear. Physical examination revealed a swollen knee and positive McMurray test for medial meniscus damage, but no significant increase in anterior translation nor a "soft end point." Stress testing with a 50-newton joint force revealed no difference in the neutral position (0.1 mm) and the following translations (in millimeters) after alignment:

	Injured	Uninjured
Total	15.1	6.2
Anterior	11.8	4.1
Posterior	3.3	2.0

Compared to the control population, this patient exhibited increased anterior and total translation in both knees. However, the injured knee exhibited two to three times greater translation than the uninjured knee. Surgical findings revealed a bucket-handle tear of the medial meniscus and complete absence of the anterior cruciate ligament.

An insufficient number of patients with rupture of the posterior cruciate ligament were tested to perform a statistical analysis. However, many of these patients had a greater posterior translation in the injured as compared to the uninjured side, and several had a greater anterior translation.

One result from this study was the importance of aligning the injured knee with the uninjured knee in the neutral position. This is illustrated by the following case:

CASE #3: This 27-year-old male sustained a right knee injury 6 weeks ago while playing squash. The knee was forced into a valgus position with subsequent swelling. Clinical examination (by three independent examiners) revealed a positive anterior translation with a poor "end point." There was a possible "pivot shift" and a negative Lachman test. However, under anesthesia the patient exhibited a positive posterior stress test, a negative Lachman test, and a negative "pivot shift." An arthrogram was negative. Stress test analysis with a 50-newton joint load revealed the right tibia was positioned 7.9 mm posteriorly to the left tibia in the neutral position. After alignment, the translations measured the following (in millimeters):

	Injured	Uninjured
Total	12.4	3.9
Anterior	1.3	2.6
Posterior	11.2	1.3

The injured knee exhibited a greatly increased posterior translation compared to the contralateral knee and compared to the normal control group. No difference was noted in anterior translation or in the translations on the uninjured side. Before alignment of the injured side, the stress test measurements indicated increased anterior translation with normal posterior displacement on the injured side. At surgery, the posterior cruciate ligament appeared lax and the anterior cruciate ligament normal.

Another important finding from in vivo tests is the frequent occurrence of a greater amount of translation occurring on the uninjured knee than the contralateral injured knee. In patients with a ruptured anterior cruciate ligament tested at 90 degrees of knee flexion, Kochan et al.[28] found that 11 of 41 (27%) had a greater amount of translation in the normal knee when compared to the injured knee, and Torzilli et al.[52] found this to occur in 6 of 25 (24%) patients. This is not an isolated finding, as it has been reported at other flexion angles and by other investigators.[20,21]

This inconsistency occurred too infrequently to be associated with patient or technical errors. It does not, however, negate the accuracy of these mechanical devices for measuring in vivo knee motion. It is more likely that any single measurement, from one particular device, will be inappropriate for diagnostic purposes. A series of biomechanical tests will have to be performed and used in conjunction with the appropriate protocol for evaluating the injured patient.

■ PATIENT EVALUATION

A systematic protocol for patient evaluation can be developed by using a unified

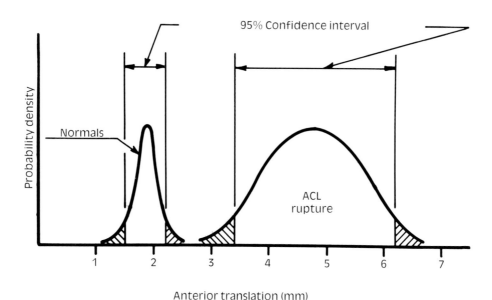

Fig. 24-35 ■ Schematic representation of probability distributions for amount of anterior translation resulting from 50-newton joint line load at 90 degrees of knee flexion for the 52 normal knees and 25 knees with anterior cruciate ligament rupture shown in Fig. 24-34.

statistical analysis of the measured parameters. One possibility is the use of confidence intervals on the measured parameters to determine patient injury status. This is illustrated schematically in Fig. 24-35. Following a biomechanical evaluation, the amount of anterior translation occurring in an injured knee can be classified according to the specific interval it is contained in, for instance, within the normal range, in a specific injury range, or between ranges. If the measured anterior translation falls within either confidence interval, it would represent a positive finding. On the other hand, if the value is outside the confidence intervals, it would be recorded as a negative or equivocal finding. Similar intervals could be determined for the other measured parameters, including differences between contralateral sides and anterior vs. posterior differences within the same knee. Shown in Figs. 24-36 and 24-37, respectively, is the probability distribution for the amount of anterior translation and the difference in the anterior translation between contralateral sides for normal subjects and patients with anterior cruciate ligament rupture. These distribu-

tions were obtained using the KT-1000 Knee Ligament Arthrometer (see Fig. 24-27) at an 89-newton anterior force at 30 degrees of knee flexion. Note that there is considerable overlap between the anterior translation distributions, while the distribution for the difference between contralateral sides demonstrates two distinct regions. The latter measurement may provide a better criterion for determining anterior cruciate ligament injuries, because there is less chance for an equivocal diagnosis.

After a multiple series of tests has been performed, all the parameters could be compared to a series of statistical distributions to determine the number of positive and negative findings. The compilation of the number of positive and negative findings could then be used to provide a statistical probabilitiy of occurrence of a particular injury. A diagnosis could then be made from the maximal likelihood or probability[57] of this particular combination of positive and negative findings occurring.

This procedure is illustrated in Fig. 24-38 using Case #3 (left knee posterior cruciate ligament rupture). Please note that

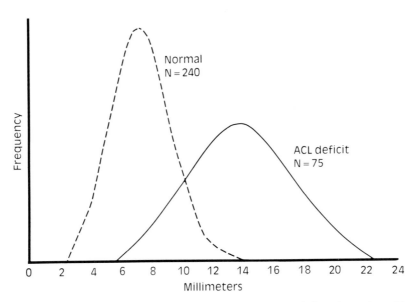

Fig. 24-36 ■ Probability distributions for amount of anterior translation (drawer) resulting from 89-newton midtibial force in 240 normal knees (120 subjects) and 75 knees with rupture of anterior cruciate ligament. All tests were performed using KT-1000 Knee Ligament Arthrometer shown in Fig. 24-27.
Data courtesy L. Malcolm, Ph. D., and D. Daniel, M.D., San Diego, Calif.

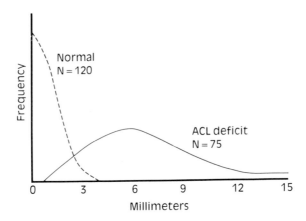

Fig. 24-37 ■ Contralateral difference in anterior translation (drawer) between contralateral knees for subject groups shown in Fig. 24-36.
Data courtesy L. Malcolm, Ph. D., and D. Daniel, M.D., San Diego, Calif.

this is a simple illustrative example based on an actual patient evaluation. Not all the abnormal probability distributions illustrated in Fig. 24-38 (particularly the posterior cruciate ligament distribution) have been fully determined.

The amount of total translation measured in the right knee (R) is far to the right of the distribution for a cruciate rupture, while the left knee (L) is normal. The difference in the neutral positions between contralateral sides is also abnormal, necessitating a shift in the anterior and posterior translation values on the right. No abnormal anterior translation is found in the left knee or shifted right knee, R_s. Before alignment, the right knee appeared to fall to the right of the distri-

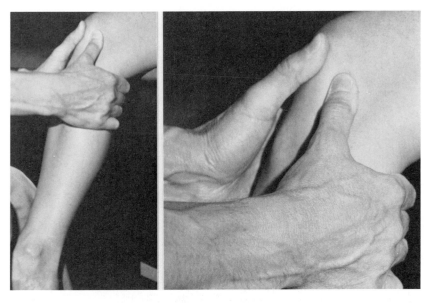

Fig. 25-15 ■ Anteromedial drawer test (for anteromedial rotary instability). Patient is seated leaning against examining room wall with hamstrings and patellar tendon relaxed. Foot is held in external rotation with examiner's legs. Tibia is pulled anteriorly with fingers. Lateral thumb applies counterpressure on inferior pole of patella. Medial thumb is used to palpate anterior displacement of medial tibial condyle. Positive test usually indicates loss of anterior cruciate ligament, failure or absence of medial meniscus, or combination. Medial meniscus may displace when high loads are used for test with patient under anesthesia. This indicates unstable tear of medial meniscus.

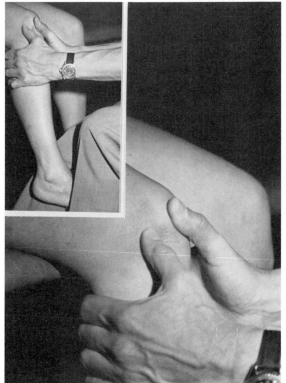

Fig. 25-16 ■ Anterolateral drawer test (for anterolateral rotary instability). Patient is seated and leaning against examining room wall. Hamstrings are relaxed. Foot is held medially rotated with examiner's legs. Fingers are used to pull tibia forward as medial thumb applies counterpressure on inferior pole of patella. Lateral thumb is used to palpate anterior displacement of lateral tibial condyle. Anterolateral rotary instability (with this test) is not as common because of powerful stabilizing affect of iliotibial band when knee is flexed and tibia internally rotated.

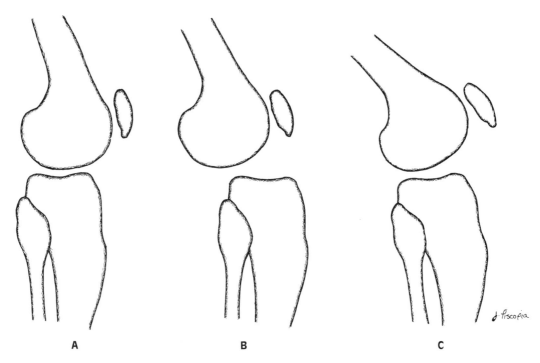

Fig. 25-17 ■ Pivot shift phenomena. **A,** Reduced 0 to 15 degrees. **B,** Subluxation 15 to 40 degrees. **C,** Reduction 40 to 135 degrees.

ing effect of the iliotibial band when the knee is flexed and the tibia internally rotated.

Pivot shift testing. The pivot shift test is a confirmatory test of the anterior cruciate ligament–deficient knee.[17,20,21,47,50] It is less frequently positive in the acute case than the Lachman's test. The pivot shift test is frequently negative for 6 weeks after the tear of the anterior cruciate ligament.[60] This may be caused by muscle spasm and edematous thickening of the capsular ligament from the hemarthrosis. The test becomes dramatically positive in the chronic anterior cruciate ligament–deficient knee, as the secondary stabilizers relax and the menisci either degrade or are torn.

With the anterior cruciate ligament torn, the tibia can be subluxed anteriorly on the femur when the knee is straighter than 15 degrees, and the tibia will spontaneously reduce to its normal position when the knee is flexed past 30 degrees (Fig. 25-17). Using one or more of the de-

scribed maneuvers, this transition can be made very sudden. It is diagnostic to the examiner and felt by the patient.

MacIntosh pivot shift test. The patient lies supine, and the examiner applies a valgus stress and internal rotation load to the extended knee. Initially, the iliotibial band passes forward to the instant center of the lateral femoral condyle, creating an anterior displacement force on the lateral tibial condyle. As the knee is flexed past 20 to 30 degrees of flexion, the iliotibial band suddenly passes behind the instant center of the lateral femoral condyle, creating a posterior displacement force on the lateral tibial condyle. The sudden reduction of the lateral tibial condyle can be felt by the patient and the examiner[21] (Fig. 25-18).

Losee test. With the patient supine, the examiner's hand is placed on the lateral side of the knee with the thumb under the head of the fibula. A valgus stress is applied. As the knee is extended, the tibia subluxes forward, and as the knee is flexed, the tibia can be seen to reduce.[48]

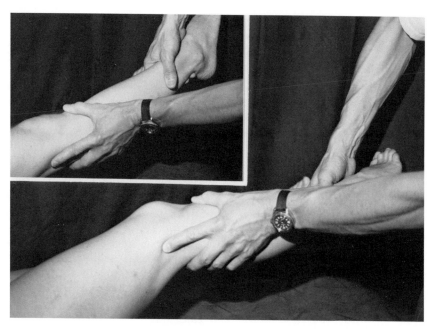

Fig. 25-18 ■ Pivot shift test. Patient is lying supine, and examiner applies valgus stress and internal rotation load to extended knee, which subluxes lateral tibial condyle anteriorly. As knee is flexed past 20 to 30 degrees of flexion, iliotibial band suddenly passes behind instant center of lateral femoral condyle (producing a sudden reduction of the lateral tibial condyle), which can be felt by patient and examiner. Test becomes more positive when medial or lateral meniscus is torn. During first 6 weeks, test may be negative or only trace positive when there is positive Lachman's test.

Jerk test. "Jerk" is a mechanical term meaning a sudden acceleration. Hughston used this term to describe the sudden acceleration noted by the patient and the examiner as the lateral tibial condyle subluxes suddenly as the knee is extended.[34] With the patient supine, the jerk test is elicited at about 30 degrees of knee flexion the moderately internally rotated tibia is brought from a position of 90 degrees of knee flexion to full extension while a mild abduction stress is applied.

Slocum test. The Slocum test[70] is done with the patient lying on the unaffected side with the affected leg up and the foot lying on the examining table. The examiner applies a valgus stress by pressing down on the tibia and femur while simultaneously flexing and extending the knee from full extension to 30 degrees of flexion. The lateral condyle of the tibia will sublux anteriorly as the knee is extended and reduce in a normal position as the knee is flexed.

Flexion-rotation drawer test. The flexion-rotation drawer test, described by Noyes et al.[62] takes advantage of the weight of the thigh to provide both a posterior and external rotation load on the femur, creating a relative anterolateral subluxation of the tibia. The test can be enhanced by axial loading of the limb by pressure on the heel. As the knee is flexed and the tibia pressed posteriorly, the tibia can be seen to suddenly reduce on the femur. This test has the advantage of not creating so much tightness in a somewhat edematous, inflexible capsule.

In our experience the flexion-rotation drawer test is the one most frequently positive in the acute injury. All of the tests are frequently positive in chronic anterior cruciate ligament injuries.

Cross-over test. Arnold and Coker[3] have described a test in which, with the patient standing, the examiner fixes the foot of the patient's affected leg by standing on it. The patient then rotates the upper body, crossing the unaffected leg over the fixed foot until he faces 90 degrees in the opposite direction. A positive test occurs when the patient describes a feeling of the knee "wanting to go out."

Posteromedial rotatory instability

Posteromedial rotatory instability test. Posteromedial rotary instability results from tearing of the posteromedial capsule complex. The knee is held in extension and a valgus stress applied. The medial side of the knee will reveal an apparent knock-knee.

Posterolateral rotatory instability

Posterolateral rotary instability results from a tear of the arcuate ligament complex with the posterior cruciate ligament left intact.[4,12,35] A number of tests can be used to identify its presence.

Posterolateral drawer test. The posterolateral drawer test described by Hughston[35] is done with the patient supine and the knee flexed 80 degrees, with the examiner sitting on the externally rotated foot. As the tibia is pushed, the lateral tibial condyle displaces posteriorly, and the tibial tubercle displaces laterally.

The posterolateral drawer test can also be done with the patient seated as for the posterior drawer test. The foot is externally rotated and the tibia pushed posteriorly. Normally, there is posterior displacement of the lateral condyle of the tibia with this maneuver, but when posterolateral rotary instability is present, the motion is greater than in the normal knee, and the tibial tubercle displaces laterally. The advantage of doing the test with the patient seated is that the examiner's thumb can be used to more accurately palpate the posture of the joint line.

External rotation recurvatum test. The external rotation recurvatum test is positive when the arcuate complex and the anteromedial and intermediate fibers of the anterior cruciate ligament are torn.[35] With the patient supine and the legs resting on the table, the examiner gently grasps the great toes of both feet at the same time and lifts the feet from the table. The test is positive when the affected knee goes into hyperextension on the lateral side and the tibia is seen to externally rotate with the posterolateral displacement of the tibial tuberosity (Fig. 25-19). The medial aspect of the knee will reveal an apparent bowleg.

Reverse pivot shift test. The Jakob test[37] is a reverse pivot shift. The tibia is reduced in extension (if the anterior cruciate ligament is intact) and subluxes posteriorly in flexion. As the fibular head is palpated and the knee passed from full extension into flexion, the fibular head can be felt to displace posteriorly and the tibia to rotate externally. For the test to be positive, the patient must sense that this reproduces his symptoms. The posterior cruciate ligament is normal or only slightly lax.

Meniscal testing
Medial meniscus instability

The patient with a chronic anterior cruciate ligament injury and the older athlete with an unstable degenerative meniscus tear will typically exhibit subtle catching and grinding over the medial joint line associated with medial joint line pain (Fig. 25-20). The classic McMurray flexion rotation test,[55,56] the Helfet test,[27] and the Apley grinding test[1,2] are useful in reproducing these symptoms. The McMurray test is done with the patient supine and the knee flexed and extended with the tibia externally rotated and valgus stress applied while the joint is simultaneously palpated. The Apley test is done with the patient prone, the knee flexed, and a downward load applied at the foot. Flexion and rotation produce a grinding sensation at the joint line. The Helfet test is performed by having the patient extend to

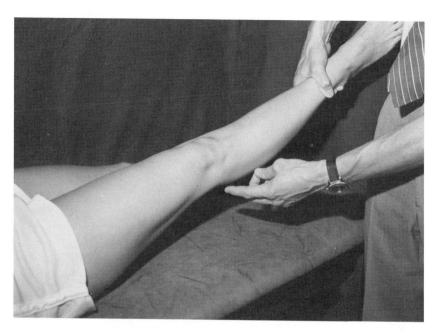

Fig. 25-19 ■ External rotation recurvatum test. Patient is supine and toe or heel is elevated. Test is positive when knee goes into hyperextension on lateral side and tibia is seen to externally rotate with posterolateral displacement of tibial tuberosity. When this test is positive, arcuate complex and anteromedial and intermediate fibers of anterior cruciate ligament are torn.

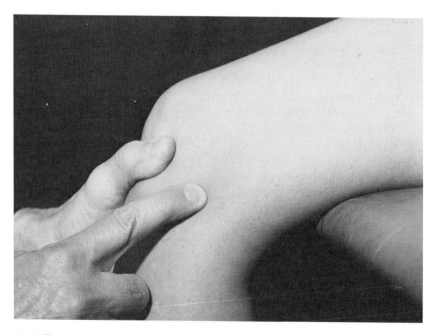

Fig. 25-20 ■ Medial meniscus instability. Medial joint line point tenderness may indicate tear of medial meniscus. Examiner must be careful to exclude inferomedial parapatellar and medial fat pad tenderness typical of patellar tendinitis from much less common medial joint line tenderness, which may indicate tear of medial meniscus.

0 degrees from a position of 90 degrees. Loss of the normal rotation relationship between the midpatella and tibial tubercle indicates a positive test.

Most of us have experienced the frustration of attempting these tests and not reproducing the symptoms at all, whereupon the patient says, "Doctor, when I do it this way it makes it pop." The patient should always be asked to attempt to reproduce the symptom or at least show the maneuver that last reproduced the symptom. In the knee with anterior cruciate ligament injury, the patient will most commonly fully flex the knee by pulling the heel up to the buttock with both hands, at which point the tibia can be seen to slip forward, and an audible "clunk" is heard.

In the knee with anterior cruciate ligament deficiency, the medial meniscus can be made to go unstable with the high-load anteromedial rotary instability test. This test is performed just as the anteromedial rotary instability test is at either 20 or 90 degrees with much higher loads (Fig. 25-21). We no longer do this test in the office, because occasionally a meniscus becomes inadvertently locked and cannot be unlocked. This test correlates well with an unstable medial meniscus tear when performed in the operating room with the patient under anesthesia. The foot is held in external rotation by an assistant, and a very high anterior drawer stress or Lachman's stress is applied by pressing posteriorly on the patella with the thumbs and pulling forward on the posterior proximal tibia with the long, ring, and little fingers. When the medial meniscus subluxes, the tibia is felt to suddenly snap forward. When the pressure is released, the tibia can be felt to suddenly reduce. The test can be done in the office with lesser loads to look only for medial joint line tenderness and apprehension by the patient.

In the knee with a deficient anterior cruciate ligament, we have accurately diagnosed 32% of medial meniscus tears in the office by clinical examination alone.[28]

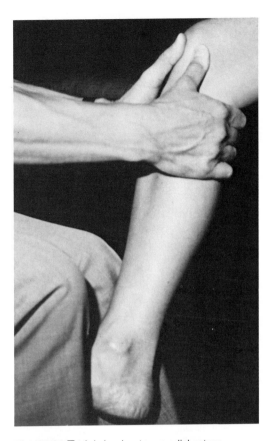

Fig. 25-21 ■ High-load anteromedial rotary instability. In anterior cruciate ligament deficiency, unstable medial meniscus may be subluxed by this test. With knee flexed either 20 or 90 degrees, tibia is pulled anteriorly with fingers and counterforce applied at inferior pole of patella with thumbs. Patient is placed under anesthesia, and examiner applies maximal force. Test is positive when meniscus displaces forward and knee suddenly subluxes. When force is released and tibia pushed posteriorly, meniscus will usually reduce. (We no longer do this test in the office because of occasional inadvertent locking of a medial meniscus.)

The arthrogram, arthroscopy, pyrophosphate scanning, and the high-load anteromedial rotary instability test performed with the patient under anesthesia are indicated to determine the status of the medial meniscus.

Lateral meniscal instability

With the patient seated and leaning back against the examining room wall, the

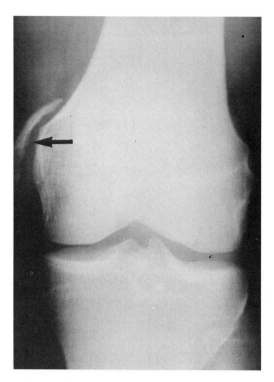

Fig. 26-16 ■ Pelligrini-Stieda disease. Note ossification of medial collateral ligament (arrow).

30 degrees of flexion. This places the patellar tendon under tension and demonstrates its functional relationship to the knee (see Fig. 26-32).

The advantages of obtaining an axial view of the patella and patellofemoral joint have been appreciated for a long time; most of the earlier techniques, such as the "skyline" and "sunrise" views, are obtained with the knee in marked flexion. However, high degrees of flexion place the patella in the distal part of the femoral groove, which is not where subluxation occurs. Recognizing this, Hughston[14] modified earlier techniques to obtain the axial view in 50 to 60 degrees of flexion (Fig. 26-17). On this view, both the sulcus angle and patellar index can provide quantitative measurements of the patella and patellofemoral joint.

Merchant et al.[28] noted three disadvantages of the Hughston technique, the most important being distortion of the image resulting from the x-ray beam striking the film at 45 degrees. In addition, rotation of the femur is not well controlled, which may alter the apparent height of the lateral femoral condyle. Third, degrees of flexion approaching 60 degrees are still relatively insensitive to subluxations.

The Merchant view, originally described by McNab,[26] is obtained with the patient supine with the knees flexed 45 degrees over the end of the x-ray table. The x-ray beam is angled caudally at an angle 30 degrees above the horizontally positioned femora (Fig. 26-18). The legs are strapped together, which controls rotation, and both knees are examined simultaneously. Employing this view, Merchant et al.[28] devised the "congruence angle," which permits measurement of the relationship of the patellar articular ridge to the intercondylar sulcus. In their series of one hundred normal subjects a congruence angle greater than +16 degrees is abnormal at the 95th percentile. We have found the Merchant view to be a convenient method for the routine axial examination of the patellofemoral relationship (Fig. 26-19).

Laurin et al.[23] further modified the axial view, enabling examination at 20 to 30 degrees of flexion (Fig. 26-20). This permits visualization of the patella at or near the proximal segment of the femoral groove where subluxation, if present, is most apparent. Using the view, the lateral patellofemoral angle devised by Laurin et al. provides a quantitative measurement, which appears to be a highly sensitive and specific indicator of subluxation of the patella. Ninety-seven percent of clinically normal knees formed a lateral patellofemoral angle that was open laterally. In all patients with proven recurrent subluxation, the lines were parallel or formed a reverse lateral patellofemoral angle. None of the normal individuals in their series had a lateral patellofemoral angle open medially.[23]

More accurate and reproducible methods of patellofemoral joint examination

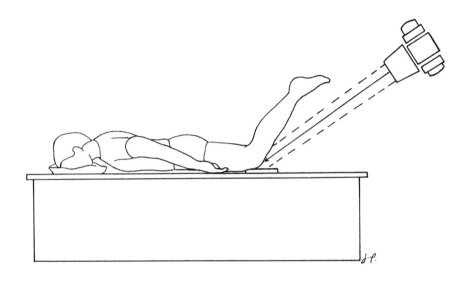

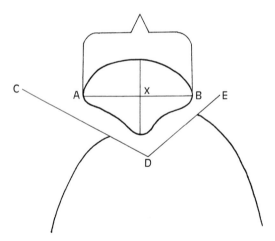

Fig. 26-17 ■ Sulcus angle is formed by lines *cd* and *de*. Patellar index is the width of the patella *(ab)* divided by the difference of the lateral facet *(ax)* and medial facet *(xb)*.
Adapted from Hughston, J.C.: J. Bone Joint Surg. **50A:**1003, 1968; with permission.

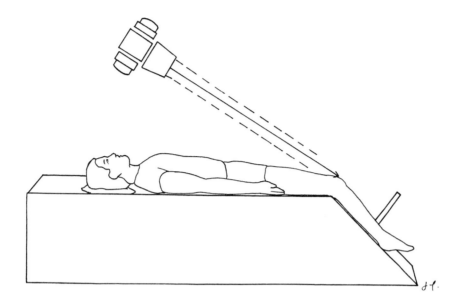

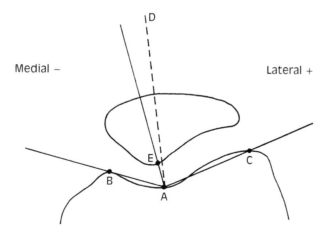

Fig. 26-18 ■ Congruence angle *(ead)* is determined by the intersection of the line *(ad)* bisecting the sulcus angle *(bac)* and a line *(ae)* drawn through lowest point on articular surface of the patella. Average congruence angle was −6 degrees with a standard deviation of 11 degrees in 100 normal subjects.

Adapted from Merchant, A.C., Mercer, R.L., Jacobson, R.H., and Cool, C.R.: J. Bone Joint Surg. **56A:**1391, 1974; with permission.

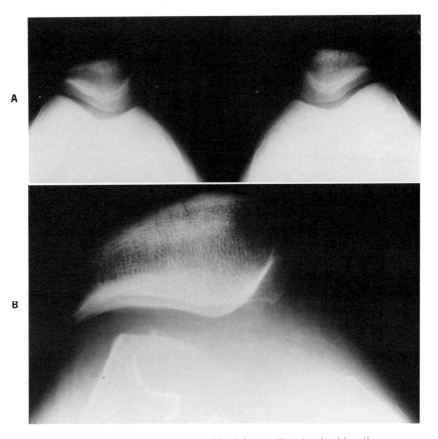

Fig. 26-19 ■ A, Normal view of both knees. **B,** Lateral subluxation.

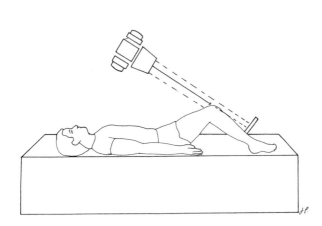

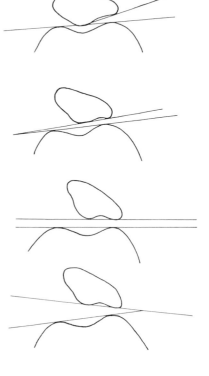

Fig. 26-20 ■ Lateral patellofemoral angle is usually open laterally and never open medially in normal individuals.
Adapted from Laurin, C.A., Levesque, H.P., Dussault, R., Labelle, H., Peides, J.P.: J. Bone Joint Surg. **60A:**55, 1978; with permission.

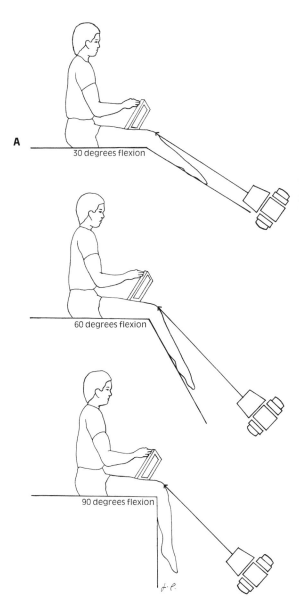

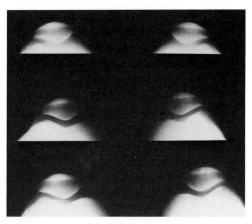

Fig. 26-21 ■ Dynamic 30-, 60-, and 90-degree flexion study positions, **A,** and roentgenograms, **B.**
Adapted from Ficat, R.P., and Hungerford, D.S.: Disorders of the patellofemoral joint, Baltimore, 1977, Williams & Wilkins Co.; with permission.

requiring special positioning apparatus and multiple exposures at different degrees of angulation have been described.[12,22,29] Ficat and Hungerford[12] have outlined a dynamic roentgenographic technique using 30, 60, and 90 degrees of flexion for more detailed examination of the patellofemoral articulation (Fig. 26-21). In a recent review of that method, the 30-degree projection was found to be most sensitive in detecting tendencies of the patella toward subluxation.[29] The axial views may reveal narrowing of the lateral patel-lofemoral joint, and there may be an increase in subchondral bone density of the lateral facet of the patella when compared with the opposite knee, indicative of a patellofemoral compression syndrome.

Complete dislocation of the patella usually does not require an axial view, because the diagnosis is quite apparent on routine frontal and lateral views (Fig. 26-22).

In more subtle cases, where there is strong clinical suspicion of patellofemoral instability, computed axial tomographic scanning through the patellofemoral joint with the knee in 15 degrees of flexion has been described to demonstrate the subluxation not readily apparent on axial radiographs[25] (Fig. 26-23). More recently, computed tomographic scanning following arthrography has been investigated and shows particular promise in the diagnosis of chondromalacia patella.[28,29]

The relatively frequent occurrence of a **bipartite patella** has occasionally caused confusion in the diagnosis of an acute patellar fracture. In the normal bipartite patella the nonunited separate ossification center occurs in the superolateral aspect of the patella and demonstrates rounded,

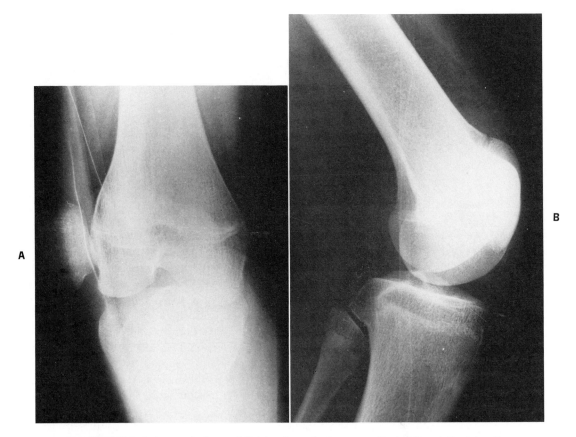

Fig. 26-22 ■ **A,** Anteroposterior, and **B,** lateral roentgenograms. Complete patella dislocation.

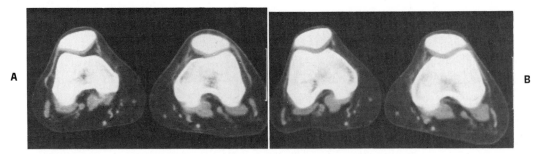

Fig. 26-23 ■ Axial CT scans at 15 degrees of flexion, **A,** and 30 degrees of flexion, **B.** Note that slight lateral subluxation of the right patella seen on the 15-degree study is missed on the 30-degree study.

smooth, and well-defined cortical margins (Fig. 26-24 and 26-25). Comparison views with the opposite leg may not be helpful, since bipartiate patellae occur both unilaterally and bilaterally (Fig 26-26). When the diagnosis of a stress fracture of the patella[8] remains in question, radionuclide bone scanning may be helpful to differentiate stress fractures from bipartite patellae.

The inferior pole of the patella is stabilized by the patellar ligament, which inserts on the tibial tuberosity. The patellar tendon, while strong, is weakest at its upper and lower attachments, which are mechanically vulnerable sites.[27]

The roentgenographic features of **Osgood-Schlatter's disease** are noted at the lower attachment of the patellar tendon (Fig. 26-27). The tibial tubercle shows frag-

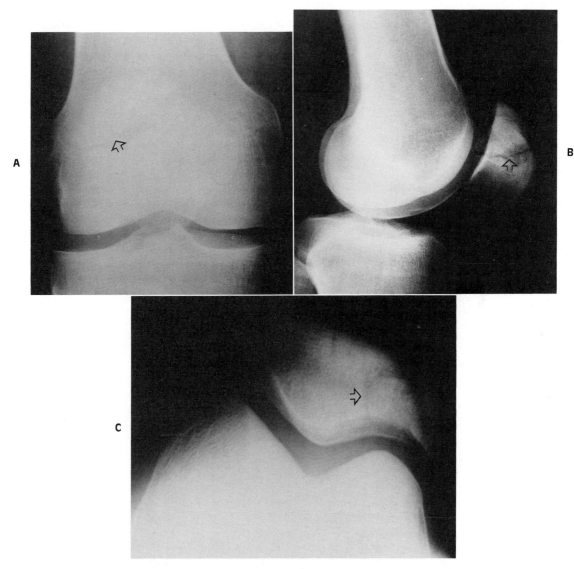

Fig. 26-24 ■ A, Anteroposterior **B,** lateral, and **C,** axial roentgenograms of a bipartate patella. Note the smooth corticated margins and typical superolateral location (arrows).

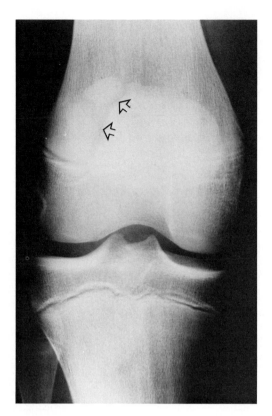

Fig. 26-25 ■ Tripartite patella *(arrows)*.

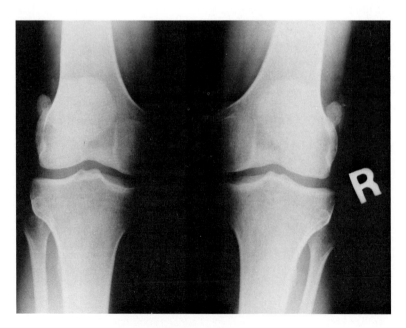

Fig. 26-26 ■ Bilateral bipartite patellae.

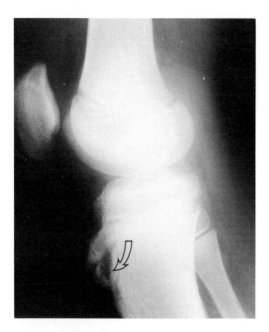

Fig. 26-27 ■ Osgood-Schlatter's disease. Note the fragmented tibial tubercle *(arrow).*

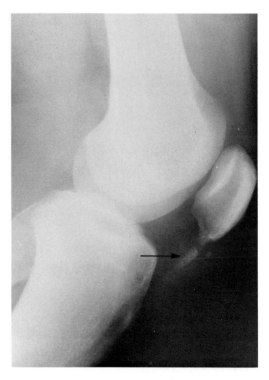

Fig. 26-28 ■ Sinding-Larsen-Johanssen syndrome. Note the organized fragment at the inferior pole of the patella *(arrow).*

mentation, and the fragments appear displaced away from the shaft. There may be no swelling of the overlying soft tissues. Sometimes the fragments of bone are increased in density. Because the tibial tubercle normally develops irregularly from either one or two ossification centers and is densely ossified, the diagnosis relies heavily on clinical correlation.[9,30] Films of the contralateral knee should be obtained for comparison.

Alternatively, the roentgenographic changes associated with **Sinding-Larsen–Johanssen** syndrome are seen at the upper portion of the patellar tendon.[18,27,34] An association with Osgood-Schlatter's disease has been noted previously.[36]

In their recent prospective study, Medlar and Lyne[27] identified four radiographic stages of the disease process. At the initial onset of symptoms (Stage I), roentgenograms show no abnormality. In 2 to 4 weeks (Stage II), irregular calcifications at the inferior pole of the patella are noted. Later (Stage III) the calcifications are seen to coalesce, and in the final stages (Stage

IV) the coalesced calcifications may either be incorporated into the patella, yielding a normal roentgenogram, or remain as a separate mass from the patella (Fig. 26-28 and 26-29).

Acute **avulsions of the patellar tendon** may be associated with a high-positioned patella because of the resultant unrestricted pull traction by the quadriceps tendon (Fig. 26–30). Partial avulsions involving the lower pole of the patella in the presence of an intact patellar ligament may result in a free osteocartilaginous fragment within the joint space (Fig. 26-31).

Patella alta may be diagnosed from the lateral roentgenogram by determining the ratio of the patellar tendon length to the greatest diagonal length of the patella, as described by Insall and Salvati[15] (Fig 26-32). This method has been confirmed by Jacobson and Berthenson,[17] and both

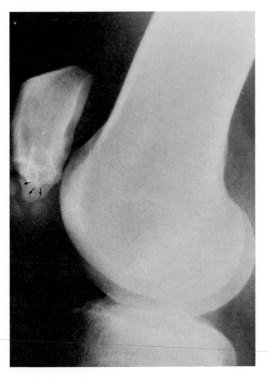

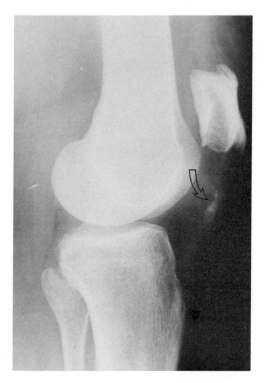

Fig. 26-29 ■ Sinding-Larsen-Johanssen syndrome. Marked fragmentation of the lower pole of the patella *(arrows)*.

Fig. 26-30 ■ Acute avulsion of the patellar tendon. Avulsed fragment *(arrow)* and high-riding patella are seen.

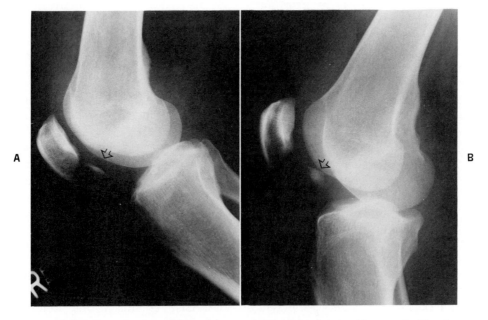

Fig. 26-31 ■ **A,** Lateral, and **B,** oblique views. Avulsed patellar fragment has resulted in a loose joint body *(arrows)*.

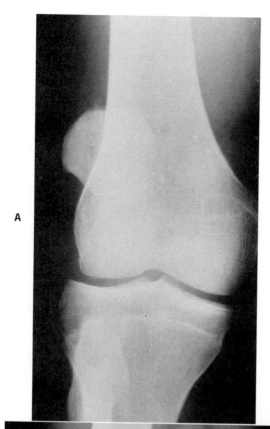

A

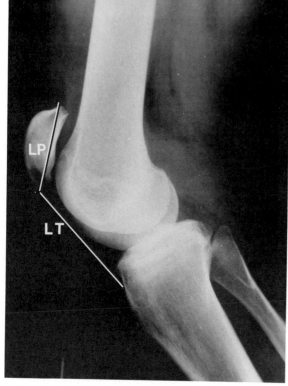

B

LP

LT

Fig. 26-32 ■ **A**, Anteroposterior, and **B**, lateral roentgenograms in patella alta. The ratio of the patellar tendon length *(LT)* to the patella length *(LP)* is 1.6, consistent with diagnosis of patella alta.

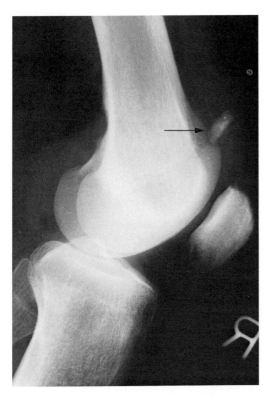

Fig. 26-33 ■ Avulsion of the superior pole of the patella *(arrow)*.

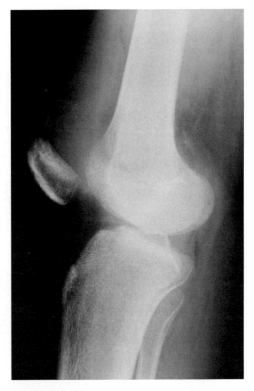

Fig. 26-34 ■ Acute rupture of the quadriceps tendon. The accumulation of blood in the suprapatellar space displaces the patella anteriorly and inferiorly.

series indicate a ratio of 1:2 as the upper limit of normal at the 98% confidence level.

The **quadriceps tendon**, which inserts into the superior pole of the patella, may also be the site of ligamentous rupture or avulsion fracture. The avulsed superior pole of the patella may be visualized on the lateral roentgenograph (Fig. 26-33). In acute rupture of the quadriceps tendon, the superior pole of the patella may be displaced anteriorly and inferiorly by the accumulation of blood within the supra-patellar space (Fig. 26–34).

■ ARTHROGRAPHY OF THE KNEE

Since its inception, arthrography has played a major role in evaluation of injuries to such joints as the knee, shoulder, and ankle. The diagnostic gains regarding internal derangement of the knee have been significantly high. Torn menisci have been clearly demonstrated in a majority of cases. Capsular and ligamentous tears have also been successfully demonstrated, except in those instances where the tear may have sealed off.

Although the recent development of arthroscopy has somewhat changed the indications for arthrography and caused a slight drop in the number of arthrographic studies of the knee, the incidence of arthrography of the shoulder and ankle remains essentially unchanged. Both arthrography and arthroscopy, however, are complementary modalities and ought to remain so.

The technique of arthrography has been very well documented in several papers and books.[1,2,8,9,21] Arthrography, if

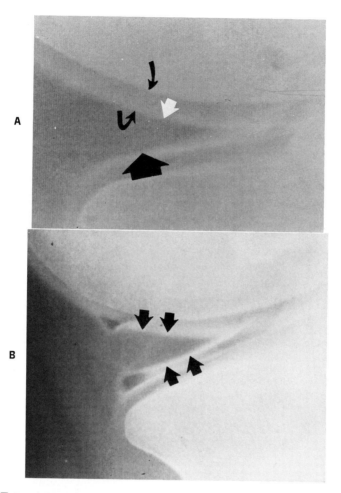

Fig. 26-35 ■ A and **B,** Normal posterior horn of medial meniscus shown in cross-section. Its normal outline is revealed by iodide contrast agent layering on its surface. Meniscus fills in space between articular surfaces of the femoral and tibial condyles. Note normal thickness of articular cartilage *(curved arrows).*

properly executed, is a relatively painless procedure that can be done on an outpatient basis. Morbidity is negligible, and reactions to contrast agents are infrequent. Joint infection is rare; when infection occurs, it is usually a result of lack of proper sterile technique.

Acute knee injuries may cause great discomfort during manipulations for optimal visualization of the menisci. However, injuries several days old should cause little undue pain or discomfort to the individual during the study. Shoulder and ankle arthrography are also relatively painless procedures.

It is beyond the scope of this chapter to include all data that have been amassed on arthrography of the knee. Only certain relevant and more commonly diagnosed conditions are included in this section.

Meniscal visualization

Normal medial and lateral menisci are demonstrated in Figs. 26-35 through 26-39. The iodide contrast agent coats the surface of the meniscus, which is demonstrated here in cross section. The outline is smooth and sharply delineated. No contrast (air or iodide) enters the

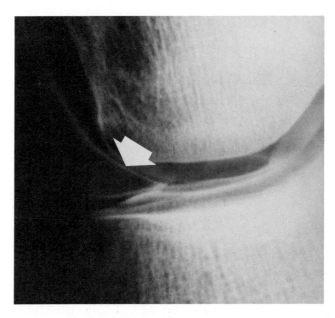

Fig. 26-36 ■ Body of normal medial meniscus is clearly outlined by double-contrast method (air and iodide). This is achieved easily by applying lateral stress to open up the medial joint space. In double-contrast arthrography, air (30 to 40 ml) and iodide contrast agent (4 to 6 ml) are instilled into knee joint.

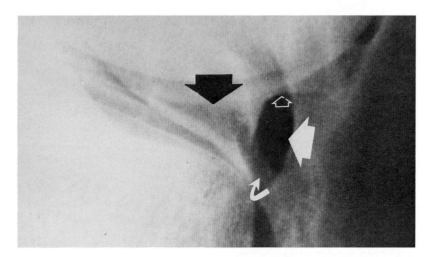

Fig. 26-37 ■ Normal posterior horn of lateral meniscus has been demonstrated on this double-contrast study. Black oval shadow *(solid white arrow)* is the hiatus for the popliteus tendon, air being present in the synovial sleeve covering the popliteus tendon. Curved white arrow points to inferior attachment of posterior horn to knee joint capsule. Superior attachment is shown depicted by the white "open" arrow. Contrast agent outlines normal posterior horn of lateral meniscus *(black arrow)*.

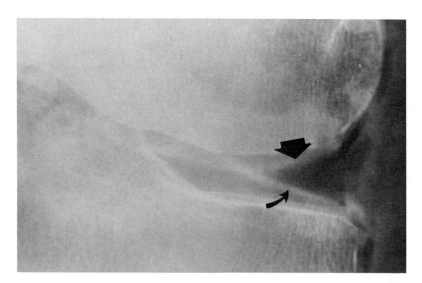

Fig. 26-38 ■ Normal body of lateral meniscus. Upper and lower surfaces of meniscus are indicated by solid and curved black arrows, respectively. Note hiatus for the popliteus tendon is no longer visible, meniscus being firmly attached to the joint capsule peripherally from this point to anterior attachment of the lateral meniscus.

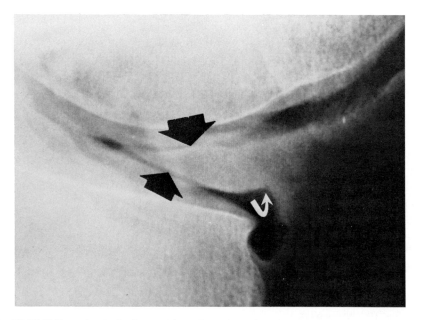

Fig. 26-39 ■ Normal anterior horn of lateral meniscus is somewhat elongated and relatively thin. Inferior, shallow recess is present at its peripheral attachment *(white arrow)*.

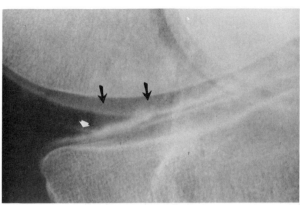 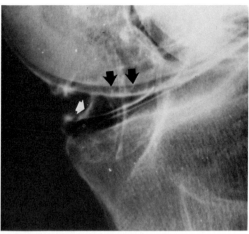

Fig. 26-40 ■ Oblique tear of posterior horn of medial meniscus. There is an oblique, linear line *(white arrow)* extending from middle undersurface of posterior horn into its substance. This line represents presence of contrast agent along an oblique tear. Solid black arrows point to normal thickness of articular cartilage.

substance of the meniscus; the free edge (apex) of the meniscus is sharp and pointed. The posterior horn of lateral meniscus demonstrated the hiatus for the popliteal tendon, air and contrast material being present in the synovial sleeve of the tendon[5,20] (see Fig. 26-37). Peripheral attachments of the posterior horn of the lateral meniscus are clearly seen as superior and inferior slings. Anteriorly the lateral meniscus is firmly attached peripherally to the capsule of the knee joint. However, the medial meniscus is attached to the joint capsule in its entire length.

The most commonly injured meniscus is the medial meniscus, although injuries to the lateral meniscus are by no means rare. Most injuries of the medial meniscus are in the posterior half of the meniscus and tend to involve the posterior horn. Arthrographic examination reveals, a tear of the meniscus, outlined by positive contrast agents like Hypaque or Renografin; in double-contrast arthrography, air and a contrast material are employed. These tears are usually oblique, horizontal, or vertical; they may even at times be complex in nature (Figs. 26-40 through

26-48). In the event of separation of torn fragments, contrast agent would lie between the torn fragments. However, in the absence of separation of the fragments, the tear of the meniscus would be indicated by the presence of a linear shadow of the contrast agent used. The medial fragment often migrates into the intercondylar region and may not be visualized clearly on arthrography, unless particular attention is paid to discerning this. These tears are often called "bucket handle" tears. Tears of the posterior third of the "lateral" meniscus are often difficult to evaluate because of the presence of the hiatus or the synovial sleeve for the popliteal tendon.[5,20] Figs. 26-40 through 26-48 show the various types of tears involving medial and lateral menisci.

Abnormalities of the articular cartilage

During arthrography for a suspected tear of a meniscus, other abnormalities, such as degenerative changes involving the articular cartilage, are often clearly demonstrated. (Figs. 26-49 through 26-51). Normally the articular cartilage in the knee is 2 to 3 millimeters thick; thinning of articular cartilage suggests degenerative

Text continued on p. 836.

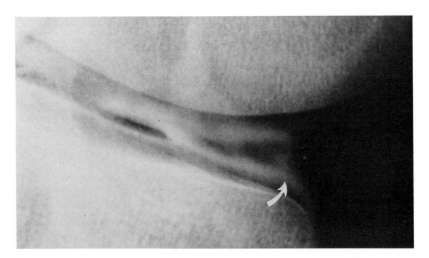

Fig. 26-41 ■ Vertical tear of posterior horn of medial meniscus. Curved white arrow points to peripheral, vertical tear in posterior horn of medial meniscus outlined by iodide contrast agent. Undersurface of meniscus has imbibed great amount of contrast, indicating associated damage to its undersurface.

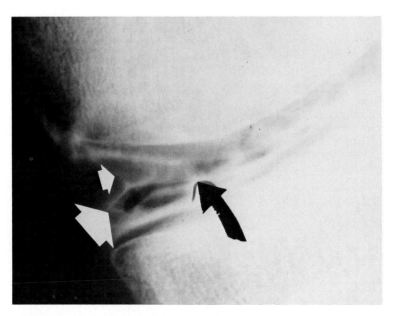

Fig. 26-42 ■ Complex tear of posterior horn of medial meniscus. Meniscus is torn in several places with marked irregularity and partial separation. Both upper and lower surfaces imbibe greater than normal amounts of contrast, probably secondary to crush injury to meniscus.

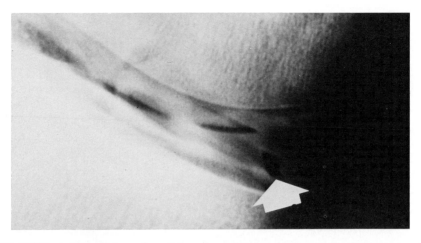

Fig. 26-43 ■ Bucket-handle tear of medial meniscus. Meniscus is torn vertically in a concentric manner, free portion having separated from peripheral segment. Often in this type of meniscal tear, the torn fragment displaces towards the intercondylar area.

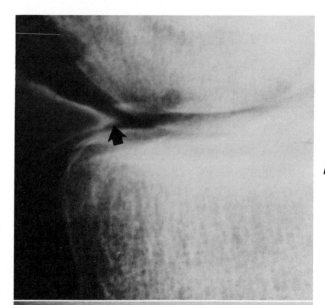

A

Fig. 26-44 ■ Torn anterior horn of medial meniscus. **A,** There is blunting of anterior portion of medial meniscus, indicating a tear. Apex of meniscus is irregular, thin, and imbibes more contrast than usual. **B,** There is loss of free portion of anterior horn of medial meniscus from a tear.

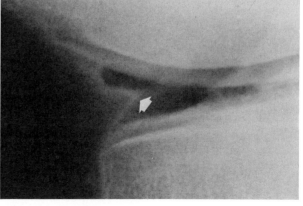

B

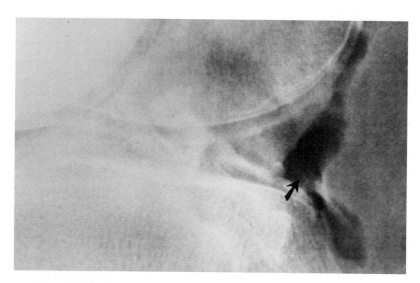

Fig. 26-45 ■ Torn posterior horn of lateral meniscus. Arrow points to torn inferior attachment of posterior horn of lateral meniscus, a difficult area for arthrographic evaluation. Rest of posterior horn is intact.

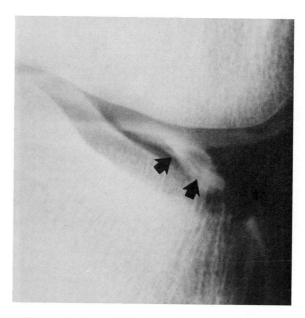

Fig. 26-46 ■ Posterior horn of lateral meniscus is crushed, deformed, and pounded. Hiatus of popliteus tendon cannot be seen.

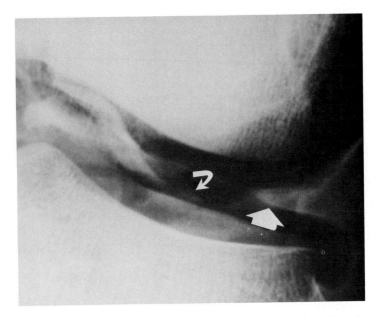

Fig. 26-47 ■ Body of lateral meniscus is deformed, short, and irregular in outline. Torn portion of meniscus is medially displaced *(curved arrow)*.

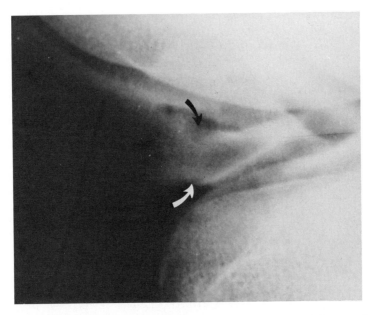

Fig. 26-48 ■ Anterior horn of lateral meniscus is "fractured" at its periphery, and medial portion is turned upward. Note site of tear *(arrows)*.

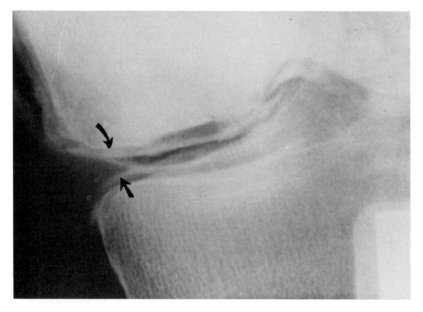

Fig. 26-49 ■ Degenerative arthritis. Curved arrow points to thinning of articular cartilage secondary to osteoarthritis. Meniscus is intact *(straight arrow)*.

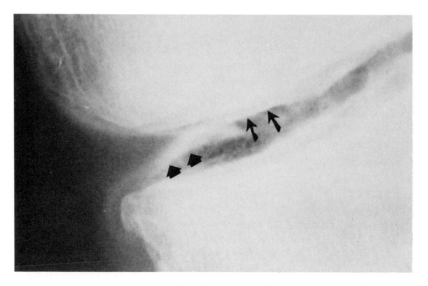

Fig. 26-50 ■ Combination of osteoarthritis with thinning of articular cartilage *(long arrows)* and degenerative change in free portion of the midthird medial meniscus, not an uncommon occurrence *(short arrows)*.

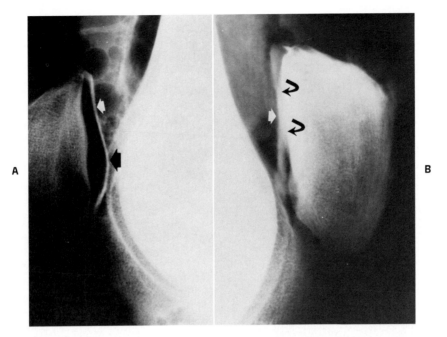

Fig. 26-51 ■ **A,** Lateral spot film study of patella shows normal articular cartilage, which is smooth and of normal thickness. **B,** In this view of patella, there is a large central erosion of articular surface of patella *(curved black arrows and small white arrow).* This appearance would be consistent with advanced case of chondromalacia or osteoarthritis.

process.[6] In osteochondritis dissecans, the nature of the cartilage over the involved area can be evaluated for a break in continuity, or the thickness of the articular cartilage overlying the lesion can be clearly assessed. If there is any break in the continuity of the articular cartilage, the contrast agent would seep into the subarticular area and surround the osteocartilaginous fragment, suggesting impending separation of the fragment.

Cruciate ligament visualization

Cruciate ligaments are easily recognized by contrast arthrography despite their extrasynovial location.[3,7,12,15-17] A normal cruciate ligament is usually very sharply delineated by the overlying synovial lining, and any change in the contour of the synovial lining in this area is indicative of a cruciate ligament injury. Fig. 26-52 demonstrates normal and torn cruciate ligaments. In an acutely injured knee, capsular tears are easily recognized by leakage

of contrast through the discontinuous capsular fibers (Fig. 26-53). However, if the examination is delayed by more than 48 to 72 hours, the tear may seal itself off and the arthrographic study may thus have a negative result. Sometimes lateral stress applied during arthrography may elicit a tear of the capsule more easily.

Popliteal cysts

Among the synovial abnormalities of the knee, popliteal cysts (often referred to as "Baker's cyst") are a frequently encountered abnormality found in arthrography (Fig. 26-54). Baker's cyst results from distention of the gastrocnemius-semimembranous bursa, which communicates with the knee joint posteriorly. On arthrography, the popliteal cyst is outlined with air or a contrast agent and is located posterior to the joint capsule in the popliteal space. The optimal position for visualization of the popliteal cyst is with the knee semiflexed, which allows contrast to enter

Arthroscopy of the knee

Barton Nisonson

Arthroscopic surgery has influenced modern orthopaedics and knee surgery more than any single advance except for total joint replacement. As in other subspecialties, endoscopic surgery has made it possible to accomplish procedures with less morbidity and more rapid recovery and rehabilitation. The technique is very different from the traditional operative skills taught to us by our masters. One must be patient and willing to try various teaching aids; once mastered, arthroscopy results in a valuable and relatively safe tool for performing diagnostic and surgical procedures.

■ HISTORY

Endoscopic surgery was attempted as early as 1877 by Max Nitze, who created a rudimentary cystoscope with the use of candlelight. Takagi is credited with inventing the first usable arthroscope in 1918. In this country, M.S. Burman from the Hospital of Joint Disease, New York, described and illustrated his experience with diagnostic knee arthroscopy in 1931. Watanabe devised a scope that had practical application; his atlas contains pathologic pictures that are still unequalled.[32,33] Fiberoptics created the breakthrough that allowed unequalled clarity and the safe use of a cold light source.

O'Connor is credited with the development of the operative arthroscope, in 1975. The use of video equipment had made this technique available to the community orthopaedist and has allowed its widespread acceptance.

■ INSTRUMENTATION

The arthroscope continues to improve, allowing more light fibers and better video reproduction as well as the refinement to a smaller size to allow successful small

---

ADVANTAGES OF ARTHROSCOPIC SURGERY
    Less morbidity
    Easier rehabilitation
    Rapid recovery
    Earlier return to sports

joint procedures. The most versatile arthroscopes for knee surgery are the 4 or 5 mm scopes with an oblique angle of about 25 to 30 degrees. The second scope that may have significant use for the amateur or expert is the 70-degree angle in the 4 to 5 mm size. This scope allows a relatively clear view of the posterior compartments through a transpatellar tendon portal.

Another important instrument is the nerve hook, or probe. Its importance lies in both diagnostic and surgical procedures. Initially it improves one's triangulation technique, which is very necessary for more advanced surgical techniques. There are various commercial brands that offer different weights, grips, and so forth. The standard, inexpensive Dandy nerve hook can be ground to various tip lengths, from 3 to 5 mm, and thus can serve the same purpose.

An array of hand instruments, including various baskets and scissors (straight or curved), are available from various manufacturers. The most versatile sizes are 4.5 and 3.4 mm. Unfortunately, they all share the problems of being expensive and easily breakable, and tending to lose sharpness rapidly. This makes it imperative to have at least two of each of the straight scissors or baskets most commonly used (3.4 mm). The more sophisticated spring-action 90-degree angle punches and 60- and 20-degree scissors help in various maneuvers but are not imperative.

Knives of various shapes complete the list of most commonly used hand instruments. I prefer the disposable double-edged knife with a slight curve because of its versatility and sharpness. Retrograde knives, both disposable and nondisposable, can smoothly detach flaps and anterior bucket handle attachments but must be used with extreme care because of the potential for breakage and damage to soft tissue and articular cartilage.

Motorized equipment needs the most improvement. Various shavers, trimmers, and meniscal cutters are available; all, un-fortunately, share the problems of rapid dulling and inadequate cutting capabilities in the 3.5 and 4.5 mm sizes. Burrs, synovectomy blades, and so forth are part of the motorized armamentarium. They are alluded to later in this chapter.

Of course, various equipment not made specifically for arthroscopy or somewhat modified can help in the more complex procedures. The skilled arthroscopists always include various pituitary rongeurs, kerasins, small osteotomes, and curettes in their array of equipment. As in other types of surgery, individual ingenuity facilitates difficult procedures.

Simplifying a seemingly difficult procedure always involves exposure, which requires the use of a leg holder. There are many on the market with or without a tourniquet. The purpose of the leg holder is to allow a valgus and varus stress without too much rotation. It is indeed possible to get a medial collateral ligament sprain on applying too much valgus, but if one is careful, it is rarely more than a Grade I. This is a reasonable price for the allowing of superior medial compartment exposure over any other technique.

■ PORTALS OF ENTRY

The arthroscopist has a choice of many portals through which he can examine the knee and operate (Fig. 27-1). The choices depend on the procedure being performed, the location of the lesion, and the surgeon's personal preference. The amount of holes made is not important and the surgeon should not hesitate in making as many as necessary for successful completion of a procedure.

I routinely start a procedure with an anterolateral portal, finding it the easiest approach to an initial examination and evaluation of the knee. The portal is usually made 1 cm lateral to the patellar tendon at about the level of the inferior tip of the patella.

The second most common portal used is the anteromedial hole. Through the use of both these approaches most of the

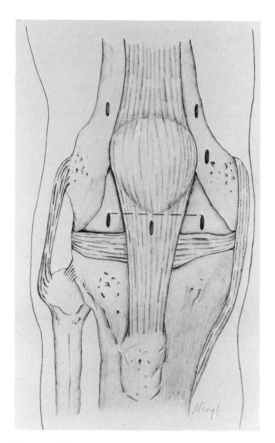

Fig. 27-1 ■ Most commonly used portals of entry to the knee.

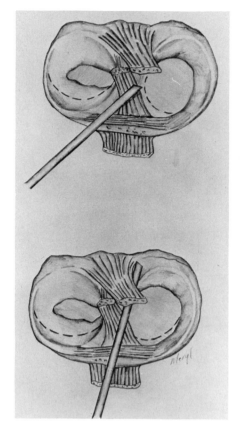

Fig. 27-2 ■ Diagram demonstrating the value of the central approach, allowing a 70-degree scope access to posterior compartments.

knee joint can be thoroughly examined except for a small portion of the posteromedial corner, an even smaller portion of the posterolateral compartment, and the most anterior portion of the knee. To view the posterior corners, one can use a posteromedial or posterolateral approach. By inserting a rapid 50 to 80 ml bolus of saline through an anterior portal, one can palpate the posterior sites of capsular bulging, make a quick stab wound, and insert the arthroscopic sheath. The alternative is to use a 70-degree scope, inserted through or close to the patellar tendon and directed posterior and lateral to the anterior cruciate ligament to view the posterolateral corner, or medial to the posterior cruciate ligament to view the

posteromedial corner (Fig. 27-2). The most anterior part of the knee can be viewed with the 70-degree scope as well or by using the lateral midpatellar approach popularized by Patel. This approach affords a clear view of the anteromedial and anterolateral menisci and prevents the crowding of instruments during the use of multiple portals. This is a difficult technique to master and may be valuable only after many attempts.

When the simultaneous use of three holes are necessary (for grasping, viewing and cutting), there are two choices. One can make anterolateral and anteromedial portals and a more medial or lateral third portal. I prefer the transpatellar, or central, technique (Swedish technique). The

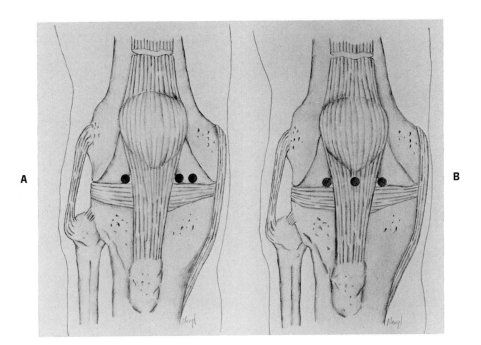

Fig. 27-3 ■ **A,** Three-portal technique, demonstrating crowding when two portals used on either side of the patellar tendon. **B,** Three-portal technique, using transpatellar or central technique, avoiding crowding because of space maintained by the bulk of the patellar tendon.

noncompressible patellar tendon between the three portals avoids crowding (Fig. 27-3), and the problem of the fat pad is easily managed by pushing the scope in rapidly toward the posterior knee and withdrawing slowly until the proper view is obtained. The transient patella tendinitis that can occur is not a significant problem. The removal of loose bodies, synovectomy, and patella procedures usually require the use of superolateral and/or superomedial portals. These are easy to master and are important additions to the above portals.

In addition to the standard portals described, I have been using an additional one. The inframeniscal approach[13] has been quite valuable for complex tears of the posterior third of the medial meniscus (Fig. 27-4). In the very tight or mildly arthritic knee this area must usually be reached by the posteromedial approach. The inframeniscal approach is an alternative to this technically difficult area.

Whatever portals are used, the spinal needle is an invaluable instrument in first locating the approach that will work best for the task. One can use it to perform the imaginary steps in a particular procedure before actually making the stab wounds.

■ DIAGNOSIS

The arthroscope's first and most important value lies in its diagnostic accuracy. Exploratory arthrotomies, with their higher morbidity, are no longer necessary. Although arthrograms may still at times be a valuable adjunct, arthroscopy offers a more accurate tool in diagnosing cruciate injuries and meniscal lesions, especially lateral menisci. The accuracy of an experienced arthroscopist should approach 98% for these lesions. Articular surface changes, not identifiable on a roentgenogram, can be well visualized with arthroscopy, and the diagnosis of chondromalacia or early arthritis can be made more precisely. Synovial disease too

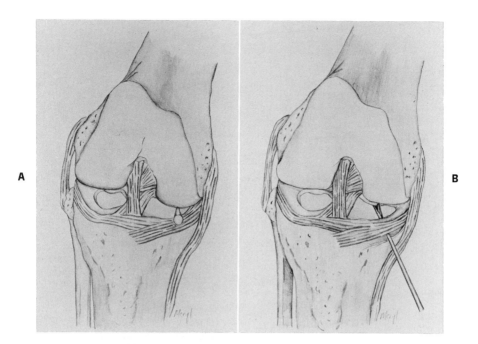

Fig. 27-4 ■ A, Standard anteromedial portal, showing how curvature of the medial femoral condyle interferes with access to the posterior one third of the medial meniscus. **B,** Inframeniscal portal, facilitating access to the posterior one third of the medial meniscus.

can be best viewed and biopsied through arthroscopy. It is therefore an important adjunct to the difficult rheumatology work-up.

The acute knee injury presents a specific use for arthroscopy that has been written about extensively.[19,26] In the young, prime athlete, the cause of an acute hemarthrosis distinctly influences the choice of treatment. Primary cruciate repair or reconstruction in the appropriate patient is felt by many to be the proper choice. In a swollen, difficult-to-examine knee, arthroscopy allows an accurate look at both cruciates as well as the ability to rule out peripheral meniscal tears and osteochondral fractures, other common causes of hemarthrosis. The surgeon can then make the decision whether to repair the meniscus or remove it, depending on the type of lesion, or to do a primary repair, augmentation, or reconstruction of the cruciates.

Examination of the cruciate ligaments

may be difficult. Hemorrhage in the synovial sleeve of both anterior and posterior cruciates makes one very suspicious of an acute tear. It is important to clear away the synovium from the ligament to allow a direct view of the fibers. This can usually be accomplished by spreading the synovial tissue with a blunt probe or by carefully using a basket forceps to remove some of the synovium. The latter technique is especially valuable in examining the femoral insertion of the posterior cruciate ligament. The use of the probe to palpate the ligament and to test continuity as well as tension is equally important in a complete examination; of course, the latter technique requires some prior experience with normal examinations. Finally, the position of the leg may facilitate this examination. For example, the figure-4 position sometimes allows easier identification of the anterior cruciate ligament in its taut position, and with the scope anterolaterally and a probe anteromedially a thorough examination of this ligament can be undertaken.

■ SURGICAL TECHNIQUE
Loose bodies

For the beginning surgical arthroscopists, loose bodies present an attractive procedure for testing one's skills (Fig. 27-5). There are a few techniques that can be used, depending on the size and location of the body. The most common location is the suprapatellar pouch and intercondylar notch. The most common way of retrieving the body is to use a grasping instrument, such as a Schlesinger pituitary rongeur, and to enlarge the portal through which the instrument is placed; or in a very large body to grasp it and push it against the opposite wall, making a counterincision. The loose body can be very elusive and it is not uncommon to lose it while attempting to grasp it. Remember to look in the gutters, both lateral and medial, the most common place where the joint mouse might float.

Posterior compartment bodies require other, more difficult techniques to retrieve them. One can either place a 70-degree scope through the notch and insert a grasping instrument via the posteromedial or posterolateral portal, or vice versa—the scope posteromedial or posterolateral and the grasping instrument, an angulated variety, through the notch. In the case of a very large, posterior compartment body, morselization may be the best means of removing it.

An elusive area where one can easily miss a joint mouse is behind the popliteus tendon. Sometimes by inserting a shaver cannula with suction attached and applying a varus stress to the knee, the fragment is sucked into the lateral compartment. Inserting a spinal needle just posterior to the popliteus tendon makes a good probe or even a skewer to trap the body or bodies. These techniques can easily be refined by practice on a wet knee model.

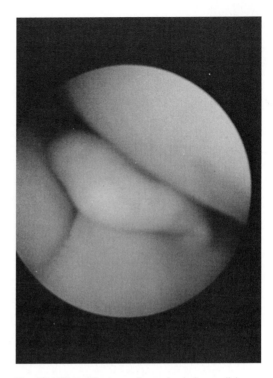

Fig. 27-5 ■ Cartilaginous loose body in medial compartment of the knee.

Meniscal lesions

The single lesion that has resulted in arthroscopy gaining such wide acceptance is the meniscal tear. Partial meniscectomies have gained wide popularity, even through open means, because of good clinical and research evidence that there may be less degenerative sequelae than in "total" meniscectomy.[7,22] The specific technique used depends on the size, type and location of the meniscal lesion.

There are, however a few basic principles that should be followed:

1. Protect the articular surfaces even in tight compartments and avoid scuffing.
2. Preserve the continuity of the remaining meniscal rim, if possible, even if it is narrow.
3. Make sure the remaining meniscal rim is stable and balanced so that there is a smooth transition between the intact and the involved areas.

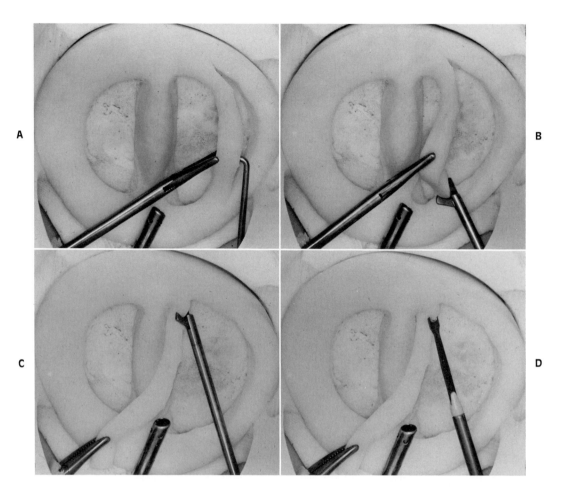

Fig. 27-6 ■ **A,** Grasping the displaceable, longitudinal tear, using probe to deliver the fragment. **B,** Cutting the anterior pole first, using hook scissors. **C,** Detaching the posterior pole with scissors, holding the fragment taut. **D,** Same as **C,** except a Smillie-type miniblade is being used to detach the posterior pole.

4. Check thoroughly for other pathology, even if the meniscal lesion seems isolated and obvious.

Classification of tears and technique

There are some basic patterns that meniscal tears follow[24] (see box). Since the type of tear dictates the technique to be used, its classification has great value.

Longitudinal or vertical tears. The longitudinal or vertical tear group also includes bucket-handle displaced or displaceable tears. The tear can also vary as to how close it is to the periphery and

---

CLASSIFICATION OF MENISCAL TEARS
Longitudinal (vertical)
Flap
Horizontal
Transverse (radial)
Degenerative (multiple plane)

---

how extensive it is. The following represents a stepwise method for a displaceable tear on the medial side (Fig 27-6):

1. If the torn segment is long enough, place the scope through the patellar tendon and the grasping instrument

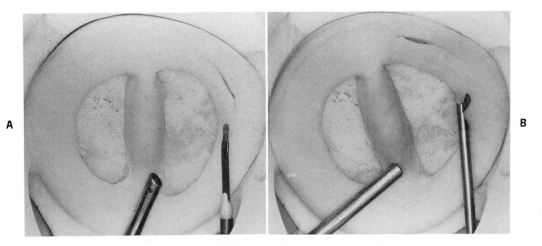

Fig. 27-7 ■ **A,** Removal of a short, posterior one-third longitudinal medial meniscal tear, using curved blade to start the plane. **B,** Scissors used in plane started by curved knife to create a flap tear based posteriorly.

(such as a meniscal clamp) through an anterolateral portal. A probe may be inserted anteromedially to help displace the tear so as to grasp it.

2. Cut the anterior pole first, using a scissors, retrograde knife, or banana-type blade through the anteromedial portal.

3. Displace the torn segment in the intercondylar notch, and, while keeping it taut, detach the posterior pole. If the tear is short, incomplete, or cannot be displaced in its most common location (the posterior third) start the cut anterior to the tear using a banana knife or blade superiorly to create a plane, then follow with a scissors or mini-Smillie blade (Fig. 27-7). Grasp the fragment, as already described as soon as possible so as to keep it taut and to facilitate the continued dissection.

4. Make sure the exit hole is large enough, and slowly tease the fragment out through the skin.

5. Probe the remaining rim to identify loose or unstable fragments that should be removed with a shaver or basket forceps and balance the rim. (Beware of the double bucket-handle tear!)

Longitudinal tears on the lateral side are treated a little differently. The tears are usually shorter and more difficult to displace. The leg should be in a figure 4 position, since that usually allows the best exposure. The scope can be placed in the transpatellar approach, but before grasping the tear through the anteromedial portal, insert a scissors and partially detach the posterior horn under direct vision. This prevents damage to both cruciates when addressing the posterior horn at the last step and allows one to avulse it if necessary. The grasping clamp is then inserted anteromedially and the meniscus grasped, if possible. The anterior attachment is cut with a scissors or retrograde blade through the anterolateral portal for short segment tears or through the anteromedial portal, without necessarily grasping the fragment, if the tear extends more anteriorly (Fig. 27-8). The posterior attachment can then be detached with a scissors through the anterolateral portal as well as avulsed as noted above.

Flap tears. Flap tears can be viewed as vertical tears already detached at one pole. If they are based posteriorly to and including the midpoint of the meniscus, grasp it from the contralateral portal (i.e., posteromedially based flaps from the an-

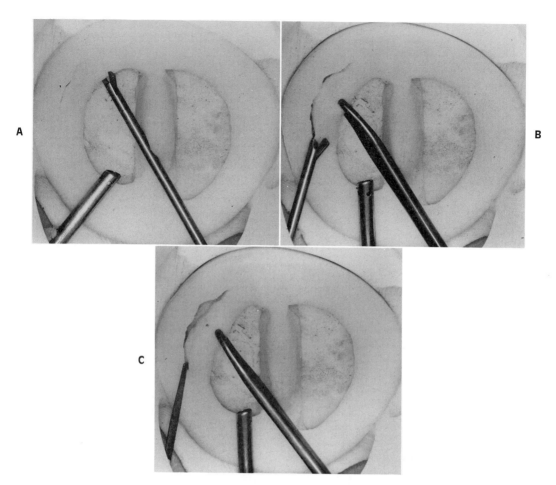

Fig. 27-8 ■ **A,** Posterior attachment of a posterolateral meniscal tear being partially cut as a first step. **B,** Posterolateral longitudinal tear being grasped through anteromedial portal, and the anterior attachment being cut with scissors. **C,** Same as **B,** except retrograde blade is being used through anterolateral portal instead of scissors.

terolateral portal), and use a scissors, knife, or basket forceps, depending on the thickness or on preference, through the ipsilateral portal (Fig. 27-9). The scope can be placed centrally or very close to the patellar tendon borders. If the flap is small, a power shaver may be used or a basket forceps to morselize it. Always probe the remaining rim to make sure that it is stable and has no tear.

A common flap tear is a flap of the superior or inferior leaf of a horizontal cleavage tear (Fig. 27-10). If this is the case, the remaining unstable portions of the horizontal tear must be appropriately handled (i.e., trimmed with a basket forceps).

Anteriorly based tears are more difficult and sometimes require more complex techniques. For example, if there is a marked synovial reaction or large fat pad, a shaver may be helpful in trimming this tissue to allow better exposure. The grasping instrument usually is placed in an ipsilateral position and the scissors contralateral, although not as anterior as usual. The scope can be central or close to the patellar tendon (Fig. 27-11). (I do not use it, but the lateral midpatellar approach of Patel for the scope may prevent crowding of instruments and allow good exposure of the fragment.) This anterior area may still be inaccessible unless the 45-degree angled forceps or scissors is used. A 90-

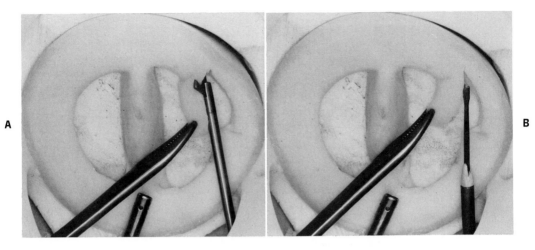

Fig. 27-9 ■ **A,** Posteromedial flap tear grasped through anterolateral portal and detached with scissors through an anteromedial portal. **B,** Same as **A,** except a Smillie miniblade is being used to detach posterior pole.

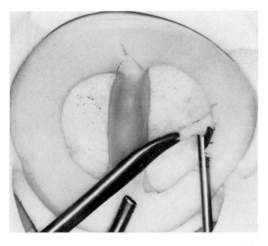

Fig. 27-10 ■ Inferior "leaf" flap tear of the medial meniscus grasped from anterolateral portal and detached from anteromedial portal.

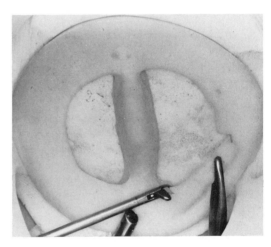

Fig. 27-11 ■ Anterior-based flap tear of the medial meniscus grasped from anteromedial portal and detached with 45 degree angled scissors from anterolateral portal.

degree punch may also be of value in the most anterior areas of both menisci.

Horizontal tears. Horizontal tears may be seen in the older individual or the remaining rim of a longitudinal tear. The first step is to probe this tear and to determine how far it extends into the periphery and whether the superior or inferior leaves have unstable elements. For the medial meniscus, the scope is placed anterolaterally, and the basket forceps is used anteromedially or inframeniscally for tears in the posterior half (Fig. 27-12). The portals are reversed for anterior tears. Lateral meniscal horizontal tears, except for the most posterior portion, are best handled with the basket forceps anteromedially and the scope anterolaterally. However, because of the side cutting blade, the shaver works best tangential to

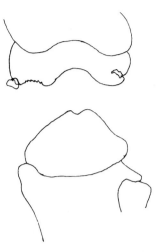

Fig. 28-1 ■ Line tracing of a roentgenogram of Group I irregularity, showing surface irregularity and separate focus of calcification.
Redrawn from Caffey, J., Madell, S.H., Royer, C., and Morales, P.: J. Bone Joint Surg. **40A:**647, 1958.

ters in the epiphyseal osseous outlines, and in Group III were found craters filled with secondary or accessory bone islands. The last group simulated the appearance of osteochondritis dissecans. These irregularities have been postulated as the precursor of osteochondritis dissecans.[164,185] More recent study[27] suggests that such an area of accessory ossification may be more vulnerable to injury but possesses reparative capabilities if the fragment remains in situ.

Pathology

The primary pathologic changes of osteochondritis dissecans are found in the bone, with secondary changes occurring in the overlying articular cartilage. Bone microscopy reveals evidence of focal avascular necrosis, often with evidence of revascularization of early repair. In the absence of healing, the interzone between the fragment and the cartilage resembles the delayed or nonunion stage of a fracture with dense fibrous tissue, and in some cases, fibrocartilage with no evidence of active vascular ingrowth or osteogenesis. The bony bed presents a simi-

---

HISTOLOGIC FINDINGS IN OSTEOCHONDRITIS

Healing lesions

Focal avascular necrosis
Revascularization/repair
Active cellular response
New bone formation

Nonhealing lesions

Dense fibrotic tissue in interzone layer similar to fracture (delayed or nonunion)
Absence of vascular ingrowth
Absence of osteogenesis
Necrotic bone

---

lar response in the early healing defect with an active cellular response, vascularization, and new bone, whereas the nonhealing defect is characterized by dense, eburnated, necrotic bone with a minimal cellular healing response, which leads in time to lack of subchondral support and secondary articular deformity with degenerative change.[144]

The overlying articular cartilage manifests normal histology and apparent viability in the early stage of the lesion but later may undergo flattening, discoloration, fissuring, or fibrillation. Following detachment, proliferation of the cartilage nourished by joint fluid may cause the fragment to enlarge.[131,147]

Clinical features

The greatest incidence is in the physiologically active adolescent, though the disease may affect those from ages 5 to 50 years.[166] The early presenting symptoms are usually knee pain and joint effusion. Complaints of giving way, catch-

---

CLINICAL FINDINGS IN OSTEOCHONDRITIS

- Knee pain
- Joint effusion
- Giving-way
- Catching
- Locking

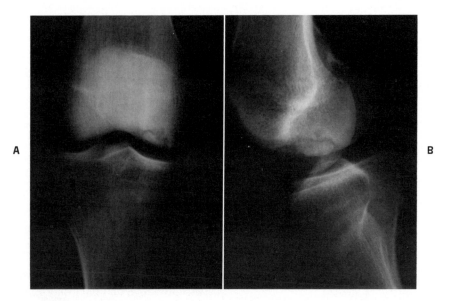

Fig. 28-2 ■ Osteochondritis dissecans of medial femoral condyle. **A,** Anteroposterior view.
B, Lateral view.

ing, or locking suggest separation of the fragment. Wilson[209] has described a diagnostic test wherein the knee on the affected side is internally rotated and flexed to 90 degrees. Pain is felt as the knee is extended. The reaction is explained by abutment of the anterior cruciate ligament from its tibial attachment with the lesion on the medial femoral condyle. However, in 2 of Wilson's 7 cases, the lesion was later found to be on the lateral condyle.

Roentgenographic findings

The lesion is usually seen as a well-circumscribed area of subchondral bone separated from the remaining femoral condyle by a crescent-shaped radiolucent line (Fig. 28-2). The fragmented bone is often similar in density to the parent condyle but occasionally may appear sclerotic. The classic location is in the lateroposterior portion of the medial femoral condyle and thus may not be visualized on the standard anteroposterior view. The defect is usually best seen on the tunnel view; the lateral view provides a second dimension that is helpful in estimating the size of the lesion. When present,

loose bodies containing sufficient bone to allow roentgenographic visualization may be found in the notch, posterior compartment, or lateral gutters.

The medial femoral condyle is affected in 75% to 85% of cases, and 20% of these may extend medially to include the weight-bearing portion of the medial femoral condyle. Another 15% to 20% of cases occur in the lateral femoral condyle, usually on the posterior surface, and the articular surface of the patella is affected in 5% of cases or less[46,97,145,165,168] (Fig. 28-3).

The potential variations in location of osteochondritis dissecans dictate that a comprehensive roentgenographic examination of the knee be performed if the disorder is suspected. This examination should include anteroposterior, lateral, right and left oblique, notch, and skyline patellar views.

When conventional films are unrevealing or equivocal and clinical suspicion remains high, technetium scan and tomography may prove helpful.

Arthrography may reveal that dye insinuates itself between the fragment and the corresponding femoral condyle, thus giving evidence of looseness.

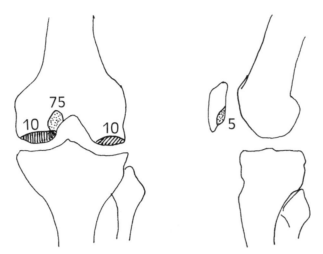

Fig. 28-3 ■ Sites of occurrence of osteochondritis dissecans. Numbers reflect percent of incidence in each location.

Treatment

The goal of treatment should be to prevent partial or complete detachment of the lesion and alteration of the articular surface leading to degenerative arthrosis.

GOALS OF TREATMENT FOR OSTEOCHONDRITIS

- Prevent detachment of lesion
- Encourage healing
- Prevent alteration of articular surface

Factors that modify the natural history of osteochondritis dissecans include age (chronologic and skeletal), whether the physis is open or closed, roentgenographic appearance of the secondary ossification centers (bilaterally for the duration of symptoms), history of onset and prior treatment, and the roentgenographic, arthrographic, and arthroscopic appearance. Based on these variables and their effect on the outcome of the disease, patients with osteochondritis dissecans may be placed into three groups.

Group I: childhood and early adolescence

Group I includes children through the age of early adolescence, skeletal age 11 for girls and 13 for boys. The most common presenting complaint is mild, nonspecific knee discomfort, with possible effusion following normal athletic activity.

Physical examination may reveal normal findings only or evidence of quadriceps atrophy, effusion, and limitation of terminal passive flexion and extension. The patient may walk with the foot of the affected extremity in external rotation. Localized tenderness to palpation over the lesion may be elicited by flexing the knee

---

IMPORTANT FACTORS IN NATURAL HISTORY OF OSTEOCHONDRITIS

- Age (chronologic and skeletal)
- Status of physis (open or closed)
- Roentgenographic appearance of secondary ossification centers
- History of onset
- Prior treatment
- Radiographic, arthrographic, and arthroscopic appearance

---

beyond 90 degrees.* Wilson's sign may be present.[209] There is a higher incidence of bilaterality in this group, ranging from 25% to 30%.

These juvenile patients still have open physes, and normal variations in the distal contour of the epiphysis may cause difficulty in establishing a diagnosis. Occasionally the lesion is found incidentally during roentgenograms obtained for other reasons.

Treatment recommendations. Treatment consists primarily of a protective regimen, since most patients in this group will respond to a few weeks of rest followed by activity modification with avoidance of symptom-related activities. Aspirin may be used in therapeutic dosages if warranted. Failure to control symptoms in this manner invites the need for crutches and cast immobilization or splinting. Rarely is traction needed to control discomfort and secondary hamstring spasm. In older Group I patients, straight-leg isometric and mild straight-leg resisted exercises in flexion, extension, and abduction are initiated to improve the tone of the hip and knee musculature. Swimming and stationary bicycle riding may be introduced when symptoms allow, followed by a standard resisted exercise program. From 6 to 12 months are usually required for healing. The prognosis for this age group is excellent.

Group II: adolescence and young adulthood

Group II includes females from skeletal age 12 and males from skeletal age 14 years, and both sexes to approximately age 20 years. The physes, though they are still seen to be open roentgenographically,

contribute minimally to further vertical growth. The patients demonstrate the physical maturation changes generally associated with approaching young adulthood.

The onset of symptoms of arthralgia and/or effusion may be insidious without antecedent trauma over a period of months or years, but an acute onset with specific trauma is more common in the older patient. These patients may also be seen initially with symptoms of a loose body such as locking, giving way, or swelling. The incidence of bilaterality in this age group is only 10%, but accompanying internal derangements are more commonly seen than in Group I.[72] Joint effusion is more likely to occur, and joint contracture and quadriceps atrophy may be present.

Arthrography and/or arthroscopy may be indicated to assess the integrity of the fragment and the condition of the overlying articular cartilage.*

Nonprogressive lesions are treated as in Group I, with rest and observation. Surgery is advised for progressive fragment formation, increasing osteosclerosis, and articular changes.

Since fragment detachment and secondary degenerative change are more common in this age group, initial treatment depends on accurate assessment of the fragment and the remainder of the joint surface. For those who are facile in its use, the arthroscope has replaced arthrography for evaluating the joint interior. It also allows the opportunity for re-

---

*Editors' note: Flexing the knee beyond 90 degrees causes the patella to drop into the lower femorotrochlear groove. The condyles are then palpable at sites normally covered by the patella. Patellar compression at 0 degrees does not tell as much and may lead to an erroneous judgment that the undersurface of the patella is at fault.

---

*Editors' note: We hold that both arthrography done first and then arthroscopy is a good approach. Many hidden Baker's cysts are associated with such conditions as disrupted articular cartilage. The arthrogram is better for this, and the arthroscope for specific visualization in the joint. However, the arthrogram should be multiplanar and read by a knowledgable orthopaedist as well as radiologist. If air is under the fragment, delaying treatment will be ineffective in this stage, and one should proceed with definitive arthroscopic treatment.

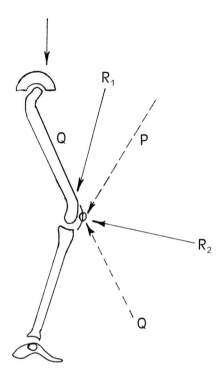

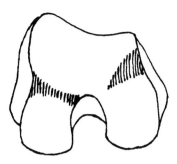

Fig. 28-21 ■ Diagram of articular surfaces of the femoral condyles. Lines triangular area on medial femoral condyle and strip on lateral condyle correspond to the areas of pannus infiltration, erosion, and osteophyte formation seen in patients with chronic flexion contracture.
Redrawn from Waugh, W., and Newton, G.: J. Bone Joint Surg. **62B:**180, 1980.

Fig. 28-20 ■ Diagrammatic representation of forces acting on the knee in the sagittal plane. *R1,* Resultant of flexor and extensor forces; *R2,* resultant of the forces of quadriceps mechanism *(Q)* and patellar tendon *(P).*
Redrawn from Maquet, P.: Clin. Orthop. **144:**70, 1979.

axes of knee flexion, producing a flexion moment that is counterbalanced by contraction of the quadriceps mechanism. The resultant (R1) of the flexor and extensor forces exerts a compressive force on the tibiofemoral joint, which is greater when the knee is loaded in flexion as opposed to extension. The extensor effect on the patellofemoral joint is produced by the forces of the quadriceps mechanism (Q) and the patellar tendon (P), and the resultant of these forces (R2) is directed in such a manner as to produce a compressive effect on the patellofemoral joint. On a clinical level, it is obvious from an analysis of these forces that weight bearing on a knee-flexion contracture brings extensive forces to bear on both the tibiofemoral and patellofemoral joint surfaces and exerts a time-related deleterious effect in terms of degenerative change. Addition-

ally, in the presence of flexion contracture, infiltration of pannus, erosion, and osteophyte formation occur in a triangular area on the medial femoral condyle and along the strip on the lateral femoral condyle corresponding to the areas normally in contact with the anterior horns of the menisci when the knee is fully extended[207] (Fig. 28-21). These lesions, occurring in areas that have no opposing articular surface when the knee cannot be fully extended, support the findings of Salter and McNeil[173] that degenerative changes develop when articular cartilage is no longer in contact with an opposing surface.

Meniscus injury and degenerative arthrosis

Long thought to be expendable or insignificant to function, the menisci of the knee are now known to play an important role in stability and the distribution of load across the joint.[176,201,206] The load-bearing function of the menisci serves to avoid concentration of compressive force over small areas of articular cartilage. Following meniscectomy, the areas of load bearing on the articular surface of the tibia are reduced to only those areas of direct contact of the tibia and femur. This leads to significant concentration of force on the articular cartilage, a circumstance favoring increased stress and wear[66,121,201,202] and leading to degenerative arthrosis.*

Surgery of the meniscus has assumed new dimensions with the advent of arthroscopy, which permits initial sparing and continued observation of meniscal lesions of questionable significance as well as low-morbidity partial resection in trained hands, a procedure that appears to be followed by less extensive degenerative change.[21,36,64,87,139]

Reports of total salvage by direct suture in cases of peripheral tears involving the meniscosynovial junction or the vascularized peripheral portion of the meniscus are favorable.† (See Chapter 29 for further information.) While logic suggests that meniscus repair is preferable to partial or complete resection insofar as continued joint function is concerned, appropriate long-term studies required to substantiate such an argument are presently lacking.

With age, the meniscus becomes fibrotic and inelastic, and its efficiency as a shock absorber and stabilizer decreases. It is arguable whether these changes are the cause or result of osteoarthrosis, or if the changes seen are merely coincidental.[138,183]

Subchondral bone

The subchondral bone is known to possess significant force-transmitting properties and, in concert with the meniscus, functions as a shock absorber to dampen incoming shock waves generated at heel strike.[159] Meniscectomy exposes the articular cartilage and subchondral bone to increased stress. Radin et al.[36,157] have demonstrated that prolonged repetitive impulse loading has an effect on the weight-bearing articular cartilage and its underlying bone, which can lead to extensive wear of the joint, fatigue microfractures of bone with increased stiffness and further compromise of its attenuation ca-

pacity, and, subsequently, degenerative arthrosis.[156,158]

Venous intraosseous hypertension and osteoarthrosis

In patients with degenerative arthrosis of the knee, there is a disturbance of venous drainage from the juxtacortical cancellous bone marrow with intraosseous stasis[129,148] and hypertension.[8,10] Clinical evidence suggests that the characteristic pain at rest of osteoarthrosis, which is usually relieved once the high medullary pressure is reduced by osteotomy or cortical fenestration, is at least partially caused by intraosseous hypertension.[9,10]

Constant aching pain of the same character that is independent of joint movement or loading occurs generally in younger patients who have no clinical or roentgenographic signs of degenerative arthrosis. Investigations have indicated that prolonged intraosseous hypertension may lead to changes in the structure of cortical and cancellous bone, such as increased bone density and osteophyte formation,[11,18] suggesting that circulatory changes in the subchondral bone may be a primary etiologic factor in some forms of degenerative arthrosis. Similarly, trabecular remodeling associated with healing of microfractures causes significant obstruction of the venous drainage in the subchondral areas. The resulting venous congestion appears to play a significant role in the production of pain.[148,154]

Degenerative arthrosis following ligamentous injury

To determine whether extensive ligament surgery should be done following injury requires statistical analysis of cases treated nonoperatively vs. those treated surgically. Long-term conclusive studies of this type are presently lacking. Funk,[60] in a retrospective study of 178 patients with degenerative knee disease severe enough to justify joint replacement or corrective osteotomy, found that 8.5% had a history compatible with significant ligamentous injury and 13.5% had undergone

---

*References 36, 39, 43, 50, 86, 90, 101, 138, and 213.
†References 25, 44, 45, 76, 152, and 188.

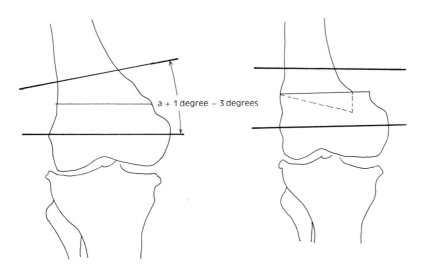

a + 1 degree – 3 degrees

Fig. 28-28 ■ Distal femoral varus osteotomy to achieve 1 to 3 degrees overcorrection of the valgus deformity.
Redrawn from Maquet, P.: Biomechanics of the knee with application to the pathogenesis and the surgical treatment of osteoarthritis, Berlin, 1976, Springer-Verlag.

to a nonoperative regimen and who for various reasons may not be candidates for major open-knee surgery. Patients with symptoms related to angular deformity or instability are not likely to benefit substantially; patients with complaints of pain, effusion, and mechanical problems such as locking and catching are more likely to be helped.

The duration of symptomatic improvement following such surgery is difficult to predict, and it is likely that slow progression of the arthrosis will ensue. What is gained is a period of varying symptomatic relief that permits more normal function by means of low-risk, low-morbidity surgery.

Unicondylar knee replacement. The state of the art unicondylar knee replacement in the treatment of unicompartmental arthrosis is presently unsettled.

Insall and Walker,[82] on the basis of their study of 24 knees that had had unicondylar replacement for 2 to 4 years, concluded that tibial osteotomy or bicondylar replacement was preferable to unicondylar knee replacement in patients with me-dial compartment disease, but that unicondylar replacement may have a role in the treatment of lateral compartment disease. Laskin[107] reported only 65% satisfactory pain relief at a minimal follow-up time of 2 years, with an absolute failure rate of 20%. All failures occurred in knees with medial compartment replacement. Marmor[122] reported good to excellent results in 75% of patients with a minimal follow-up time of 4 years, with no difference between medial and lateral joint disease.

However, Scott and Santore[175] experienced 92% good to excellent results in 100 patients with an average follow-up time of 3.5 years. They found no significant difference in the success rate between medial and lateral unicompartmental replacements, and concluded that unicompartmental knee replacement is a suitable alternative to proximal tibial osteotomy or bicompartmental knee replacement in elderly patients with unicompartmental osteoarthrosis. They reported that unicondylar knee replacement provides a higher incidence of satisfactory pain relief with greater range of motion, less risk of phlebitis, and less infection and peroneal palsy. The presence of obesity, however, is a strong argument against its use.

Total prosthetic knee replacement. Total prosthetic knee replacement should be reserved for those knees in which the state of destruction is bad enough to exclude other forms of treatment. There are numerous designs of artificial knee joints, which fall into four groups[80]:

1. Surface replacements, which replace one or more joint surfaces, possess no inherent stability, and require intact ligaments.[24,95,106,161]
2. Semiconstrained nonlinked condylar replacement, which provide some stability by virtue of the shape of the articular component. These are often cruciate-sacrificing prostheses.[24,56,95]
3. Linked units, which provide stability without a fixed axis motion and permit some rotary movement.[12,160,184]
4. Rigid hinges, which permit single-plane, fixed-axis motion.[24,40,95]

The semiconstrained prosthesis is presently the most popular type and provides the most suitable design elements from a biomechanical standpoint, while surface replacements and rigid hinges have very limited application.

Patellofemoral osteoarthrosis
Clinical and roentgenographic findings

Patellofemoral osteoarthrosis may be defined as Grade IV chondromalacia exhibiting erosive change with exposure of subchondral bone. The patella is usually involved in its lateral or central portion.[78,155]

Pain is usually anteromedial in location, though it may occasionally be anterolateral or popliteal. It is aggravated by activity, particularly stair climbing and walking downhill. Periods of extended inactivity, such as when sitting with the knee flexed, produce discomfort and a sense of stiffness. Additional symptoms include clicking, catching or pseudolocking, and giving-way.

The major clinical sign is retropatellar pain elicited by patellofemoral compression with the knee flexed. Patellar crepitus is present in most cases. However, these signs are not helpful in differentiating this condition from chondromalacia.

The roentgenographic findings of joint space narrowing, sclerosis, and spurring most often involve the lateral facets, and mirror changes are often present on the opposing surface of the femur.

Nonoperative management

The initial treatment is nonoperative and consists of weight loss when appropriate and gentle quadriceps stretching and straight leg isometric exercises performed within the limits of comfort. Further strength gain may be achieved by adding weights. Short arc resisted quadriceps exercises may be attempted by some patients but should be discontinued if they produce discomfort. An elasticized brace with horseshoe padding may be quite helpful in reducing symptoms if worn continuously. Mild analgesics, nonsteroidal oral antiinflammatory medication, and occasional intraarticular corticosteroids compliment the physical therapy treatment program.

Surgical management

The usual indication for surgery is intractable pain of intensity sufficient to alter the patient's life-style that persists for longer than 6 months and is unresponsive to nonoperative measures.

Lateral release. Lateral retinacular release is technically a simple procedure that can be performed with the patient under local anesthesia. The procedure produces a decompressive effect on the patellofemoral joint and can be useful when there is evidence that the degenerative changes are caused by excessive lateral compartment pressure. Despite its usefulness in certain cases of patellalgia, results when used alone for patellofemoral osteoarthrosis have not fostered a great deal of optimism.

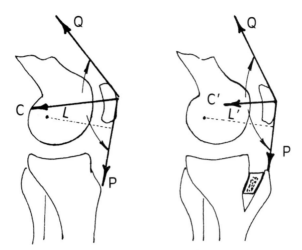

Fig. 28-29 ■ Force vectors about the patellofemoral joint. *Q*, quadriceps force; *P*, force transmitted by patellar tendon; *C*, resultant compressive force acting on patellofemoral joint; Left, before, and right, after anterior displacement of tibial tubercle. Opening the angle formed by the pull of the quadriceps and patellar tendons increases the extensor lever arm from L to L', thus augmenting the efficiency of the quadriceps muscle while decreasing the resultant compressive force C' acting across the patellofemoral joint.
Redrawn from Maquet, P.: Biomechanics of the knee with application to the pathogenesis and the surgical treatment of osteoarthritis, Berlin, 1976, Springer-Verlag.

Tibial tubercle elevation—Maquet procedure. Anterior displacement of the tibial tubercle reduces the force vector coapting the patella to the femur by opening the angle of application of the quadriceps pull through the patella to the tibia and increasing the moment arm of the patellar tendon. The effect is to relieve focal overload on the patellofemoral joint by increasing the mechanical advantage of the patellofemoral mechanism[118,120] (Figs. 28-29 and 28-30). Maquet recommended elevating the tubercle at least 2 cm, but Ferguson's work[51] suggests that 1 cm of elevation is sufficient and that further elevation does not increase the effectiveness of the operation. Leach and Radin[108] have reported better than 90% excellent results with this operation, while others have been less sanguine.[170]

When both medial and patellofemoral compartments are involved, performing high tibial osteotomy without attention to a diseased patellofemoral joint may result in persistent symptoms, which may worsen as the Q angle is increased by the

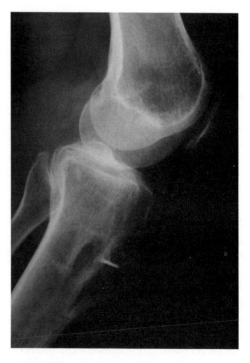

Fig. 28-30 ■ Postoperative film showing tibial tubercle elevation. Defect in tibia posterior to elevated tubercle marks graft donor site.

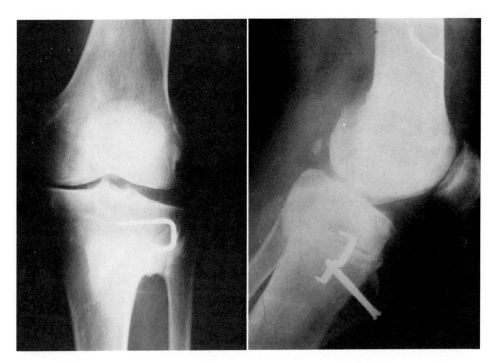

Fig. 28-31 ■ Postoperative films showing combined high tibial valgus osteotomy and tibial tubercle elevation. Internal fixation devices are often not necessary.

valgus osteotomy. Combining the Maquet procedure and proximal valgus tibial osteotomy is advantageous; only one incision is necessary, the need for a separate donor site is obviated since the tibial wedge provides excellent grafting material to augment the tubercle, and the sagittal alignment of the tibial shaft with the plateau is preserved[16] (Fig. 28-31).

Spongialization

Perforation of the subchondral plate to allow ingrowth of fibrous tissue was described by Pridie[153] as a method of resurfacing joints devoid of normal cartilage. The modification of this procedure by Ficat et al.[53] is to resect en bloc all diseased cartilage and its corresponding subchondral bone, creating a completely exposed cancellous bony bed. Ficat et al. termed this procedure "spongialization" to connote complete exposure of the spongiosa. Their rationale rests with the belief that the subchondral plate in osteoarthrosis,

which is dense and ischemic, is itself abnormal and a source of pain, since it is well innervated and sensitive to pressure transmitted by softened cartilage. The structure of the material that regenerates at the site varies from fibrous to fibrocartilage to cartilage. It is yet undetermined how the ensuing metaplasia may be directed at the clinical level during rehabilitation to favor the development of cartilage over fibrous tissue and fibrocartilage, but it may be stated that joint decompression by lateral release and Maquet tubercle plasty in conjunction with active mobilization of the extremity appear to be the most important factors favoring the regeneration of functional tissue in the defect.

Patelloplasty—prosthetic resurfacing

Prosthetic resurfacing or hemiarthroplasty of the patellofemoral joint is an alternative to patellectomy in the treatment of selected cases of patellofemoral os-

ament tears that were also treated surgically. There have been no recurrent tears to date in any of these acute meniscus repairs. The remaining 60% of peripheral meniscus repairs were late, averaging 6 months following injury, and approximately half of these cases also had chronic anterior cruciate ligament tears, some of which were stabilized at the time of meniscus repair. All were athletes who returned to at least recreational athletics, and the elite amateur or professional athletes have been able to return to their original sports at their previous level of competition. There have been no instances of neurovascular complications or infection.

To date, with 8 years maximum of follow-up, there are seven patients who have torn the meniscus again and all have occurred in the late repair group. Two of these were individuals who were permitted to return to soccer too soon (4 to 5 months) and who sustained tears through the repair site with a hard cutting maneuver. Of the remaining five patients with these tears, four had chronic anterior cruciate ligament tears that were not stabilized and with continued instability, again tore the meniscus.

In all, three of these seven tears have occurred through the previous repair site and none of them have been amenable to a second repair, although this has been reported by Cassidy to be successful. The other four cases sustained the subsequent tear through a different portion of the meniscus, were treated by arthroscopic partial meniscectomy, and the remaining peripheral rim was well healed to the capsule at the site of the previous repair (Fig. 29-9). Patients with chronic anterior cruciate ligament tears who underwent meniscus repair without stabilization have suffered subsequent tear rates of 30%, whereas only one patient who underwent ligamentous reconstruction at the time of meniscus repair has encountered a recurrent tear (7%). I still repair menisci in selected cases without ligamentous reconstruction, but the selection parameters are much more strict than several years ago. Since making this change, and at approximately the same time imposing the 6-month moratorium on hard running and agility activities following meniscus repair, I have not encountered a recurrent tear of any type during the past 3 years.

Second-look arthroscopy has been performed in 19 patients who have not sustained recurrent rupture of repaired menisci, and all demonstrated excellent healing of the repair site, normal appearance of the meniscus, and no evidence of damage of the articular cartilage (Fig. 29-10). The remaining patients have been followed clinically, and in spite of returning to athletic activities and placing significant stresses on the repaired menisci, they are free of meniscal symptoms and signs. In addition, all patients to date 5 years or more following successful repair have had normal weight-bearing roentgenograms providing evidence that the repaired menisci are biomechanically functional. Long-term follow-up on these patients will be necessary to be certain that the repaired menisci will continue to survive, function effectively, and prevent the late degenerative changes seen following meniscectomy.

The results of repair of anterior central lesions have not been quite as consistent. Stone has reported no case in which he has resorted to meniscectomy, but 8 of 30 patients continued to have pain. Goletz and Clancy reported that some of their repairs continued to have disabling symptoms and required partial or total meniscectomy to relieve the symptoms. None of the three repairs of this type I have performed have had any clinical symptoms or findings, and none have required any subsequent treatment.

Arthroscopic meniscus repair

Several techniques have been developed and are being evaluated that carry out meniscus repair under arthroscopic control.

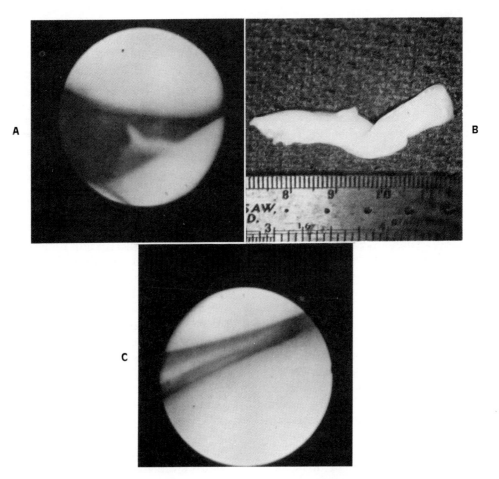

Fig. 29-9 ■ Retear of a previously repaired medial meniscus. **A,** The arthroscopic picture of a medial meniscus repaired 14 months previously that retore as a displaced bucket-handle tear. The medial femoral condyle is seen superiorly, and the displaced fragment of medial meniscus inferiorly. **B,** This photograph shows the displaced portion of the meniscus that was excised arthroscopically. **C,** The arthroscopic appearance of the remaining posterior peripheral rim following resection of the retorn and displaced fragment. The femoral condyle is seen superiorly, the tibial plateau is seen inferiorly, and in between is a substantial posterior rim, which was well attached to the capsule in the area of the previous repair.
From Casscells, S.W.: Arthroscopy: diagnostic and surgical practice, Philadelphia, 1984, Lea & Febiger.

Current techniques include the passage of long needles through the inner fragment of the meniscus across the site of the tear and through the peripheral rim, capsule, subcutaneous tissues, and skin. Cannula systems have been developed to facilitate passage of the needles. The ends of the sutures are then tied externally over bolsters or small skin incisions are used to permit tying the sutures beneath the skin. There are theoretic and real concerns re-garding the use of this procedure for pe-ripheral tears that can be repaired by the open techniques described.

The theoretic concerns are that rim preparation cannot be performed as well (particularly the rim of the body of the meniscus), that it is difficult if not impos-sible to place the sutures in a vertical ori-entation, and that it requires perforation of the avascular but intact inner segment of the meniscus. These theoretic con-

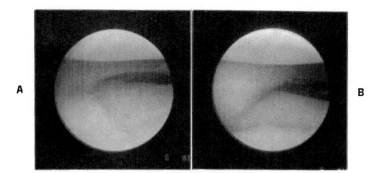

Fig. 29-10 ■ **A,** A previously repaired lateral meniscus is examined arthroscopically 14 months following repair at the time of subsequent anterior cruciate ligament reconstruction; this photograph demonstrates a normal appearance of the meniscus and articular cartilage of the lateral femoral and tibial condyles. **B,** A probe introduced to evaluate the posterior horn demonstrates the normal stability provided by the previous repair.
From Casscells, S.W.: Arthroscopy: diagnostic and surgical practice, Philadelphia, 1984, Lea & Febiger.

cerns raise the possibility that arthroscopic repair of this type may not prove to be as effective as open techniques, and only careful evaluation of clinical trials currently in progress will determine whether these theoretic concerns are valid.

The real concerns about these techniques relate to several serious complications that have been reported by experienced arthroscopic surgeons in a relatively small number of cases. These include popliteal artery lacerations, peroneal and saphenous nerve injuries, and superficial and deep infections. At present, the recommendation is to continue with open repair of peripheral lesions until it has been documented that arthroscopic techniques are just as effective and safe and are easier for the patient or surgeon.

However, certain repairable lesions are encountered that are too far in from the periphery to be accessible to open techniques, and arthroscopic repair offers the only possibility for repair rather than performing partial meniscectomy. In these instances, arthroscopic repair is preferable, but it is recommended that the technique include a posteromedial or posterolateral skin incision is advocated by Henning and Jakob, so the needles can be retrieved under direct vision as they perforate the capsule and thereby ensure protection of the neurovascular structures.

The concept of creating vascular access channels to permit a healing response for lesions in the avascular zone of the meniscus has been studied in the laboratory by Arnoczky.[1] It is possible that arthroscopic repair techniques using the concept of vascular access channels may permit repair of increasing numbers of meniscus lesions currently believed to be nonrepairable. It is a concern, however, that Arnoczky's work in dogs has demonstrated the necessity of creating a full-thickness access channel to allow effective healing. A full-thickness channel totally disrupts the peripheral circumferential fibers that have been shown to be essential for much of the biomechanical load-bearing functions of the meniscus. It is possible that these techniques will produce a healed, but biomechanically ineffective meniscus, and the entire concept requires further study before widespread clinical application is warranted. The potential application of these techniques in the future provides great promise, however, and it should be interesting and exciting to observe future developments in this area.

Partial meniscectomy

Lesions unsuitable for leaving alone or repair are considered for partial meniscectomy. Unfortunately, in my experience over the past several years the vast majority (75%) of meniscus lesions treated have required partial meniscectomy. The general concept of partial meniscectomy is to remove the torn or abnormally mobile fragment and leave behind a rim that is intact, stable, and well contoured. When these guidelines are followed, reoperation rates for recurrent tears of the residual meniscus rim are less than 5%. The goals of partial as compared to total meniscectomy are to relieve the symptoms and improve the long-term results.

Arthroscopic techniques permit partial meniscectomy to be carried out under direct vision, including posteriorly through small skin and capsular incisions that decrease the morbidity and improve the cosmetic results compared to arthrotomy. However, partial meniscectomy can frequently be well performed as an open procedure, especially if the small arthroscopic instruments are used through the arthrotomy incision. The arthrotomy will result in greater initial morbidity, but the long-term result should be the same.

Arthroscopic surgical techniques should be superimposed directly on the advanced diagnostic system that each individual surgeon has become accustomed to, using triagulation skills and multiple portals, including proximal and posterior approaches. It should be emphasized that the development of arthroscopic surgical skills is an evolutionary process passing through easy, intermediate, and advanced phases. All partial meniscectomies cannot be performed arthroscopically during this evolutionary process, and the surgeon should not be reluctant to abandon the arthroscopic procedure, prep and drape the knee again, and proceed to arthrotomy. It is frequently possible to complete the partial meniscectomy as an open procedure using the arthroscopic intruments. Even if this is not possible, a well-done, tradi-tional meniscectomy is better than a poor attempt at arthroscopic partial meniscectomy that is left that way.

Only general aspects of arthroscopic partial meniscectomy will be discussed, since details of various arthroscopic techniques have been published elsewhere.[4,6,19] Most surgeons use triangulation techniques exclusively, viewing through a 4 or 5 mm telescope with 25- or 30-degree optics. Operative instruments are inserted through separate portals as two-puncture or three-puncture procedures as necessary (Fig. 29-11). The most frequently employed operative instruments are basket forceps, grasping instruments, knives, and powered instrumentation. Arthroscopic instruments should be available in large (3.4 to 4 mm) and small (2.75 to 3 mm) sizes. Individual experience and preference of the surgeon will dictate the exact techniques and choice of instruments. The use of television has been helpful in providing more effective assistance, allowing the surgeon to assume a more comfortable body position and facilitating more effective teaching. I prefer to attach the video camera to the arthroscope with a beam splitter so there is always the option of working off the television monitor or looking directly down the arthroscope without disconnecting the camera (Fig. 29-12).

The most recent 400 cases of partial meniscectomy I have performed include 63% medial menisci and 37% lateral menisci. Of these cases, 96% were done arthroscopically and 4% were done as open procedures.

Several studies have documented the dramatic reduction of morbidity and early return of function provided by arthroscopic partial meniscectomy. Athletes are usually able to return to unsupported ambulation in 1 to 3 days, return to strenuous training in 7 to 14 days, and return to competition in 3 to 4 weeks. Exceptional patients have been able to return to competition in 10 days or less. Intermediate (5-year) results have recently been pre-

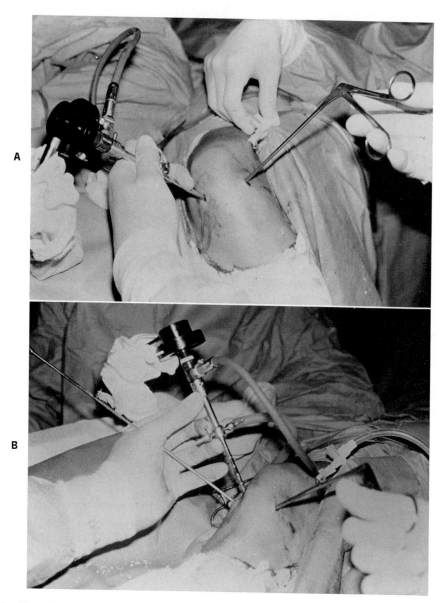

Fig. 29-11 ■ Arthroscopic partial meniscectomy. **A,** Using two-puncture technique with arthroscope in one portal and operating instrument in the other, and **B,** using three-puncture technique with grasping instrument in the anterolateral portal, arthroscope in the anteromedial portal, and cutting instrument in an accessory medial portal.

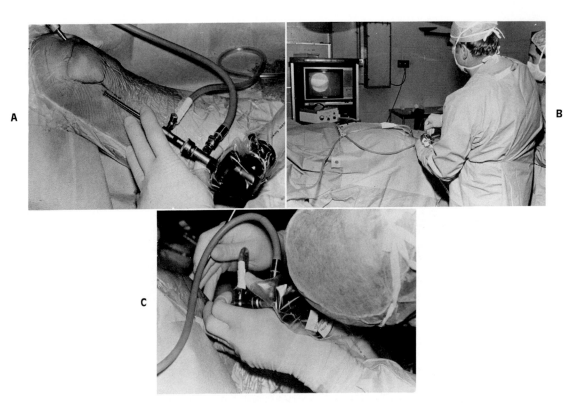

Fig. 29-12 ■ Video camera is attached to the arthroscope by means of a beam splitter so that surgeon always has the option of working with use of the television monitor or looking directly down the arthroscope, without having to disconnect the camera.

sented by Metcalf et al. and document good to excellent results in 89% of cases. Jackson has compared partial to total meniscectomy in a reasonably well-matched series of patients, and the results of partial meniscectomy were significantly better at 7 years' average follow-up. Whether long-term results will continue to be superior to total meniscectomy results remains unknown at this time, but 10- to 15-year results will soon be available.

Because of the greatly decreased morbidity associated with arthroscopic surgery as compared to open procedures, there has sometimes been a naive tendency to feel that the traditional emphasis on rehabilitation following meniscus surgery is not necessary if arthroscopy is done, even for active athletes. Nothing could be further from the truth. The need for proper rehabilitation following menis-

cus surgery is not changed just because the surgery happens to be performed arthroscopically. The only difference is that rehabilitation can usually progress faster and be completed in a shorter period of time.

> After arthroscopic partial meniscectomy
> ↓
> Rehabilitate patient

Athletes with chronic lesions will have thigh atrophy, weakness, and often contractures that will be increased to some degree by the procedure; even patients with acute cases experience some degree of the same deficiencies. We employ the same type of flexibility and progressive resistance exercises for arthroscopic cases that were used in the past for open meniscus surgery, use the same milestones

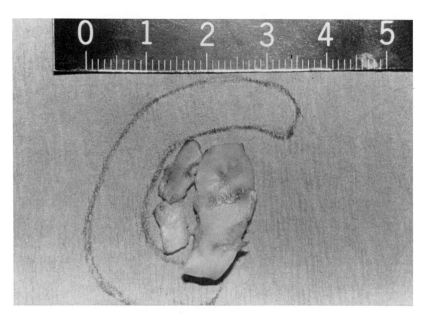

Fig. 29-13 ■ Resected central portion of torn discoid lateral meniscus that was treated by open partial meniscectomy.

for progressing through a graduated running program, and apply the same criteria for return to full activity. Again, the only difference is that the entire process can be accomplished in approximately one half the time.

Meniscus cysts

Peripheral parameniscal cysts are occasionally encountered (almost always involving the lateral meniscus) and are usually associated with a radial or horizontal cleavage tear of the meniscus in the area adjacent to the cyst. If the cyst is not large, arthroscopic partial meniscectomy of the associated meniscus lesion generally allows the cyst to spontaneously resolve without requiring surgical resection. If no meniscus lesion is identified at arthroscopy, the cyst is exposed through a local incision and resected, leaving the meniscus in situ.

Discoid menisci

Discoid menisci are occasionally encountered in athletes. If the discoid meniscus is not torn and is an incidental finding, it can be left alone, but the pa-

tient should be advised that compared to a normal meniscus there is some increased risk of a tear developing in the future. If torn, the central zone is usually involved, and partial meniscectomy can be carried out (either arthroscopically or open), leaving behind a peripheral rim that approximates the size of a normal lateral meniscus (Fig. 29-13). If the residual rim is intact, stable, and well contoured, the risk of additional tears developing has not been higher than for other types of meniscus lesions.

Total meniscectomy

While total meniscectomy has become an extremely rare procedure in recent years for surgeons employing the other options already discussed in this chapter, a few indications remain. One indication is major tears in association with large parameniscal cysts, where open, en bloc resection of the meniscus and cyst remains the procedure of choice (Fig. 29-14). Another indication is when the meniscus has been torn into two separate pieces with all circumferential fibers disrupted in a young individual with normal

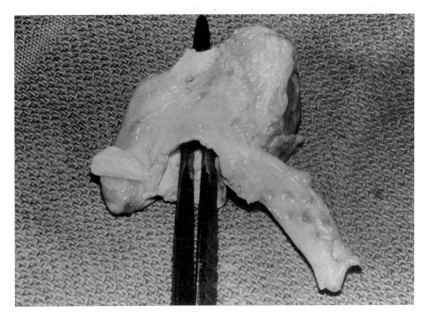

Fig. 29-14 ■ Operative specimen of large meniscal cyst associated with an extensive tear of the medial meniscus. Open en bloc excision of the meniscus and cyst remains the treatment of choice for this unusual lesion.

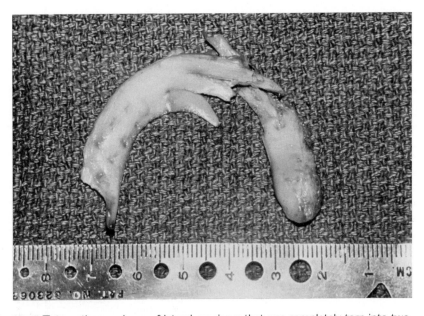

Fig. 29-15 ■ Operative specimen of lateral meniscus that was completely torn into two separate pieces through the region of the popliteus tendon in a young athlete. At the same time, the athlete sustained a complete rupture of the anterior cruciate ligament.

tory instability. This terminology* is widely used today but has recently been challenged by Noyes, because the terms do not accurately describe the abnormal motion that is occurring in the knee.[103,111] For example, anterolateral rotatory instability is primarily a translational laxity,

*Editors' note: The American Orthopaedic Society for Sports Medicine introduced, after years of study, a classification system that is used today. Until a new research committee studies these differences, we think it best to hold to the AOSSM Research and Education Committee nomenclature. (See Nicholas, J.A.: Am. J. Sports Med. **6:**295, 1978.) Whatever the description and classification of these instabilities, the classification system devised in the early 1970s was a major accomplishment, serving as a basis for both accurate diagnosis and treatment.

with only a small rotatory component.

In evaluating a knee, the physician conducts a laxity examination of the injured and normal knees to determine the presence of an anatomic lesion. The classification system that has been interposed between the interpretation of the physical examination and the understanding of which ligaments are disrupted sometimes confuses the physician. In some instances treatment can be directed toward the correction of an event described by the classification term rather than what is actually occuring in the knee, especially in a knee instability that does not fit into the system. Although we recognize the value of the classification system and use it, we agree with Apley's "plea for plain words."[3];

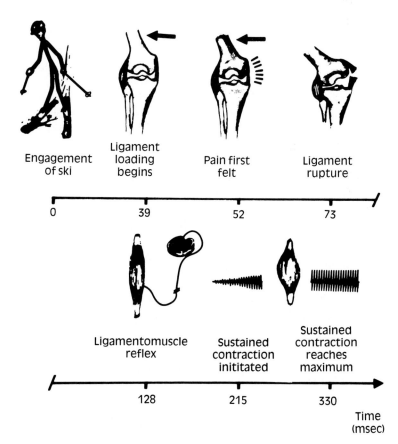

| Engagement of ski | Ligament loading begins | Pain first felt | Ligament rupture |

| 0 | 39 | 52 | 73 |

| Ligamentomuscle reflex | Sustained contraction inititated | Sustained contraction reaches maximum |

| 128 | 215 | 330 |

Time (msec)

Fig. 30-2 ■ Experimental study by Pope et al. showing that muscle contraction occurs too late to protect the knee from injury in a typical sports situation.
From Pope, M.H., Johnson, R.J., Brown, D.W., and Tighe, C.: J. Bone Joint Surg. **61A:**398, 1979.

we will try to simplify this chapter by organizing it around the treatment of specific anatomic lesions rather than types of instabilities.

We believe all ligament operations to correct functional instability resulting from capsular or ligamentous lesions should be static and that "dynamic" operations are not truely effective. The efficacy of dynamic repairs has never been proved. Although subjective improvement is commonly reported by patients who have had these operations, a great deal of indirect evidence argues against the validity of the concept of dynamic repairs (1) A transferred muscle or tendon loses one grade in strength on being transferred.[95] (2) Advancing a musculotendinous insertion weakens its muscle by elongating the muscle beyond its optimal length. (3) Knee injury occurs so quickly that there is insufficient time for the reflex arc to initiate muscle contraction[120] (Fig. 30-2). (4) The mechanical advantage of musculotendinous units about the knee is stronger at 90 degrees of flexion than in extension. As the knee approaches extension and the tendons lie more parallel to the axis of the joint, the mechanical advantage is diminished. Most knee injuries occur in the relatively extended position rather than in flexion.* (5) The transferred tendon has a tendency to scar down and become a static restraint. In our opinion, "dynamic" repairs may very well help stabilize the knee but do so in the static mode.

■ TORN MEDIAL COLLATERAL LIGAMENT

This section will deal with the diagnosis and treatment of injuries that involve only the medial ligaments and capsule and spare other major restraints. The correct anatomic terms for the medial ligamentous restraints of the knee are "tibial col-

lateral ligament" and "mid-third medial capsule" (Figs. 30-3 and 30-4). The mid-third medial capsule is often referred to as the "deep" portion of the medial collateral ligament. Last[76] introduced the terms "superficial and deep portions of the medial collateral ligament" in 1948 as a functional, not anatomic, description. In current usage the functional and anatomic descriptions are sometimes used interchangeably. We prefer the correct anatomic nomenclature and believe the terms "superficial and deep portions of the medial collateral ligament" should be abandoned. We will use the term "medial collateral ligament" when referring to the tibial collateral ligament and the mid-third medial capsule in a general (nonanatomic) sense only.

The medial capsule can be subdivided into a thin anterior third, a strong mid-third, and a moderately strong posterior third. The posteromedial capsule is also called the "posterior oblique ligament"[51] (Fig. 30-5).

The tibial collateral ligament is the primary restraint to medial joint opening.[40,134] The mid-third medial capsule is a secondary restraint to valgus stress and is usually torn with more force than necessary to tear the tibial collateral ligament alone. The extent of tearing of the posteromedial capsule depends on the amount of force to which the knee is subjected and the relative position of knee in terms of flexion at the time of injury.

The menisci usually tear when subjected to compression and shear forces. Therefore the medial mensicus is not usually torn when the knee receives a valgus stress that tears the medial collateral ligament. However, the medial meniscus can be torn *away* from its tibial attachments when the meniscotibial ligament tears[121] (Fig. 30-6). This type of injury should be viewed as a detached meniscus rather than a torn meniscus.

The mechanism of injury to the medial collateral ligament is most commonly a contact force to the lateral or posterolat-

*Editors' note: This has not been the case in our experience. Many injuries do occur as an athlete is struck on the knee while falling, with the knee at 60 to 90 degrees of flexion.

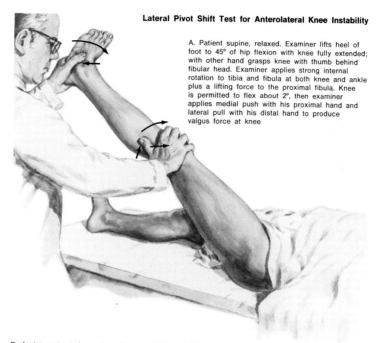

Lateral Pivot Shift Test for Anterolateral Knee Instability

A. Patient supine, relaxed. Examiner lifts heel of foot to 45° of hip flexion with knee fully extended; with other hand grasps knee with thumb behind fibular head. Examiner applies strong internal rotation to tibia and fibula at both knee and ankle plus a lifting force to the proximal fibula. Knee is permitted to flex about 2°, then examiner applies medial push with his proximal hand and lateral pull with his distal hand to produce valgus force at knee

B. As internal rotation, valgus force, and forward displacement of lateral tibial condyle are maintained, knee is passively flexed. If anterior subluxation of tibia (anterolateral instability) is present, sudden visible, audible, and palpable reduction occurs at about 20° to 40° of flexion

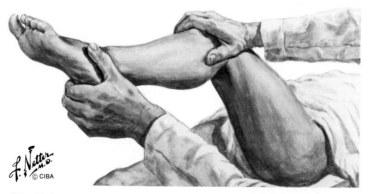

Skiing Injuries — Dr. Ellison

Reg. No. 2739

Fig. 30-21 ■ Lateral pivot shift test for anterior tibial subluxation.

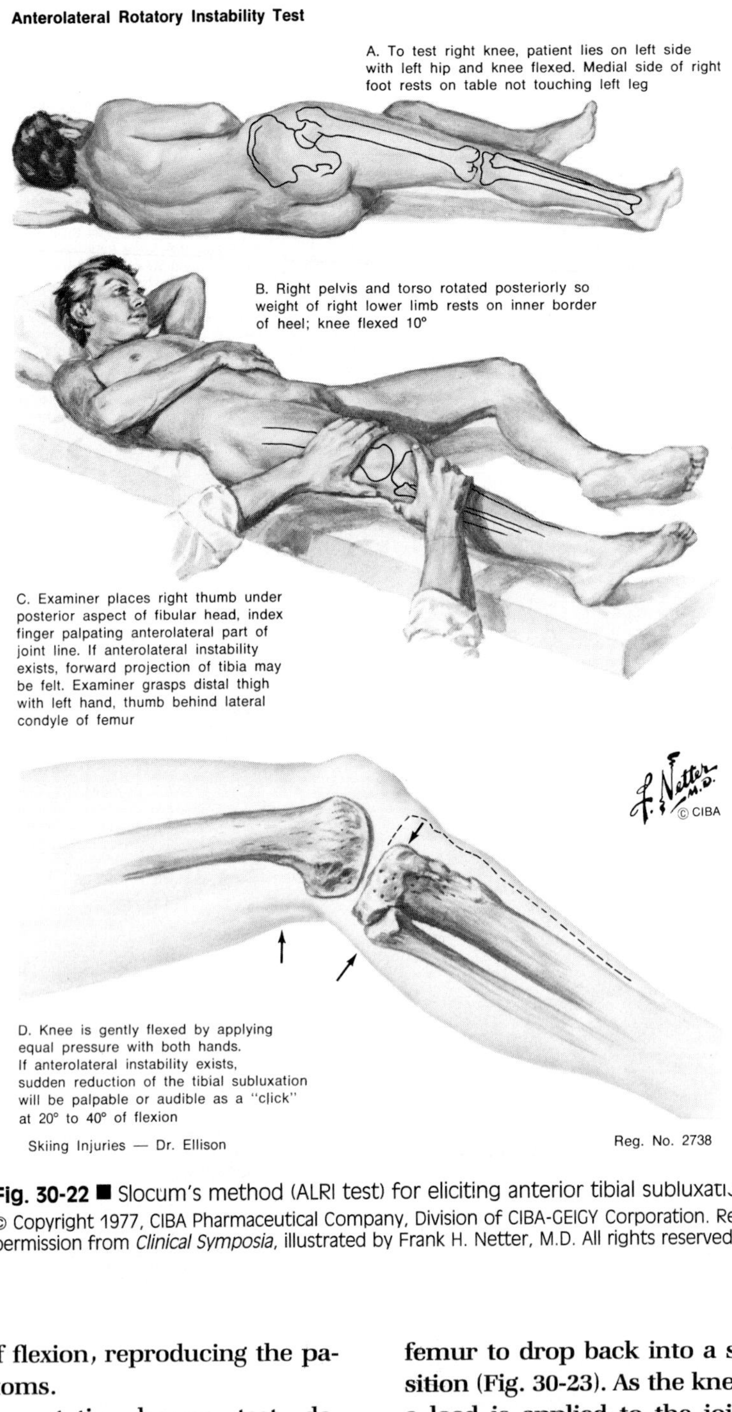

Anterolateral Rotatory Instability Test

A. To test right knee, patient lies on left side with left hip and knee flexed. Medial side of right foot rests on table not touching left leg

B. Right pelvis and torso rotated posteriorly so weight of right lower limb rests on inner border of heel; knee flexed 10°

C. Examiner places right thumb under posterior aspect of fibular head, index finger palpating anterolateral part of joint line. If anterolateral instability exists, forward projection of tibia may be felt. Examiner grasps distal thigh with left hand, thumb behind lateral condyle of femur

D. Knee is gently flexed by applying equal pressure with both hands. If anterolateral instability exists, sudden reduction of the tibial subluxation will be palpable or audible as a "click" at 20° to 40° of flexion

Skiing Injuries — Dr. Ellison

Reg. No. 2738

Fig. 30-22 ■ Slocum's method (ALRI test) for eliciting anterior tibial subluxation.

40 degrees of flexion, reproducing the patient's symptoms.

The flexion-rotation-drawer test described by Noyes et al.[104] is another modification of the MacIntosh technique designed to elicit the pivot shift phenomenon. The leg is held in 20 degrees of flexion and neutral rotation, which allows the femur to drop back into a subluxated position (Fig. 30-23). As the knee is flexed and a load is applied to the joint, the lateral femoral condyle reduces and rolls into internal rotation. We have found this test to be most useful for detecting small amounts of subluxation that can be missed using other methods.

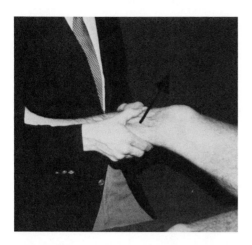

Fig. 30-23 ■ The flexion-rotation-drawer (FRD) test for eliciting the pivot shift phenomenon. The examiner holds the leg, cradling the proximal tibia in the hands and supporting the ankle between the elbow and iliac crest. The leg is held at 20 degrees of flexion and the femur is allowed to drop back into a subluxated position. With an axial load applied and the tibia kept subluxated, the knee is flexed. As the knee reaches 25 to 30 degrees of flexion, the subluxated position can no longer be maintained and sudden reduction occurs. A posteriorly directed force and external rotation of the tibia at the time of reduction accentuates the test.

The anterior drawer sign at 20 degrees of flexion (Lachman test) and the pivot shift are basically the same phenomenon occurring in the knee: a forward displacement (subluxation) and/or reduction of the tibia on the femur. The basic difference is that in the pivot shift the knee is *loaded.* Loading can be accomplished by axial compression, valgus stress (which loads the lateral compartment) and/or internal rotation. The tibial subluxation is primarily a translocation rather than a rotation phenomenon. In other words, both medial and lateral tibial surfaces slide forward on the femoral condyles and back again.[111,126]

Subluxation is more apparent in the lateral than medial compartment for a number of reasons. The lateral femoral condyle is rounder and shorter in the anteroposterior direction compared to a larger, longer medial femoral condyle. Furthermore, the lateral tibial condyle is relatively flat or even convex compared to a more concave medial condyle. Both situations favor greater motion in the lateral compartment. If the lateral capsular restraints are stretched in addition to a torn anterior cruciate ligament, the subluxation of the lateral tibial condyle can be increased even further. The iliotibial tract does not directly cause the pivot shift phenomenon, although it does tend to maintain the tibia in a reduced position until it can no longer do so. The tibia then subluxates forward with a sudden jerk. Galway and MacIntosh[37] and Jakob et al.[58] experimentally divided the iliotibial tract and found that the tibia remained subluxated in all positions and subsequently did not reduce with a sudden jerk.

A term that has been used to describe the abnormal knee motion that occurs following loss of the anterior cruciate ligament for the past decade is "anterolateral rotatory instability (ALRI)."[47,48,67,100] Because the instability appears to be primarily an abnormal or excessive translation rather than rotation,[103,111] we will use the descriptive phrase **anterior tibial subluxation** to describe the laxity tested by the pivot shift phenomenon.

Mild anterior tibial subluxation can be a physiologic event, such as in loose-jointed persons who have generalized ligamentous laxity. These people have excessive physiologic hyperextension of the knees and therefore a normally lax anterior cruciate ligament.* It is possible to elicit mild subluxation (up to 5 mm of the tibia) with pivot shift testing using the flexion-rotation drawer (FRD) method.[104] This is referred to as **pivot slip.**[111] Therefore it is very important to examine the opposite (normal) knee to determine the degree of physiologic laxity. If the opposite knee has not been injured, the difference between right and left knee laxity can be inter-

*Editors' note: Anyone who cares for athletes should always remember this fact in the preparticipation profile examination and record these laxities so as not to mistake it later, after a twist, as a necessarily surgical knee.

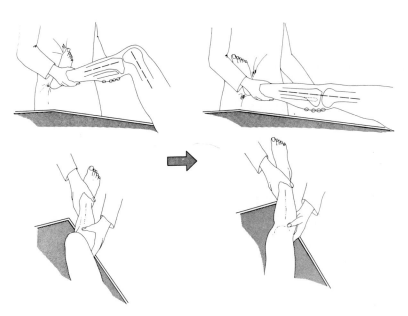

Fig. 30-24 ■ Examination for reverse pivot shift sign. In examining the right knee, the examiner supports the foot on the right side of the pelvis. The left hand supports the lateral side of the calf with the palm on the proximal fibula. Flex the knee to 70 or 80 degrees, at which position external rotation of the tibia causes the lateral tibial plateau to subluxate posteriorly in relation to the lateral femoral condyle. This is visualized as a posterior sag of the tibia. The knee is allowed to extend and an axial load and valgus force are applied. As the knee approaches a position of 20 degrees of flexion, the lateral tibial plateau suddenly reduces from a position of posterior subluxation and external rotation to a position of reduction and neutral rotation.
From Jakob, R.P., Hassler, H., and Steubli, H.-U.: Acta Orthop. Scand. (Suppl. 191) **52**:19, 1981.

preted as abnormally excessive laxity (i.e., instability). If the knee gives out when the patient pivots on the leg, this can be called "functional instability." **The functional instability resulting from a torn anterior cruciate ligament is directly related to the severity of tibial subluxation (i.e., the degree of pivot shift).**

The pivot shift phenomenon should be differentiated from the "reverse pivot shift"[58,80] (Fig. 30-24). In the latter case, the tibia subluxates posterior rather than anterior to the lateral femoral condyle (Fig. 30-25).

Roentgenograms are usually normal or may demonstrate an effusion. A small avulsion fracture from the lateral margin of the tibial condyle can be seen on anteroposterior view; this implies avulsion of the meniscotibial portion of the mid-third lateral capsule from the tibia (Fig.

30-26). This "lateral capsular sign" was described by Woods et al.[119] and is usually associated with a torn anterior cruciate ligament. Arthrography is reported to have an accuracy of 90% to 95% in diagnosing tears of the anterior cruciate ligament[119] but is not widely used for this purpose.

Arthroscopy combined with examination under anesthesia is an accurate way to diagnose a torn anterior cruciate ligament; it may be indicated in the case in which the diagnosis is suspected from the patient's history but is not evident on clinical examination. The main value of using arthroscopy in evaluating a knee that has an obvious anterior cruciate ligament injury on the basis of examination is to diagnose associated joint pathologic conditions such as meniscal tears or chondral fractures.[24,104]

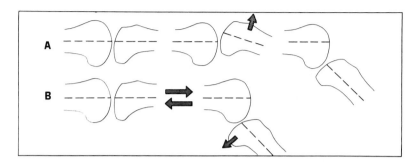

Fig. 30-25 ■ The displacement of the lateral tibial plateau during **A,** the true pivot shift test and **B,** the reversed pivot shift test. In the true pivot shift test the lateral tibial plateau shifts from a reduced position in extension into anterior subluxation in slight flexion and reduces again at 30 degrees of flexion. In the reversed pivot shift test the lateral tibial plateau falls from a reduced position in extension into posterior subluxation and flexion.
From Jakob, R.P., Hassler, H., and Steubli, H.-U.: Acta. Orthop. Scand. (Suppl. 191) **52:**24, 1981.

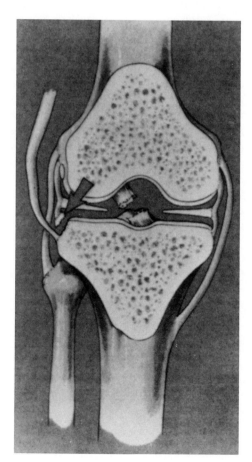

Fig. 30-26 ■ Lateral capsular sign: avulsion of the meniscotibial portion of the mid-third of the lateral capsule that can be seen on anteroposterior radiographs. This indicated severe lateral capsular injury and should alert the examiner to the high probability of injury to the anterior cruciate and medial ligaments.
From Woods, G.W., Stanley, R.F., and Tullos, H.S.: Am. J. Sports Med. **7:**27, 1979.

Natural history of the knee with a torn anterior cruciate ligament

In 1938 Palmer[117] described the clinical picture and natural history of a knee with a torn anterior cruciate ligament:

Ligamentous insufficiency generally makes itself felt as a sensation of insecurity when weight is applied. However, in isolated injuries to the crucial bands the sensation is not experienced when the patient is just walking or standing, but only when more difficult movements are made. . . Thus the ligamentous insufficiency is revealed in the forms of complicated joint action with a flexion-rotation movement which the muscles do not completely control. In addition, we have the deteriorating effects on the joint. "Sprains," which should be regarded as subluxations of the 'drawer' type, stretch and irritate the capsule which responds with recurring exudates. Pinching with "locking," caused by a fold of the capsule being sucked into the joint, meniscal dislocation and remnants of crucial bands cloud the picture of ligamentous insufficiency. Due to the instability and loosening of the joint, the pinching is often a short duration but of frequent occurrence.

The natural history of a knee with a torn anterior cruciate ligament is that of repeated episodes of "giving way" especially on pivoting or twisting motions. The patient has a "trick knee" and a predictable instability. The phenomenon that occurs when the knee gives way can be reproduced by the various pivot shift tests.*

---

*References 27, 37, 38, 47, 48, 77, 80, 104, and 123.

When the tibia subluxates forward under load, the posterior horns of the medial and/or lateral menisci get wedged between the femoral and tibial condyles, which can result in circumferential (vertical longitudinal) meniscal tears. If the torn central part of the meniscus remains forward of the femoral condyle when the tibia reduces, a displaced "bucket-handle" tear of the meniscus results (Fig. 30-27). Shearing forces under load are probably also responsible for chondral fractures of the femoral condyles that eventually result in degenerative changes (Fig. 30-28). Degenerative arthritis has been shown to be a long-term sequela of loss of the anterior cruciate ligament[57,85] and meniscectomy.[31]

Anterior tibial subluxation results in a predictable functional instability: recurrent giving way of the knee on pivoting motions. It should *not* cause other symptoms such as pain (except after acute injury or reinjury), swelling, locking, or popping. These additional symptoms of internal derangement are caused by secondary joint pathologic conditions such as torn menisci, chondral fractures, or posttraumatic changes of the articular surfaces. The symptoms of instability should be clearly separated from other symptoms resulting from additional joint pathologic conditions. Symptoms should be correlated with physical examination, radiographic findings and arthroscopy, and treatment directed accordingly.

Not all patients who tear the anterior cruciate ligament have significant functional instability. Palmer[117] stated in 1938:

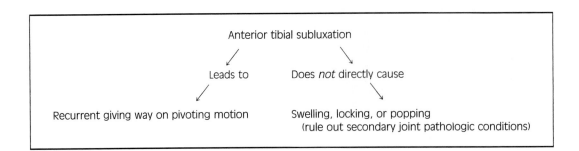

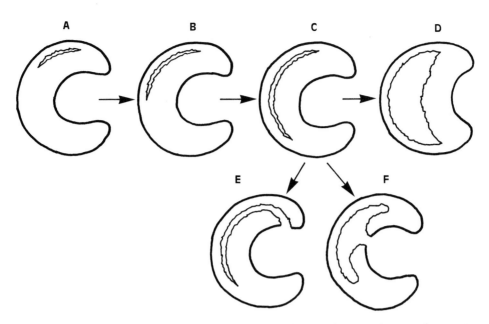

Fig. 30-27 ■ A circumferential (vertical longitudinal) tear in a meniscus can become longer with repeated injuries **(A** to **D)** or a split causing flap tears **(E** and **F)**. If the displaced portion remains forward of the femoral condyle following reduction of the tibia (i.e., displaced into the intercondylar notch), it is commonly called a "bucket-handle" tear **(D)**.

In some cases—generally young, healthy individuals—the patient eventually learns to 'control the joint'. As the muscular atrophy disappears after the period of fixation, the patient gradually regains one form of stability—the active. And in addition, he learns to use his muscles to check and put back into position subluxations in the sagittal plane. This, however, does not mean that he is free from troubles. He may be relatively incapacitated since the muscles are not able to cope with all situations.

In a study on the functional disability in athletically active individuals with tears of the anterior cruciate ligament, Noyes et al.[108,109] analyzed 103 patients with long-term follow-up of symptomatic chronic laxity of the anterior cruciate ligament uncomplicated by other associated ligament deficiency. He found that approximately one-third of patients with tears of the anterior cruciate ligament did well with nonoperative management and could compensate for absence of the anterior cruciate ligament. A third of the patients

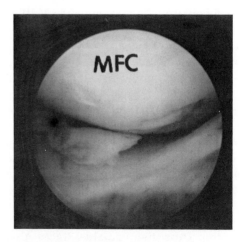

Fig. 30-28 ■ Arthroscopic view of a chondral fracture fragment of the medial femoral condyle in a knee with an acute tear of the anterior cruciate ligament. The defect in the femoral condyle can be seen.

were borderline and a third became progressively worse with increasing functional instability that prevented recreational sports activities and often interferred with daily activities.

Chick and Jackson[15] followed 30 competitive athletes who had an absent or nonfunctioning anterior cruciate ligament treated by meniscectomy without ligament reconstruction. Twenty-five (83%) returned to full athletic activity, but six developed increased instability.

McDaniel and Dameron[90] reviewed the status of 53 knees with surgically verified "isolated" tears of the anterior cruciate ligament at an average of 10 years following injury. All but eight had had a meniscectomy. Only one knee was completely stable to anterior and rotatory stress. Eighty percent of these knees were diagnosed as having chronic anterolateral rotatory instability and 60% either a varus or valgus instability. Pain, swelling, and weakness were symptoms in 70% to 85%, and giving way was a complaint in 83%.

Fetto and Marshall[34] studied the natural history of anterior cruciate ligament tears and found uniformly poor results at 5 year follow-up with a seemingly relentless course of deterioration toward a common end state condition (i.e., clinical and functional instability).

On the other hand, Hughston[49] reported on the results of treatment in 93 knees with acute anteromedial rotatory instability. He found that the knee with a torn and unrepaired anterior cruciate ligament did not progress to the subsequent disability and deterioration as has been commonly reported. This study, however, excluded knees with a torn anterior cruciate ligament that had acute anterolateral instability. Thus the unstable knees that would be expected to have progressive instability were not followed in this study.

Evidence suggests that meniscectomy can result in increased instability as well as long term disability due to degenerative changes.[49,57,64,91] Therefore the meniscus should be saved and repaired whenever possible.

Treatment of acute anterior cruciate ligament tears

Treatment of acute tears of the anterior cruciate ligament should be individualized based on current knowledge of factors that will affect the final outcome. A poor prognosis can be expected in untreated patients who are young, very active in sports, and loose jointed (having laxity of secondary restraints). The coexistence of torn menisci and injured articular carti-

---

FACTORS TO CONSIDER IN THE TREATMENT OF ACL INJURY

Age
Activity level
Secondary restraint integrity
Meniscal status
Articular cartilage status
Rehabilitation potential
Patient goals and expectations

---

lage are other factors that worsen the prognosis. Rehabilitation potential and patient goals and expectations should also be considered.

In young patients a more aggressive surgical approach should be taken since this group tends to be more active and thus the chances of reinjury are higher. Young children rarely sustain midsubstance tears of the anterior cruciate ligament but rather avulse the tibial attachment with a bone fragment.[9] If the tibial attachment is elevated and displaced, open reduction and internal fixation of the tibial spine is recommended.[94]

Activity level is an important factor since athletic individuals are more prone to reinjury than sedentary ones. Those participating in high-risk sports are more prone to reinjury, especially in sports requiring sudden pivoting, such as basketball and football.

The severity of anterior tibial subluxation (anterolateral rotatory laxity) as measured by various tests for the pivot shift phemenon (Fig. 30-29) seems to correlate directly with the amount of functional instability. If the knee has mild (Grade I) an-

Classification of anterolateral rotatory laxity

Severity (Grade)	Amount of abnormal tibial motion	Positive test	Comment
Mild (Grade I)	1 + (< 5 mm)	Lachman, FRD	May be present with generalized joint laxity (physiologic)
Moderate (Grade II)	2 + (5-10 mm)	Lachman, FRD, Losee, ALRI, pivot "slide" but not "jerk"	No obvious jump with jerk and PS
Severe (Grade III)	3 + (11-15 mm)	Lachman, FRD, Losee, ALRI, jerk, PS	Obvious jump with jerk and PS and gross subluxation-reduction with test
Gross (Grade IV)	4 + (> 15 mm)	Lachman, FRD, Losee ALRI, jerk, PS	Impingement of lateral tibial plateau in subluxated position which requires examiner to backoff during pivot shift test to effect reduction

Fig. 30-29 ■ Grading severity of anterior tibial subluxation (anterolateral rotatory laxity). (See text for explanation of tests.) FRD, Flexion rotation drawer; ALRI, anterolateral rotatory instability; PS, pivot shift.
Adapted from Noyes, F.R., Grood, E.S., Suntay, W.J., and Butler, D.L.: Iowa Orthop. J. **3**:32, 1982.

terior tibial subluxation, with slightly positive Lachman and FRD tests but other tests negative, the patient can be expected to have little or no functional instability. This degree of laxity can be physiologic, such as in loose-jointed persons. This group generally does well with a nonoperative regimen. The knee with moderate

---

Functional instability relates to anterior tibial subluxation (anterolateral rotatory laxity)

(Grade II) anterior tibial subluxation, manifested by positive Lachman and FRD tests, and a pivot "slide" or "slip" but negative pivot shift and jerk tests, usually has little short-term functional impairment but is at a higher risk for reinjury as the secondary restraints stretch. This group can be treated nonoperatively unless there are injuries to other ligaments (such

as an acute tear of the medial collateral ligament) or reparable meniscal tears. Patients in this group who have generalized ligamentous laxity tend to do less well with a nonoperative approach, especially those whose activities place high demands on their knees.

Patients with Grade III or IV anterior tibial subluxation, manifested by markedly positive pivot shift and jerk tests, usually will have functional instability manifested by giving way of the knee. Operative treatment is usually indicated, especially in patients in the high-risk categories.

The prevalence of meniscal tears associated with an acutely torn anterior cruciate ligament is 60% to 70%.[24,104,129] The meniscal tears usually are circumferential (vertical longitudinal).[136] Peripheral tears (i.e., at meniscosynovial junction or within the peripheral third of the meniscus), should be repaired whenever possible.[14] Arthrotomy offers considerable advantage over arthroscopic attempts, since a more secure repair can be obtained. Furthermore, the instability can be corrected at the same time. If the meniscus is repaired but the instability is *not* corrected, the meniscus will probably retear for the same reason it tore originally (i.e., compression and shear during anterior subluxation of the tibia under the femur).

Nonoperative treatment of acute anterior cruciate ligament tears

Initial treatment consists of ice, immobilization with an external splint, and a partial weight-bearing gait using crutches. Arthroscopy and examination under anesthesia are carried out if the diagnosis is not clear from the history and clinical examination. Rigid immobilization for a long period of time in a cast is probably not indicated, since the deleterious effects of joint immobilization outweigh potential benefit.

As the pain diminishes and the hemarthrosis resolves over 2 to 3 weeks, gentle range of motion exercises can be initiated. If a partial tear of the anterior cruciate ligament is suspected, active quadriceps exercises should probably be avoided, since they tend to pull the tibia forward. This is especially true from 45 degrees of flexion to full extension.[66] There is some evidence that the hamstrings might help control anterior subluxation of the tibia and therefore hamstring strengthening exercises could be of benefit.[122] As the patient regains full knee range of motion and muscular control and gradually increases functional activity, an external support or knee brace can be ordered. Simple elastic bandages probably have a beneficial effect, since they remind the patient to be cautious of pivoting on the leg, and they probably facilitate proprioception by sensory cutaneous feedback. Custom-made braces such as the Lenox Hill or Can-Am are more effective but will not completely stabilize the knee to anterior subluxation in extension.

Operative treatment of acute anterior cruciate ligament tears

Primary repair of a torn anterior cruciate ligament alone results in a high percentage of failures. Feagin and Curl[32] carried out a 5-year follow-up study on 32 knees following this form of treatment. More than two thirds had pain, swelling, stiffness, and giving way of the knee. We do not recommend primary repair of a torn anterior cruciate ligament alone except in the rare instances in which the ligament itself appears to be uninjured but avulsed from its femoral or tibial attachment.

Augmentation of a primary repair with a transferred autogenous tissue graft has been shown to improve the percentage of stable knees following surgical repair. Marshall and associates carried out primary anterior cruciate ligament repairs, which were reinforced with a tube of the iliotibial tract based distally on Gerdy's tubercle and brought over-the-top of the lateral femoral condyle.[87] At an average 2½ years' follow-up, no patient was troubled by giving way and 93% were active in sports. Warren[132] later looked at those patients with a 5-year or greater follow-up and found that none complained of giving way and 99% were participating in sports.

Other techniques use the same principles but different tissues, such as the semitendinosus tendon,[97] gracilis tendon,[92] or a slip of patellar tendon to act as a stent or graft.[30] The operation thus becomes a primary reconstruction in addition to primary repair. Therefore the same technique used for late reconstruction can be applied to primary reconstruction (see p. 962). The urgency of primary repair within the first week following injury thus becomes less important.

In summary, the knee with a typical history of a noncontact pivoting injury resulting in a "pop" and rapid severe swelling most likely has a torn anterior cruciate ligament. Diagnosis can be confirmed by arthroscopy and examination under anesthesia, at which time associ-

---

TREATMENT OF ACUTE ACL INJURY

Nonoperative	Operative
No or minimal anterior tibial subluxation	Marked anterior tibial subluxation
No additional intraarticular pathology	Additional intraarticular pathology
Middle or older age group	Young age group
Minimal athletic participation	Active in sports

NOTE: The majority of patients fall between these two extremes, and treatment should always be individualized.

---

ated intraarticular injury can be diagnosed. If the patient has little or no anterior tibial subluxation on examination, no additional intraarticular pathologic condition, is in the older age group, and is not active in athletics, the knee can be treated nonoperatively with a good success rate. On the other hand, if the patient is young, active in sports, and the knee has a marked instability, primary repair augmented by a primary reconstructive procedure should be carried out. This is especially true if a meniscus is torn but reparable. The majority of injuries fall between these extremes and should be treated individually, taking into consideration the degree of knee instability, associated intraarticular injury, the functional demands that will be placed on the knee, and the surgeon's experience in treating these injuries.

Chronic instability resulting from torn anterior cruciate ligament

The primary indication for surgical stabilization of a knee with recurrent anterior tibial subluxation is functional instability, despite rehabilitative efforts, that can be reproduced by pivot shift testing.

INDICATIONS FOR SURGERY IN CHRONIC ACL TEAR INSTABILITY

- Functional instability reproducible by pivot shift testing despite rehabilitation
- Young athlete with high demands
- Knee with reparable meniscus
- Progression from mild to moderate instability in a short time despite rehabilitation

---

The patient who has a torn anterior cruciate ligament and mild instability should also be considered for surgery if he is in a high-risk category (young, high functional demands, and a history of torn anterior cruciate ligament in the contralateral knee with previously demonstrated progressive disability). Surgical reconstruction should also be considered in the knee with a reparable meniscus (as documented by arthrogram and/or arthroscopy) or if reexamination shows that there has been a progression from mild to moderate instability in a short time.

Relative contraindications to surgery are advanced degenerative joint disease in a patient for whom compliance to the postoperative rehabilitation protocol is anticipated to be poor. If the symptoms of giving way are the predominant cause of disability, however, a knee with severe degenerative changes can be improved functionally by surgery, although little or no improvement of the symptoms resulting from degenerative changes would be anticipated.

The success of surgical reconstruction is directly related to the amount of reduction of anterior tibial subluxation. The goal of surgery, therefore, is to eliminate the pivot shift. If the pivot shift is eliminated, the anterior drawer sign at 25 degrees of flexion should also be eliminated or significantly diminished. The anterior drawer sign at 90 degrees of flexion is of little functional importance, since very few activities are done at this degree of knee flexion. Furthermore, at 90 degrees flexion the hamstring muscles have considerable mechanical advantage to dynamically stabilize the joint.

General principles of anterior cruciate reconstruction

The goals of reconstructive surgery are to restore stability yet maintain a full range of motion. To achieve these goals, it is essential that all ligament and capsular restraints are *isometric* within a full range of motion. The medial collateral ligament accomplishes this by virtue of its long fibers that originate proximally at the medial femoral epicondyle. The parallel fiber

---

GOALS OF RECONSTRUCTIVE SURGERY

Restored stability
Maintenance of full range of motion
Isometric ligament and capsular function

---

arrangement anterior and posterior to the instant center of rotation provides constant tension in at least some portion of the ligament in all joint positions.[4,134] Isometric function of the anterior cruciate ligament is achieved through its unique configuration of fiber bundles and their attachments. The anterior cruciate ligament is not a single cord, but rather a bundle of individual fibers that assume a spiral configuration and fan out over broad attachment areas. Because of this complex structure, ligament attachment sites should not be altered.[5]

Material and biologic properties of tissue used for anterior cruciate reconstruction must be taken into consideration when deciding which to transfer. The tensile strength of various tissues commonly used for anterior cruciate ligament reconstruction have been determined by Noyes et al.[112] One must consider that the strength of the tissue will probably diminish after it is transferred as a result of loss of vascular and/or nerve supply. It is doubtful that the graft will gain in strength following surgery. Therefore we believe that the tensile strength used to

reconstruct the anterior cruciate ligament should be at least as great as, if not greater than, the tensile strength of the anterior cruciate ligament. Anything less can result in failure if excessive tension is placed on the reconstructed ligament. With the exception of patellar tendon, most structures when used alone cannot match the tensile strength of the anterior cruciate ligament, according to Noyes et al.[112] For this reason we recommend using the combined strength of two graft tissues such as both the iliotibial tract and semitendinosus tendon when not using patellar tendon for anterior cruciate reconstruction.

There are two basically different techniques used in anterior cruciate ligament reconstruction: intraarticular and extraarticular. Both are designed to decrease anterior subluxation of the tibia and thereby eliminate the pivot shift. Unlike their extraarticular counterpart, intraarticular procedures attempt to anatomically replace the torn anterior cruciate ligament, usually with some sort of graft.

Extraarticular procedures

Static lateral extraarticular reconstructive procedures are commonly performed alone for anterior tibial subluxation. These operations are designed to functionally eliminate the pivot shift by creating a static restraint to anterior tibial subluxation. This is accomplished by connecting the lateral femoral epicondyle to Gerdy's tubercle, with the collagenous restraint lying parallel to the intraarticular course of the anterior cruciate ligament.

MacIntosh and Darby[82] were among the first to describe a method of lateral extraarticular substitution repair. A strip of distally based iliotibial tract was fashioned and released proximally. The strip was then passed deep to the fibular collateral ligament and either passed "over-the-top" of the lateral femoral condyle (intraarticular) or "return lateral loop" (extraarticular). Arnold et al.[7] modified this technique slightly by looping the strip back on itself

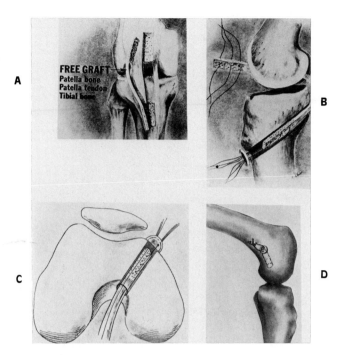

Fig. 30-42 ■ Clancy's method of posterior cruciate ligament reconstruction using a free patellar tendon graft with its tibial and patellar bone attachments. A free graft is taken from the central third patella tendon **(A)** and passed through drill holes in the tibia **(B)** and femur **(C)**. It is sewn over a button placed over the tibial and femoral **(D)** tunnels.
From Clancy, W.G., Nelson, D.A., Reider, B., and Narechania, R.G.: J. Bone Joint Surg. **65A:**310, 1983.

with chronic posterior instability with an average follow-up of 31 months.[21] The overall objective and functional results were good or excellent in 11 knees. The advantages reported by Clancy for using this method are bone-to-bone healing and "adequate" tensile strength of the graft.

The results of dynamic reconstruction using a bone block transfer of the origin of the medial head of the gastrocnemius were reported by Insall and Hood.[53] Eight knees with chronic posterior instability, followed from 29 to 48 months, were all reported to have objective improvements in stability using this method. Six out of eight were reported to have good or excellent overall results, with ability to return to sports. Insall and Hood believe this acts as a "dynamic" reconstruction, with the tibia moving forward on the femur with active plantar flexion of the foot.

Kennedy and Galpin[69] recommended transfer of the medial head of the gastrocnemius with a diamond-braided polypropylene leader through a femoral drill hole. Postoperatively a posterior sag was still present in all patients, although the reported posterior displacement was less. Despite failure of the procedure to significantly improve laxity, Kennedy and Galpin reported a functional improvement in 80%.

Our current approach is to transfer both the semitendinosus and gracilis tendon through a drill hole in the tibia and femur and to staple the grafts to the femur in the area of the medial epicondyle. We have transferred the medial head of the gastrocnemius in conjunction with the above-mentioned reconstructive procedures in several cases to act as a vascularized muscle pedicle for the transferred tendons. Our experience with transfer of the medial head of the gastrocnemius alone has been consistent failure of this technique to hold the tibia in the reduced position. In several cases we have also used a prosthetic ligament stent in addition to the tissue transfers.

■ OTHER TORN LIGAMENT COMBINATIONS

More severe knee injuries with disruption of multiple knee ligaments can occur with the application of even greater forces. When multiple ligaments are completely torn, one should suspect that knee dislocation with subsequent reduction has occurred, and treatment should procede with appropriate precautions.

A severe knee injury will often appear less swollen and less painful on stress testing than a knee with a less severe ligament injury. This is because the extreme degrees of joint displacement that cause multiple ligament disruptions usually rupture the synovium and capsule as well, allowing the blood inside the joint to dissipate into the soft tissues; therefore a tense hemarthrosis will not be present. In addition, application of stress to a completely torn ligament results in no tension in the structure (Fig. 30-43).

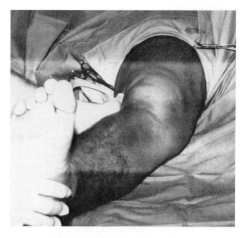

Fig. 30-43 ■ Valgus stress of right knee shows marked laxity in extension. Both cruciate ligaments and the entire medial capsule and tibial collateral ligament were torn.

```
Knee dislocation
        ↓
Assume vascular injury until proven
        otherwise
```

The prime consideration in knees with complete disruption of multiple ligaments and suspected dislocation (Fig. 30-44) should be for the neurovascular structures. The incidence of disruption of the popliteal artery has been reported to be greater than 50%.[45] Therefore a dislocated knee should be assumed to have a popliteal artery injury until proven otherwise. If the injury is open and requires immediate surgery, a femoral arteriogram should be performed even in the presence of good pulses, especially if a tourniquet will be used. This can be done in the operating room using ipsilateral femoral arteriography with single-film recording on the operating table. With a closed injury, absence or weakening of the distal pulses are definite indications for obtaining an arteriogram before consideration of definitive treatment of the knee injury. Because of the good collateral network about the knee, capallary pulsation and even weakly palpable pedal pulses can be present even in the presence of severe vessel damage. Fasciotomy of the anterior, lateral, and deep posterior compartments should be considered in the face of arterial insufficiency and subsequent repair.

If the dorsalis pedis and posterior tibialis pulses are strong, we recommend waiting several days for the status of the lower extremity to stabilize before primary repair of injured ligaments. Surgical considerations in repairing multiple ligament disruptions, especially if both cruciate ligaments are torn, should include the use of internal or external fixation to maintain reduction. This should be applied before final repair of the ligaments. We prefer a large, smooth Steinman pin that crosses the joint in the intercondylar area (Fig. 30-45). We recommend that both

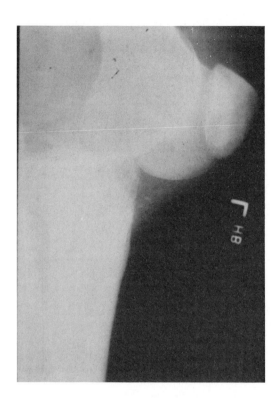

Fig. 30-44 ■ Left knee roentgenogram showing posterior dislocation. The probability of injury to the popliteal artery is very high in this type of injury.

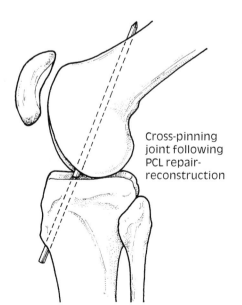

Cross-pinning joint following PCL repair-reconstruction

Fig. 30-45 ■ A large, smooth pin is used to stabilize the knee to prevent posterior tibial subluxation after repair of the posterior cruciate ligament. This should be left protruding from the femur as well as the tibia to allow extraction of both pieces in case of fatigue failure and breakage of the pin.

ends of the pin protrude through the bone to allow removal in case of breakage of the intraarticular section of the pin. A solid long leg cast is required. The cross-pin fixation can be removed at 6 to 8 weeks after surgery.

If both cruciate ligaments are torn, we try to repair both ligaments primarily, but usually augment only the posterior cruciate ligament repair.

REFERENCES

1. Andrews, J.R., Sanders, R.A., and Morin, B.: Surgical treatment of anterolateral rotatory instability: a follow-up study, Am. J. Sports Med. **13**:112, 1985.

2. Andrews, J.R., and Sanders, R.: A "mini-reconstruction" technique in treating anterolateral rotatory instability (ALRI), Clin. Orthop. **172**:93, 1983.

3. Apley, A.G.: Instability of the knee resulting from ligamentous injury: a plea for plain words, J. Bone Joint Surg. **62B**:515, 1980.

4. Arms, S., Boyle, J., Johnson, R., and Pope, M.: Strain measurement in the medial collateral ligament of the human knee: an autopsy study, J. Biomech. **16**:491, 1983.

5. Arms, S.W., Pope, M.H., Johnson, R.J., Fischer, R.A., Arvidsson, I., and Eriksson, E.: The biomechanics of anterior cruciate ligament rehabilitation and reconstruction, Am. J. Sports Med. **12**:8, 1984.

6. Arnoczky, S.P., Tarvin, G.B., and Marshall, J.L.: Anterior cruciate ligament replacement using patellar tendon, J. Bone Joint Surg. **64A**:217, 1982.

7. Arnold, J.A., Coker, T.P., Heaton, L.M., Park, J.P., and Harris, W.D.: Natural history of anterior cruciate tears, Am. J. Sports Med. **7**:305, 1979.

8. Bianchi, M.: Acute tears of the posterior cruciate ligament: clinical study and results of operative treatment in 27 cases, Am. J. Sports Med. **11**:308, 1983.

9. Bradley, G.W., Shives, T.C., and Samuelson, K.M.: Ligament injuries in the knees of children, J. Bone Joint Surg. **61A**:588, 1979.

10. Brody, G.A., Eisinger, M., Arnoczky, S.P., and Warren, K.S.: In vitro fibroblast seeding of a prosthetic anterior cruciate ligament, Orthop. Trans. **7**:254, 1983.

11. Butler, D.L., Noyes, F.R., and Grood, E.S.: Ligamentous restraints to anterior-posterior drawer in the human knee, J. Bone Joint Surg. **62A**:259, 1980.

12. Cabaud, H.E.: Biomechanics of the anterior cruciate ligament, Clin. Orthop. **172**:26, 1983.

13. Carrell, W.B.: Use of fascia lata in knee-joint instability, J. Bone Joint Surg. **19**:1018, 1937.

14. Cassidy, R.E., and Shaffer, A.J.: Repair of peripheral meniscus tears: a preliminary report, Am. J. Sports Med. **9**:209, 1981.

15. Chick, R.R., and Jackson, D.W.: Tears of the anterior cruciate ligament in young athlete, J. Bone Joint Surg. **60A**:970, 1978.

16. Cho, K.O.: Reconstruction of the anterior cruciate ligament by semitendinosus tenodesis, J. Bone Joint Surg. **57A**:608, 1975.

17. Clancy, W.G.: Functional rehabilitation of isolated medial collateral ligament sprains (symposium), Am. J. Sports Med. **7**:206, 1979.

18. Clancy, W.G.: Anterior cruciate ligament functional instability: a static intra-articular and dynamic extra-articular procedure, Clin. Orthop. **172**:102, 1983.

19. Clancy, W.G., Jr., Narechania, R.G., Rosenberg, T.D., Gmeiner, J.G., Wisnefske, D.D., and Lange, T.A.: Anterior and posterior cruciate ligament reconstruction in rhesus monkeys: a histological, microangiographic, and biomechanical analysis, J. Bone Joint Surg. **63A**:1270, 1981.

20. Clancy, W.G., Nelson, D.A., Reider, B., and Narechania, R.G.: Anterior cruciate ligament reconstruction using one-third of the patellar ligament, augmented by extra-articular tendon transfers, J. Bone Joint Surg. **64A**:352, 1982.

21. Clancy, W.G., Nelson, D.A., Reider, B., and Narechania, R.G.: Treatment of knee joint instability secondary to rupture of the posterior cruciate ligament. Report of a new procedure. J. Bone Surg. **65A**:310, 1983.

22. Collins, H.R., Hughston, J.C., DeHaven, K.E., Bergfeld, J.A., and Evarts, C.M.: The meniscus as a cruciate ligament substitute. J. Sports Med. **2**:11, 1974.

23. Dandy, D.J., and Pusey, R.J.: The long-term results of unrepaired tears of the posterior cruciate ligament, J. Bone Joint Surg. **64A**:92, 1982.

24. DeHaven, K.E.: Diagnosis of acute knee injuries with hemarthrosis, Am. J. Sports Med. **8**:9, 1980.

25. DeLee, J.C., Riley, M.B., and Rockwood, C.A.: Acute straight lateral instability of the knee, Am. J. Sports Med. **11**:404, 1983.

26. Drez, D.: Modified Eriksson procedure for chronic anterior cruciate instability, Orthopaedics **1**:30, 1978.

27. Ellison, A.E.: Skiing injuries, Clin. Symp. **29**:543, 1977.

28. Ellison, A.E.: Distal iliotibial-band transfer for anterolateral rotatory instability of the knee, J. Bone Joint Surg. **61A**:330, 1979.

29. Ellsasser, J.C., Reynolds, F.C., and Omohundro, J.R.: The nonoperative treatment of collateral ligament injuries of the knee in professional football players: an analysis of 74 injuries

treated nonoperatively and 24 injuries treated surgically, J. Bone Joint Surg. **56A:**1185, 1974.

30. Eriksson, E.: Reconstruction of the anterior cruciate ligament, Orthop. Clin. North Am. **7:**167, 1976.

31. Fairbank, T.J.: Knee joint changes after meniscectomy, J. Bone Joint Surg. **30B:**664, 1948.

32. Feagin, J.A., and Curl, W.W.: Isolated tear of the anterior cruciate ligament: 5-year follow-up study, Am. J. Sports Med. **4:**95, 1976.

33. Fetto, J.F., and Marshall, J.L.: Medial collateral ligament injuries of the knee: a rationale for treatment, Clin. Orthop. **132:**206, 1978.

34. Fetto, J.F., and Marshall, J.L.: The natural history and diagnosis of anterior cruciate ligament insufficiency, Clin. Orthop. **147:**29, 1980.

35. Fleming, R.E., Blatz, D.J., and McCarroll, J.R.: Posterior problems in the knee: posterior cruciate insufficiency and posterolateral rotatory insufficiency, Am. J. Sports Med. **9:**107, 1981.

36. Frank, C., Woo, S.L-Y., Amiel, D., Harwood, F., Gomez, M., and Akeson, W.: Medial collateral ligament healing. a multidisciplinary assessment in rabbits, Am. J. Sports Med. **11:**379, 1983.

37. Galway, H.R., and MacIntosh, D.L.: The lateral pivot shift: a symptom and sign of anterior cruciate ligament insufficiency, Clin. Orthop. **147:**45, 1980.

38. Galway, R.D., Beaupre, A., and MacIntosh, D.L.: Pivot shift: a clinical sign of symptomatic anterior cruciate insufficiency, J. Bone Joint Surg. **54B:**763, 1972.

39. Girgis, F.G., Marshall, J.L., and Monajem, A.R.S.: The cruciate ligaments of the knee joint: anatomical, functional, and experimental analysis, Clin. Orthop. **106:**216, 1975.

40. Grood, E.S., Noyes, F.R., Butler, D.L., and Suntay, W.J.: Ligamentous and capsular restraints preventing straight medial and lateral laxity in intact human cadaver knees, J. Bone Joint Surg. **63A:**1257, 1981.

41. Hanks, G.A., Joyner, D.M., and Kalenak, A.: Anterolateral rotatory instability of the knee: an analysis of the Ellison procedure, Am. J. Sports Med. **9:**225, 1981.

42. Hewson, G.F.: Drill guides for improving accuracy in anterior cruciate ligament repair and reconstruction, Clin. Orthop. **172:**119, 1981.

43. Hey-Groves, E.W. The crucial ligaments of the knee joint: their function, rupture, and the operative treatment of the same, Br. J. Surg. **7:**505, 1920.

44. Holden, D.L., Eggert, A.W., and Butler, J.E.: The nonoperative treatment of Grade I and II medial collateral ligament injuries to the knee, Am. J. Sports Med. **11:**340, 1983.

45. Hoover, N.W.: Injuries of the popliteal artery associated with fractures and dislocations, Surg. Clin. North Am. **41:**1099, 1961.

46. Horne, J.G., and Parsons, C.J.: The anterior cruciate ligament: its anatomy and a new method of reconstruction, Can. J. Surg. **20:**214, 1977.

47. Hughston, J.C., Andrews, J.A., Cross, M.J., and Moschi, A.: Classification of knee ligament instabilities; Part I, The medial compartment and cruciate ligaments, J. Bone Joint Surg. **58A:**159, 1976.

48. Hughston, J.C., Andrews, J.R., Cross, M.J., and Moschi, A.: Classification of knee ligament instability; Part II, The lateral compartment, J. Bone Joint Surg. **58A:**173, 1976.

49. Hughston, J.C., and Barrett, G.R.: Acute anteromedial rotatory instability—long term results of surgical repair, J. Bone Joint Surg. **65A:**145, 1983.

50. Hughston, J.C., Bowden, J.A., Andrews, J.R., and Norwood, L.A.: Acute tears of the posterior cruciate ligament, J. Bone Joint Surg. **62A:**438, 1980.

51. Hughston, J.C., and Eilers, A.F.: The role of the posterior oblique ligament in repairs of acute medial ligament tears of the knee, J. Bone Joint Surg. **55A:**923, 1973.

52. Indelicato, P.A.: Non-operative treatment of complete tears of the medial collateral ligament of the knee, J. Bone Joint Surg. **65A:**323, 1983.

53. Insall, J., and Hood, R.W.: Bone-block transfer of the medial head of the gastrocnemius for posterior cruciate insufficiency, J. Bone Joint Surg. **64A:**691, 1982.

54. Insall, J., Joseph, D.M., Aglietti, P., and Campbell, R.D.: Bone-block iliotibial-band transfer for anterior cruciate insufficiency, J. Bone Joint Surg. **63A:**560, 1981.

55. Ireland, J., and Trickey, E.L.: MacIntosh tenodesis for anterolateral instability of the knee, J. Bone Joint Surg. **62B:**340, 1980.

56. Ivey, F.M., Blazina, M.E., Fox, J.M., and DelPizzo, W.: Intraarticular substitution for anterior cruciate insufficiency: a clinical comparison between patellar tendon and meniscus, Am. J. Sports Med. **8:**405, 1980.

57. Jacobsen, K.: Osteoarthritis following insufficiency of the cruciate ligaments in man, Acta Orthop. Scand. **48:**520, 1977.

58. Jacob, R.P., Hassler, H., and Staeubli, H.-U.: Observations on rotatory instability of the lateral compartment of the knee: experimental studies on the functional anatomy and the pathomechanism of the true and reversed pivot shift sign, Acta Orthop. Scand. (Suppl. 191), **52:**1, 1981.

59. James, S.L.: Biomechanics of knee ligament reconstruction, Clin. Orthop. **146:**90, 1980.

60. James, S.: Knee ligament reconstruction. In Evarts, C.M., ed.: Surgery of the musculoskeletal system, vol. 3, New York, 1983 Churchill-Livingstone.

61. Jenkins, D.H.R.: The repair of cruciate liga-

ments with flexible carbon fibre: a longer term study of the induction of new ligaments and the fate of the implanted carbon, J. Bone Joint Surg. **60B**:520, 1978.

62. Jenkins, D.H.R., Forster, I.W., McKibbin, B., and Ralis, Z.: Induction of tendon and ligament formation by carbon implants, J. Bone Joint Surg. **59B**:53, 1977.

63. Jenkins, D.H.R., and McKibbin, B.: The role of flexible carbon fiber implants as tendon and ligament substitutes in clinical practice, J. Bone Joint Surg. **62B**:497, 1980.

64. Johnson, R.J., Kettlekamp, D.B., Clark, W., and Leaverton, P.: Factors affecting late results after meniscectomy, J. Bone Joint Surg. **56A**:719, 1974.

65. Jones, K.G.: Reconstruction of the anterior cruciate ligament: a technique using the central one-third of the patellar ligament, J. Bone Joint Surg. **45A**:925, 1973.

66. Jonsson, T., Althoff, B., Peterson, L., and Renstrom, P.: Clinical diagnosis of ruptures of the anterior cruciate ligament: a comparative study of the Lachman test and the anterior drawer sign, Am. J. Sports Med. **10**:100, 1982.

67. Kennedy, J.C., ed.: The injured adolescent knee, Baltimore, 1979, Williams & Wilkins, p. 142.

68. Kennedy, J.C., and Fowler, P.J.: Medial and anterior instability of the knee: an anatomic and clinical study using stress machines, J. Bone Joint Surg. **53A**:1257, 1971.

69. Kennedy, J.C., and Galpin, R.D.: The use of the medial head of the gastrocnemius muscle in the posterior cruciate deficient knee: indications—technique—results, Am. J. Sports Med. **10**:63, 1982.

70. Kennedy, J.C., and Grainger, R.W.: The posterior cruciate ligament, J. Trauma **7**:367, 1967.

71. Kennedy, J.C., Roth, J.H., and Mendenhall, H.V.: Intraarticular replacement in anterior cruciate ligament deficient knees, Am. J. Sports Med. **8**:1-14, 1980.

72. Kennedy, J.C., Roth, J.H., and Walder, D.M.: Posterior cruciate ligament injuries, Orthop. Digest **7**:19, 1979.

73. Kennedy, J.C., Stewart, R., and Walker, D.M.: Anterolateral rotatory instability of the knee joint: an early analysis of the Ellison procedure, J. Bone Joint Surg. **60A**:1031, 1978.

74. Kennedy, J.C., Weinberg, H.W., and Wilson, A.S.: The anatomy and function of the anterior cruciate ligament, J. Bone Joint Surg. **56A**:223, 1974.

75. Lam, S.J.S.: Reconstruction of the anterior cruciate ligament using the Jones procedure and its Guy's Hospital modification, J. Bone Joint Surg. **50A**:1213, 1968.

76. Last, R.J.: Some anatomical details of the knee joint, J. Bone Joint Surg. **30B**:683, 1948.

77. Lemaire, M.: Instabilité chronique de genou: techniques et résultats des plasties ligamentaires en traumatologie sportive, J. Chir. (Paris) **110**:20, 1975.

78. Lipscomb, A.B., Johnston, R.K., Snyder, R.B., and Brothers, J.C.: Secondary reconstruction of anterior cruciate ligament in athletes by using the semitendinosus tendon, Am. J. Sports Med. **7**:81, 1979.

79. Loos, W.C., Fox, J.M., Blazina, M.E., Del Pizzo, W., and Friedman, M.J.: Acute posterior cruciate ligament injuries, Am. J. Sports Med. **9**:86, 1981.

80. Losee, R.E., Johnson, T.R., and Southwick, W.O.: Anterior subluxation of the lateral tibial plateau, J. Bone Joint Surg. **60A**:1015, 1978.

81. Lysholm, J., and Gillquist, J.: Arthroscopic examination of the posterior cruciate ligament, J. Bone Joint Surg. **63A**:363, 1981.

82. MacIntosh, D.L., and Darby, T.A.: Lateral substitution reconstruction. In Proceedings and reports of universities, colleges, councils and associations, J. Bone Joint Surg. **58B**:142, 1976.

83. MacIntosh, D.L., and Tregonning, R.J.A.: A follow-up study and evaluation of "over-the-top" repair of acute tears of the anterior cruciate ligament. In Proceedings and reports of universities, colleges, councils and associations, J. Bone Joint Surg. **59B**:511, 1977.

84. Manske, P.R., Bridwell, K., and Lesker, P.A.: Nutrient pathways to flexor tendons of chickens using tritiated preline, J. Hand Surg. **3**:352, 1978.

85. Marshall, J.L., and Olsson, S.E.: Instability of the knee: a long-term experimental study in dogs, J. Bone Joint Surg. **53A**:1561, 1971.

86. Marshall, J.L., Rubin, R.M., Wang, J.B., Fetto, J.F., and Arnoczky, S.P.: The anterior cruciate ligament: the diagnosis and treatment of its injuries and their serious prognostic implications. Orthop. Rev. **VII**:35, 1978.

87. Marshall, J.L., Warren, R.F., and Wickiewicz, T.L.: Primary surgical treatment of anterior cruciate ligament lesions, Am. J. Sports Med. **10**:103, 1982.

88. Marshall, J.L., Warren, R.F., Wickiewicz, T.L., and Fetto, J.F.: Reconstruction of functioning anterior cruciate ligament: preliminary report using quadriceps tendon, Orthop. Rev. **VIII**:49, 1979.

89. Marshall, J.L., Warren, R.F., and Wickiewicz, T.L.: The anterior cruciate ligament: a technique of repair and reconstruction, Clin. Orthop. **143**:97, 1979.

90. McDaniel, W.J., and Dameron, T.B.: Untreated ruptures of the anterior cruciate ligament, J. Bone Joint Surg. **62A**:696, 1980.

91. McDaniel, W.J., and Dameron, T.B.: The untreated anterior cruciate ligament rupture, Clin. Orthop. **172**:158, 1983.

Certainly the repeated stresses applied to the patellofemoral joint in deceleration maneuvers[44] in sports are the most common cause of injuries to this joint (Fig. 32-3).

■ DIAGNOSIS—HISTORY AND PHYSICAL EXAMINATION

Hughston[42] pointed out that patellofemoral subluxation is a major cause of internal derangements of the knee joint. He also noted that the diagnosis is based primarily on the patient's history and on physical examination.

The history of an injury to the knee joint is very easily overlooked when the physician sees the patient point to a painful area. However, the history in patellofemoral subluxation is very crucial. The patellofemoral mechanism and anatomy have been present long before the symptoms occurred; however, most patients will say that one particular injury caused the trouble with the knee.

Sometimes the history will be of chronic pain over a prolonged period. However, frequently a history of patellofemoral subluxation reveals that the patient's knee is giving way, and on further questioning the physician discovers that the knee gives way when the patient is cutting away from the affected side (Fig. 32-4)—that is, the femur is internally rotated on a tibia that is fixed in external rotation, allowing the patella to sublux laterally. Characteristically there would be no physical contact that produced the giving-way sensation.

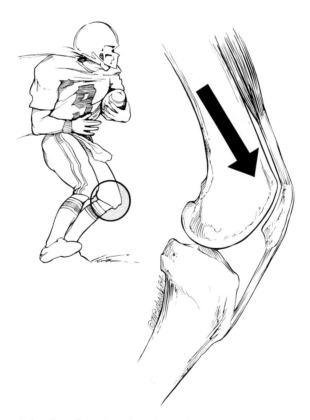

Fig. 32-4 ■ The patella often dislocates when the patient cuts back to the contralateral side—that is, the foot is planted and the femur internally rotates, thereby dislocating the patella laterally.

Occasionally the patient will remember that the patella slid over and that he or she felt a "click" as it subluxed. Some patients describe this phenomenon as "locking," but the subsequent normal range of motion after the injury should help rule out true locking. A history of an effusion that occurs within 12 hours after the injury is common. If an osteochondral fracture of the patella or femur has occurred, effusion may collect more rapidly—within 2 hours. According to Bassett,[2] if the hemarthrosis is aspirated and fat droplets are noted, in a large percentage of cases an osteochondral fracture is present. If there has been no osteochondral fracture, effusion is usually serosanguinous. This effusion will usually resolve within 7 to 10 days if no aspiration is done and if no internal derangement has occurred.

The patient often complains of weakness of the leg, especially during running, cutting, and stair climbing. Frequently the patient is not aware that the patella slid out of joint but will complain of this symptom by saying that something "jumped out." Certainly the most common symptom of a pathologic condition of the patellofemoral joint is pain on flexion, accentuated by stair climbing. It is more common for the patient to have pain going down stairs than up stairs.

Localization of the pain is significant (Fig. 32-5). Most patients will have pain inferiorly on the patellar tendon, medially or laterally on the quadriceps retinaculum, or superiorly on the quadriceps tendon. The pain may migrate; that is, the initial complaint may be of pain medially, then laterally. Pain of a patellar origin may also be referred to the popliteal fossa.[103] One should remember that although patellofemoral subluxation may be suggested by the patient's history, it is common to find associated lesions with the patellofemoral subluxation, such as torn medial or lateral meniscus or the anterior cruciate ligament.

Table 32-1 summarizes the tests and measurements that should be included in the physical examination. The physical ex-

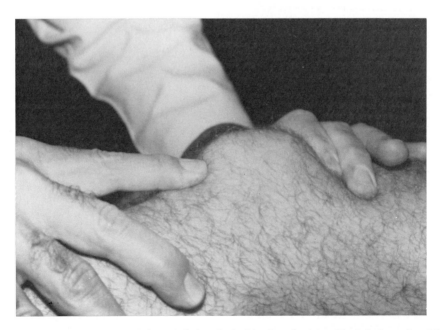

Fig. 32-5 ■ Tenderness around the patella is palpated by the physician. The inferior pole of the patella is palpated by "tipping" the apex anterior for better access. Tenderness distally is called the patellar tip sign.

amination should include examination of the gait. By watching the patient walk in shorts in the examination room, one is aware of the general alignment of the lower extremity. Evaluation includes femoral neck anteversion, tibial torsion, genu valgum, and pronation of the feet.

James et al. described the "miserable malalignment syndrome" of runners (Fig. 32-6). It should be noted that the patella is the central part of the malalignment syndrome. Buchbinder et al.[11] felt that pronation of the feet is the primary cause of chondromalacia. Jackson[52] noted that the patient with patellofemoral subluxation has a higher incidence of arthritis associated with the decreased quadriceps

strength. Quadriceps atrophy should be evaluated during physical examination as the patient ambulates in the office. It is almost universally present in an injured knee of long-standing nature.

The patient should then be asked to kneel and sit back on the heels[81]* (Fig. 32-7). This allows the examiner to check for quadriceps atrophy, and if the patient describes pain around the knee, this will

---

*Editors' note: More often, visible atrophy of other muscles, particularly the adductors, is demonstrated by this test. Also, joint motion can be evaluated roughly if the patient cannot sit symmetrically. This is a quick, revealing diagnostic test for anterior knee pain, meniscal derangement, patellofemoral disease, and weakened thigh musculature.

Table 32-1 ■ Summary of physical examination: extremity measurements frequently associated with patellofemoral disorders

Description of test, measurement, comments	Normal	Patient position	Degree of knee flexion	Patellofemoral disorder or malalignment
Quadriceps or Q angle—angle formed between the line from the anterior iliac spine to center of the patella and a line from center of patella to tibial tubercle	M, 10 degrees F, 15 degrees	Supine	0	Increased Q angle with excessive femoral anteversion, genu valgum, external tibial torsion, chrondromalacia; may have decreased Q angle with chronic subluxation of patella
Quadriceps mass–circumference 10 cm proximal to patella with active straight leg raising	Equal bilaterally	Supine	0	Associated with vastus medialis obliquus dysplasia, congenital hypoplasia, or generalized atrophy
Hip range of motion; internal and external rotation	Usually have greater external rotation; abnormal if internal exceeds external rotation by more than 30 degrees	Prone	90	Abnormal femoral anteversion or retroversion (may have increased Q-angle with excessive femoral anteversion)

From Carson, W.G., et al.: Clin. Orthop. **185**:165, 1984.

Continued.

Table 32-1 ■ Summary of physical examination: extremity measurements frequently associated with patellofemoral disorders—cont'd

Description of test, measurement, comments	Normal	Patient position	Degree of knee flexion	Patellofemoral disorder or malalignment			
Leg–ground angle—evaluation of tibia vara	Less than 10 degrees	Standing	0	Genu vara, tibia vara	Triceps surae contracture	Hindfoot varus	Forefoot supination
Neutral position of subtalar joint; patient lifts medial edge of heel—palpate talar head medially and laterally and check for hyperpronated foot	Subtalar joint should be close to neutral while standing	Standing	0	↘ ↓ ↓ ↙ Compensatory subtalar joint pronation			
Ankle dorsiflexion	More than 10 degrees	Supine	0 0	Primary subtalar joint pronation → Obligatory internal tibial rotation (may be increased or prolonged)			
Leg–heel alignment—longitudinal axis of leg to heel (with foot in neutral position)	2-3 degrees of varus	Prone (feet hanging from table edge)					
Hindfoot–forefoot alignment—long axis of heel to transverse axis of forefoot (with foot in neutral position)	Long axis of heel normally 90 degrees perpendicular to transverse axis forefoot	Prone (feet hanging from table edge)	0	Abnormal rotational stress absorbed by soft tissues at knee joint ↓ Peripatellar and anterior knee pain			

suggest the site of the injury. For instance, patients with patellofemoral subluxation often complain of pain behind the patella or in the popliteal fossa. If the pain is medial or lateral, the appropriate meniscus is suggested.

Next have the patient sit on the edge of the table and observe the site for a high-riding patella or patella alta, which, according to Smillie,[100] is the most consistent sign of patellofemoral subluxation. Hughston[44] noted the lateral tilt of the patella and named this the "grasshopper eye" patella (Fig. 32-8).

The patient is then asked to extend the knee, and the oblique head of the vastus medialis is examined. The dysplastic vastus medialis obliquus will reveal a dimple; this may be palpated medially (Fig. 32-9). The vastus lateralis is often hypertrophied and may show a hyperactive electromyogram (EMG) pattern.

The tibial tubercle may be observed with the patient sitting on the table; a large tibial tubercle indicates existing Osgood-Schlatter's disease. The patient then lies supine, and the knee is flexed approximately 30 degrees and evaluated. The fat

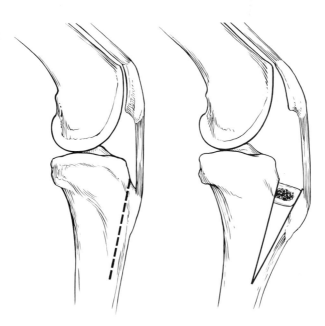

Fig. 32-16 ■ Anterior displacement of the tibial tubercle to decrease patellofemoral pressure.

of the patella should touch a projected line from the intercondylar notch of the femur with the knee flexed to 30 degrees (Fig. 32-17); if it did not, patella alta was present.*

Merchant et al.[76] (see Fig. 26-18) described an axial view with the knee flexed 45 degrees over the end of the table. The central x-ray beam is inclined 30 degrees from horizontal to strike the film cassette at a right angle. Using this method, Merchant et al. described the congruence angle, with a normal angle of 16 degrees.

Hughston[44] described a sunrise view (Fig. 32-18): with the patient prone and the knee flexed 55 degrees, the intercondylar notch of the femur should have an angle of 125 degrees (Fig. 32-19). However, occult changes in position and quadriceps tone make roentgenographic critera difficult to evaluate. The diagnosis of subluxation of the patella by roentgenographic evaluation alone is difficult. One of the most important uses of roentgenography

*Editors' note: Too many exceptions to the rule make Blumensaat's line an unreliable sign.

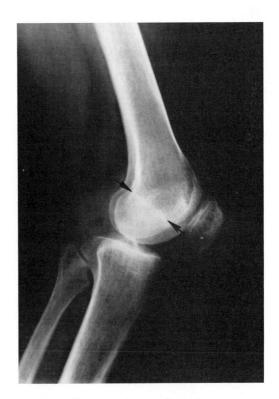

Fig. 32-17 ■ Roentgenogram illustrating Blumensaat's line.

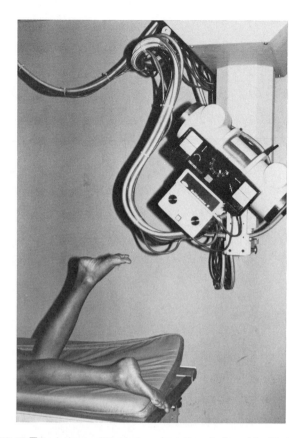

Fig. 32-18 ■ Technique of Hughston view. Knee is flexed to 55 degrees.

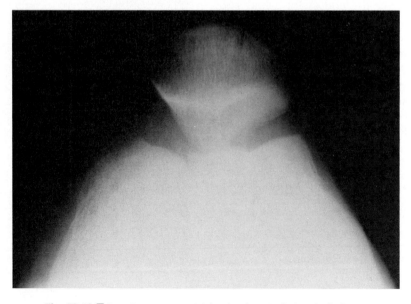

Fig. 32-19 ■ Roentgenogram obtained using Hughston technique.

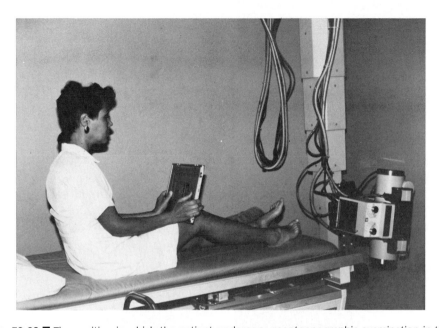

Fig. 32-20 ■ The position in which the patient undergoes roentgenographic examination in the Laurin technique. The knee is flexed 20 degrees. In this position the patella lies in the proximal—potentially unstable—segment of the femoral sulcus.

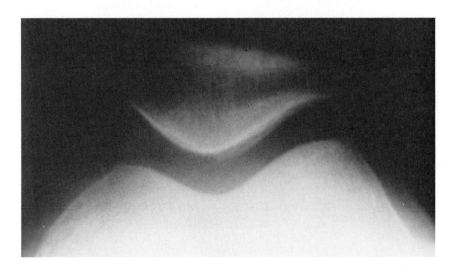

Fig. 32-21 ■ A patellofemoral roentgenogram using the Laurin technique.

is to rule out a concomitant osteochondral fracture.

Laurin et al.[62,63] described the lateral patellofemoral angle in diagnosis of subluxation of the patella. The knee is flexed 20 degrees (Fig. 32-20). They pointed out that in this position the patella lies in the proximal—potentially unstable—segment of the femoral sulcus (Fig. 32-21).

Insall and Salvati[49] compared the length of the patella and the ligamentum patellae on lateral roentgenograms (Fig. 32-22). Measurements were approximately equal, and normal variation did not exceed 20%. They suggested that a diagnosis of patella alta could be made with a ratio of less than 1:1. Lancourt and Cristini[60] used the Insall-Salvati criteria to evaluate patellofemoral programs. They found that patients with patellar dislocation had an index of 0.8, patients with chondromalacia of the patella had 0.86, and for those with apophysitis of the tibial tubercle the index was 1.2. They again noted the ratio of patellar length to patellar ligament length was 1.0 in normal patients.

Horns[41] used double-contrast arthrography to diagnose chondromalacia. He had a success rate of 90%, as proved by open operation.

■ TREATMENT
Medication

Cathepsin, a lysosomal protease, is a major factor in the degradation of cartilage matrix. Mankin[69] injected cortisol (hydrocortisone) in the joints of rabbits and found that the cortisol caused a de-

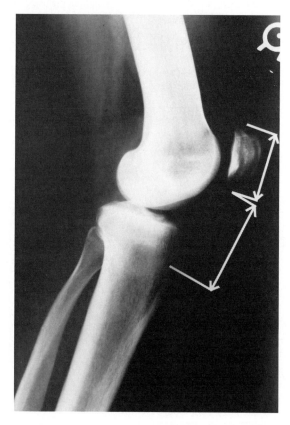

Fig. 32-22 ■ Insall-Salvati method of measuring patella alta; the patellar measurement and the ligamentum patella measurement should be roughly equal. Ratio of less than 1:1 represents patella alta, according to Insall and Salvati.

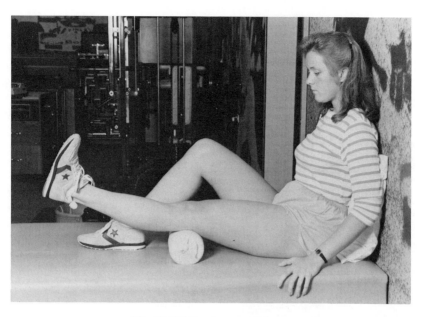

Fig. 33-7 ■ Short arc quadriceps.

ors. The patient tightens the quadriceps and holds for 2 seconds, then lifts the entire leg until the heel is 6 inches above the mat. The extremity is held in that position for 2 seconds, and then lowered and held for 2 seconds and repeated for 2 sets of 10.

Short arc quadriceps exercises are added once the patient can tolerate 2 pounds on the straight leg raises (Fig. 33-7). With the patient sitting, a firm pad is placed under the knee to limit flexion to less than 45 degrees. The back of the thigh is pressed into the pad as the knee extends, and the heel is raised and held for 2 seconds, then slowly lowered. The patient completes 2 sets of 10 repetitions. This produces a concentric contraction, because the muscle shortens as the knee extends.

Hamstring setting exercises are performed sitting with 50 to 60 degrees of knee flexion (Fig. 33-8). The patient attempts to dig the heel into the mat while pulling downward on the leg. The hamstring contraction is sustained for 10 seconds, followed by a 2-second period of relaxation, and repeated for two sets of 10.

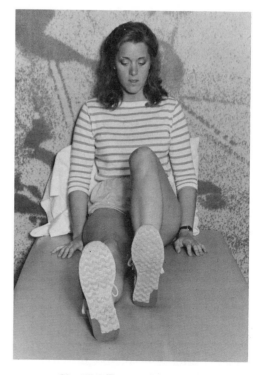

Fig. 33-8 ■ Hamstring setting.

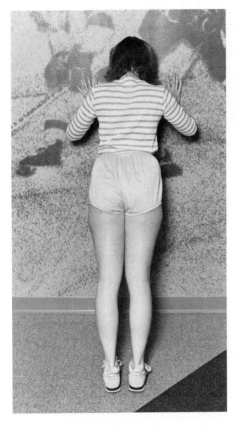

Fig. 33-9 ■ Toe raise.

Calf exercises

Toe raises are initiated with body weight alone, equally distributed on both legs. The patient stands on the floor, braced against the wall for support (Fig. 33-9). The plantar flexors of the ankle are held in contraction for 10 seconds and then slowly relaxed as the body weight returns to the heel. For each set, 25 repetitions are done. As these hip and knee ex-

---

CALF EXERCISE FOR *DISTAL* MUSCLE STRENGTH DEVELOPMENT
Toe raises

---

ercises are repeated, weights are increased at approximately 2-pound increments until the patient can handle 10 pounds. The resistance is added to the an-

kle with a weighted boot. A transfer to the Universal Gym or Nautilus equipment usually occurs smoothly once this plateau has been reached. A 5-pound slotted weight can be added to either system, allowing the increases to be in units of 5 rather than 10 pounds. The repetitions are gradually increased up to three sets of 10.

Stretching

Stretching is added when the patient has gained full knee extension. During rehabilitation, stretching should always be performed before the athlete is "warmed-up" to permit maximal muscle length development and plastic deformation of the muscle. Stretching after warming up will lead to elastic deformation. This is more

---

STRETCHING
Calf
Hamstring

---

desirable before athlete participation, when maximal flexibility may be required. Lengthening of the calf and hamstring muscles are added along with resistance exercises (Fig. 33-10). A towel stretch is performed by sitting against the wall with the involved leg extended. The towel is looped around the ball of the involved foot, which is pulled slowly into dorsiflexion, thus stretching the calf if the knee is kept as flat as possible. Standing gastrocnemius stretches are added as tolerated by the patient (Fig. 33-11). The patient stands approximately 18 inches from the wall with both feet flat on the floor and leans forward while keeping the knees extended, holding the position for 20 seconds, and then relaxing 5 seconds. Both stretches are repeated until two sets of 10 have been accomplished.

Cool-down

At the end of the workout, the knee is iced for 10 minutes to control soreness and swelling.

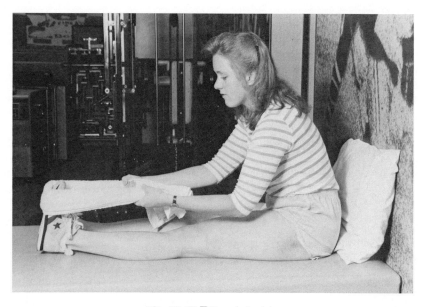

Fig. 33-10 ■ Towel stretch.

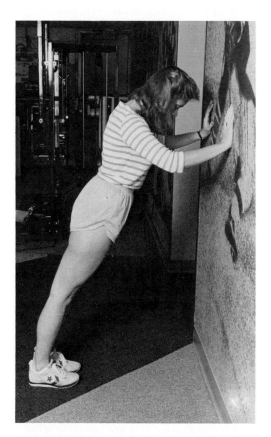

Fig. 33-11 ■ Standing gastrocnemius stretch.

Methods for achieving knee flexion and extension strength

Cybex. The Cybex II Dynamometer (Lumex, Bayshore, N.Y.) can be used as a training device. Several studies have shown that isokinetic rehabilitation is safe and effective, because the resistance is never greater than the produced muscular tension.[34,43,48,50] Both Coyle et al.[11] and Costill et al.[9] demonstrated hypertrophy of Type II muscle fibers and glycolytic enzyme enhancement following isokinetic training. Coyle et al. also showed that training at high velocity (300 degrees/sec) will also improve torque output at slower velocities.

Our requirements for isokinetic training are (1) the patient can lift two sets of 10 pounds for 10 repetitions per set, and (2) the patient has a minimum of 110 degrees of knee motion. The athlete is started at an angular velocity of 300 degrees per second and will produce 10 maximal quadriceps contractions, with the range limited from 100 degrees to as close to a full extension as possible. This is repeated three times with two-minute rest periods. The program is performed 3

ISOKINETIC TRAINING

Requirements

Patient can lift two sets of 10 repetitions of 10 pounds
Patient has 110 degrees of knee motion

Program

Initial
300 degrees/sec—10 repetitions from 100 degrees to maximal extension
Rest 2 minutes
Repeat
Rest 2 minutes
Repeat
Advanced
Decrease velocity in 30-degree increments until 90 degrees/sec
NOTE: Hamstrings can also be trained in the same fashion, using a range of 0 to 90 degrees of knee flexion.

---

days per week. Once the patient is able to perform three sets of 10 maximal contractions with 1-minute intervals of rest, the velocity is gradually decreased in 30-degree increments until 90 degrees per second. The patient will then train at the lower velocity. The hamstrings can be trained in a similar manner, using the range of 0 to 90 degrees of knee flexion.

Free weights. Ankle weights can be used for isotonic training with straight leg

---

FREE WEIGHT TRAINING

Exercises

Straight leg raises
Short arc quadriceps

Program

10 repetitions
Rest 2 minutes
10 repetitions
Rest 2 minutes
10 repetitions
Rest 2 minutes
10 repetitions

Weights

Begin at maximal tolerated for 10 repetitions
Increase at 2-pound increments
Goal is maximal strength level of normal leg

---

raises. In the short arc quadriceps exercises, the range is from 60 degrees to maximal extension. Weights are added in 2-pound increments for both exercises. The patient performs a set of 10 contractions with the weight followed by a 2-minute rest period and then repeated three times. The weights are increased until the strength level of the other leg is reached. This is the maximal weight that the patient can lift and control for 10 repetitions in the same range of motion. The hamstrings can be trained by having the patient lie in the prone position. The leg is worked from maximal allowable extension to 90 degrees of flexion with the same weight increases. Again the goal is the maximal weight that can be handled for 10 repetitions in the normal leg. Several authors have outlined isotonic weight protocols.[9,33,50] At any sign of patellofemoral problems, short arc exercises are eliminated and concentration is placed on straight leg raising.*

Home program

Performance of the home program is alternated with therapy visits. Active range of motion exercises are done in the bathtub or pool; the hip exercises are performed without weights, and the knee is worked isometrically and iced afterwards. The stretches and toe raises are also practiced along with normal gait motion. Vigorous pool walking in waist-level water will strengthen the upper thigh and lower abdominal muscles.

A summary of the starting phase program is presented in the box on p. 1067.

Intermediate phase
Warm-up

Warm-up is begun with 10 minutes of riding on a stationary bicycle with no resistance, once the patient has reached 110 degrees of knee flexion. In this phase of

---

*Editors' note: If all exercises that use the quadriceps are painful, we resort to straight leg raising in abduction, adduction, and hip flexion. We often find that these are weak, but they can be strengthened to permit quadriceps exercises to proceed.

STARTING PHASE PROGRAM

Warm-up

Hot/cold contrast

Exercises	Repetitions	Sets	Weight increase (pounds)
Wall slides (ROM)	10	2	NA
Hip flexion	10	2	5
Hip abduction	10	2	5
Hip extension	10	2	5
Hip adduction	10	2	5
Quadriceps setting	10	2	0
Short arc quadriceps	10	2	2
Hamstring setting	10	2	0
Toe raises	25	2	2

Stretching

Calf
Hamstring

Home program

Isometrics
Pool walking

---

the rehabilitation, the quadriceps and hamstring musculature are not very well conditioned, and it would be painful to add resistance on the bicycle. It is very important to adjust the seat height so that there is no more than 90 degrees of flexion at the hip and 110 degrees of flexion at the knee on the upstroke of the pedal.[37]

INTERMEDIATE PHASE

Warm-up
Range of motion
Stretching
Isotonic training
Functional activity
Home program

The higher seat level decreases the force on the extensor mechanism. At the downstroke of the pedal, the ankle should have the maximal dorsiflexion that the patient can tolerate.

Wall slides are continued until the patient has a full range of knee flexion.

Isotonic training

Hip adduction and abduction are performed on the Nautilus or Universal Gym equipment (Fig. 33-12). Hip extension is

---

ISOTONIC TRAINING

Hip abduction/adduction
Hip extension/flexion
Hamstring curls
Short arc quadriceps

---

done on the Nautilus and hip flexion on the Universal. The resistance is added in 10-pound increments until the strength has reached that of a normal extremity. This is defined as a maximal weight with which a patient can perform two sets of 25 repetitions with a 2-minute rest period between sets. Hamstring curls are done on the Nautilus or Universal Gym equipment (Fig. 33-13). Eccentric contractions are added as the patient progresses on the Nautilus. The weight is lifted with both legs, but the involved leg holds the weight for 2 seconds and slowly lowers the weight. This allows the hamstrings to contract while lengthening. Several studies have shown that more weight can be handled with less effort in an eccentric contraction than in a concentric contraction.[4,36,52]

Quadriceps resisted exercises are performed in the short arc of 0 to 50 degrees

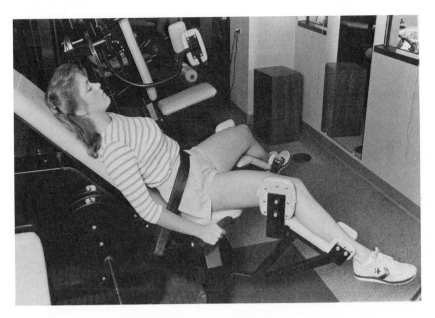

Fig. 33-12 ■ Nautilus hip abductor.

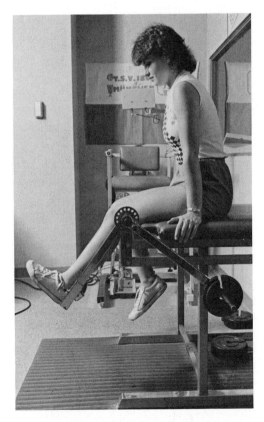

Fig. 33-13 ■ Hamstring curl.

to hold the patellar compressive forces to one and one-half times body weight.[41] Eccentric quadriceps contractions are done on the Universal Gym by pulling the upper pad by hand so that the lower pad is resting on the involved leg with the knee as straight as possible (Fig. 33-14). The upper pad is released, and the weight is held for 2 seconds by the involved leg and slowly released. These exercises can also be performed on the Nautilus leg extension machine by raising the weight with both legs and holding for 2 seconds with the involved leg, then lowering.

Toe raises are continued with weights on the Universal Gym or Nautilus machine (Fig. 33-15).

Stretching

In the stretching phase of the rehabilitation, it is important to check for a tight iliotibial band. This is accomplished by the performance of the Ober test. The patient lies with the unaffected side down, and with hip and knee maximally flexed on the down side to flatten the lumbar

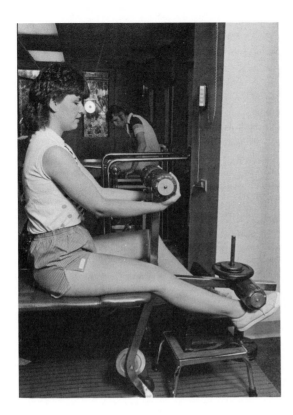

Fig. 33-14 ■ Universal gym eccentric quadriceps exercise.

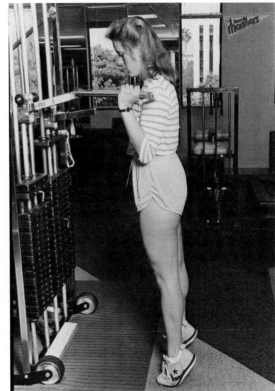

Fig. 33-15 ■ Universal gym toe raise.

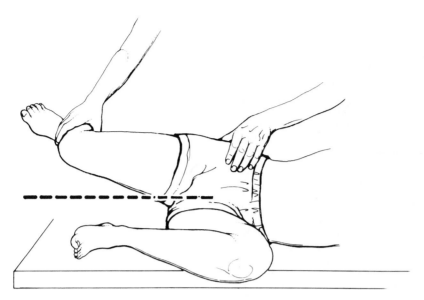

Fig. 33-16 ■ Ober test.

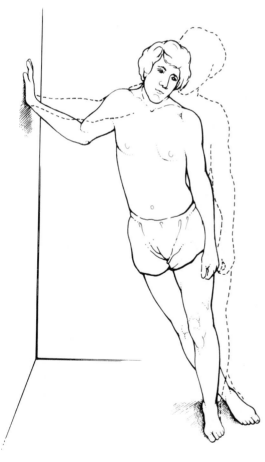

Fig. 33-17 ■ Abductor and iliotibial tract stretching.

spine. The involved knee is flexed to 90 degrees. The hip is abducted and hyperextended, then allowed to adduct maximally. The knee on the tested extremity should always be kept at 90 degrees of flexion. The angle that the thigh makes with the horizontal line parallel to the table represents the degree of abduction contracture. Normally, the extremity drops well below the horizontal (Fig. 33-16). Abductor and iliotibial tract stretching is performed with the individual standing. The patients stands at arm's distance from the wall. The leg closest to the wall is placed behind the outside leg, and then the patient leans the body closer to the wall while keeping the knee and hip extended. This will stretch the iliotibial band (Fig. 33-17). This stretch is maintained for 10 seconds with a 5-second rest period and then repeated for two sets of 10.

Calf stretches are performed from the standing position over a 2-inch wooden block or a tilt board (Fig. 33-18).

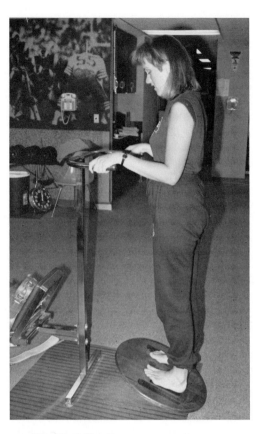

Fig. 33-18 ■ Calf stretches on tilt board.

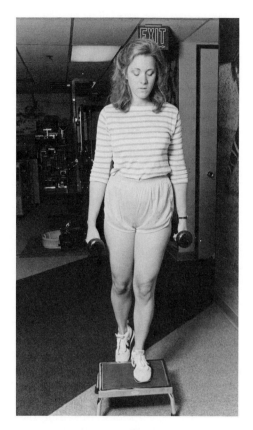

Fig. 33-19 ■ Step-up.

Functional activity

Step-ups are a form of functional activity that employs several muscle groups* (Fig. 33-19). The height of the step should not require more than 70 degrees of knee flexion. This will keep the patellar compressive forces less than two times the body weight. The patient slowly steps up onto the platform with the involved leg first, trying not to push off with the normal leg. In stepping down, the normal leg proceeds first. This exercise is started with just the patient's body weight. Additional weights are added in 10-pound increments until one third of the patient's

---

*Dr. Joseph Godfrey of Buffalo, N.Y. deserves the credit for step-ups. He described them in 1964 and showed lateral step-ups as well, for when pain is present in regular step-ups.

STEP-UPS

Keep step low!
Height should not require more than 70 degrees of knee flexion to keep patellofemoral compression forces below twice body weight.
Discontinue at sign of patellofemoral pain!

---

body weight can be handled in two sets of 25 repetitions. The patient should carry dumbbells in either hand as a simple method to perform step-ups.

Home program

The home program continues with strengthening of the hip, knee, and calf musculature. The patient is instructed to use ankle weights but to keep them at least 10 pounds lighter than the weights

---

INTERMEDIATE PHASE PROGRAM

Warm-up

Bike
Stretching
  Calf-tilt board
  Hamstring
  ITB (if indicated)

Exercise	Repetitions	Sets	Weight increase (pounds)
Hip adduction	10	2	10
Hip abduction	10	2	10
Hip flexion	10	2	10
Hamstring curls	10	2	10
Short arc quadriceps	10	2	10
Step-ups	25	2	10

Home program

Resisted exercises
Swimming
Bicycling

---

handled in therapy. The patients are warned not to lift weights at home if pain and swelling develop. Toe raises are added along with step-ups. Swimming is beneficial, but straight leg kicks should be used only with caution, since patellar pain may develop. Bicycling is also added, because both bicycling and swimming are functional exercises. At this point, the patient should have enough range of motion for normal gait, but the therapist should observe the gait and correct any deficiencies.

A summary of the intermediate phase program is shown in the box above.

Advanced phase

The advanced phase concentrates on the gradual return to functional activities. Strength and endurance are maximized, using isokinetic machines to train the

---

ADVANCED PHASE

Warm-up
Isokinetic training
Agility drills
Trampoline jogging
Treadmill
Home program

---

limb to move at the fast speeds required in athletic competition.

Warm-up

The warm-up and stretching routines are continued as in the intermediate phase.

Isokinetic training

Wyatt and Edwards suggest that the quadriceps need to be exercised at work rates of 200 to 300 degrees per second to be functionally rehabilitated for just walking.[57] The hip, knee, and calf musculature are trained isotonically until normal strength is achieved. The hip, quadriceps, and hamstring exercises are performed on the Cybex machine at a speed of 300 degrees per second for two sets of 20 repetitions (Fig. 33-20). If the Orthotron equipment is used, it is set at a speed of 10, which is equal to 300 degrees per-second on the Cybex. In both machines, the speed of the exercises is controlled, either electronically in the former or hydraulically in the latter. Also, the resistance accommodates to the patient's pain, since no resistance will be met if the limb moves slower than the set speed. The repetitions and sets are kept the same as the

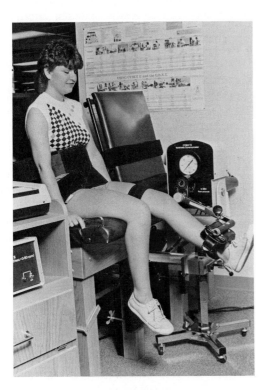

Fig. 33-20 ■ Cybex.

isotonic routine and the speed reduced at increments of 30 degrees per second until 180 degrees per second is reached.

Agility drills

Agility drills are incorporated to aid regaining lateral and rotational mobility.

Trampoline jogging and treadmill

Jogging is started on the trampoline in therapy to minimize the stresses on the knee. This can begin when the injured knee has achieved 80% of quadriceps and hamstring strength of the normal extremity on Cybex testing. This usually corresponds to 1 cm of thigh atrophy at 20 cm above the superior pole of the patella. Jogging on the trampoline is started in 5-minute segments and continued until 10 minutes can be tolerated. Then the treadmill is used, beginning with 2-minute sessions and continuing until the patient can tolerate 10 minutes of continuous running.

Home program

The home program described for the intermediate phase is expanded to include 5 minutes of running and 5 minutes of walking until the total distance of 1 mile can be covered. Running gradually replaces all of the walking, provided there is no swelling or pain. Agility exercises are begun with figure-8 running on a basket-

AGILITY DRILLS	
Running (straight ahead)	Vertical jumps
Figure-8 running	Lateral running
Backward running	Crossovers
Rope skipping	

ball half-court and progressing to Figure-8s inside the center key. Backward running, rope skipping, vertical jumps, lateral running, and crossovers are started at a slow pace. When this can be accomplished without pain and swelling, the athlete can begin practicing the skills necessary for the specific sport. Racquetball is started with doubles play to regain total body coordination. These agility drills should not cause pain and can be performed with increasing speed as the athlete's power and endurance improve. See the box on p. 1074 for a summary of the advanced phase program.*

Termination of therapy

Cybex testing is used to decide when to terminate therapy. Prior training on isokinetic equipment has been shown to improve the athlete's scores as well as motor-performance skills.[44,45] The test protocol includes measurements of **strength** as the peak torque develops, at speeds of 180, 240, and 300 degrees per second. The amount of time it takes to develop this torque is the **power. Endurance**, recorded at 240

---

*Editors' note: We cannot overstress the importance of the authors' remarks on the home program. The fitness and rehabilitation center should not be an "umbilical cord" for the patient. Goals to substitute an excellent rehabilitation program at home should be of primary importance ultimately.

ADVANCED PHASE PROGRAM

Warm-up
Bike
Trampoline
Treadmill

Exercise	Repetitions	Sets	Speed reductions (degrees/second)
Hip	20	2	30
Quadriceps	20	2	30
Hamstring	20	2	30

Home program
Jog-walk
Agility drills

---

degrees per second, is the point at which the patient can no longer produce 50% of the original peak torque for this speed. The athlete can return to full athletic activity when strength, power, and endurance are 85% of the normal leg. It is very useful to have a preseason Cybex test, because the strength level of both legs may drop after an injury. This visual record of the strength of the involved leg helps in counseling the athlete.

TERMINATION OF THERAPY EVALUATION

Isokinetic strength
Peak torque at 180, 240, and 300 degrees per second

Isokinetic endurance
Continuous, repeated maximal efforts (240 degrees per second) until the torque developed is 50% of original peak torque

Isokinetic power
Amount of time to develop peak torque

Sport-specific training

Once the competitor realizes that strength in the leg has returned to normal, a vigorous training program can be begun for that athlete's sport. This allows the athlete to regain confidence in the injured extremity. The competitor is also instructed in an isotonic program to main-

tain strength levels over the next 6 months. The maintenance level is 85% of the maximal weight level that the patient achieved at the termination of formal therapy. This requires lifting twice a week in addition to the usual training routine. Bicycle riding or running are good methods of maintaining cardiovascular endurance. Wearing a Neoprene rubber sleeve for competition appears to decrease some of the sensitivity experienced on return to activity. Finally, the patient is instructed in a proper warm-up and stretching technique.

■ IMMEDIATE POSTOPERATIVE REHABILITATION

The adverse effects of immobilization have been demonstrated at the tissue level by several authors. Costill et al.[10] demonstrated a significant decrease in oxidative enzyme systems. Haggmark and Eriksson[19] described the selective atrophy of type I slow-twitch muscle fibers with casting. Eriksson and Haggmark[15] demonstrated that electrical stimulation can alter these changes. They concluded that electrical stimulation not only reduces atrophy and weakness but also augments oxidative enzyme activity in the muscle. When electrical stimulation is to be used during the immobilization period,[17] it is important to have the patient go through a trial of electrical stimulation to allay apprehension and to ensure proper electrode placement. One electrode is placed proximally at the femoral triangle, and the other is placed in the middle or distal portion of the vastus medialis muscle. The distal motor point varies, and therefore the distal electrode is moved until the strongest and most comfortable quadriceps contraction is elicited.

Studies have indicated that static or isometric exercise can produce strength gains.[18,46] These benefits are not as dramatic as those achieved by isotonic exercises but are very practical during immobilization. Isometric exercises can be started in the immediate postoperative period. When leg lifts are comfortable, hip abduction, hip adduction, and hip extension leg exercises can be added even while the extremity is still immobilized.[53] If the ankle is not included in the cast, the patient can be instructed in toe raises. Toe raises are performed with the patient standing with support of either a table or a wall in front. They are initiated with body weight alone. The patient is then instructed to add equal amounts of weight in each hand, and this can gradually be increased from 10 to 20 pounds with two sets of 25 repetitions.

Vigorous exercise of the contralateral extremity has been shown to produce a "cross-over" strengthening effect in the casted limb. Animal studies have demonstrated as much as a 30% increase in strength because of this effect.[21-23] Upper body conditioning can be maintained by circuit training on the Nautilus or Universal Gym equipment. Single leg stationary bicycle riding can also be used for cardiac endurance.[10]

■ INJURY DEPENDENT REHABILITATION VARIATIONS
Collateral ligament sprains

Rehabilitation after injury to the collateral ligaments is shorter and progresses with fewer problems than the program for cruciate ligament injury. This is because of the decreased severity of the injury as well as the fact that there are no specific strengthening exercises to mod-

ify. For medial-side lesions, care must be taken during hip exercises to avoid valgus stress at the knee. Conversely, for lateral ligament injuries, varus stress should not be allowed. Placing the weights above the knee for the hip exercises will alleviate these loads. The one major problem that

---

COLLATERAL LIGAMENT INJURIES

During isotonic training of hip musculature, place weights proximal to knee to avoid valgus/varus stress (as necessary)

---

occurs during rehabilitation in collateral ligament injuries is limited range of motion. This occurs because of adherence of the ligament at the injury site. It may be seen as a block to flexion or extension and is more common on the medial side. The therapist must pay close attention to range of motion changes until the full arc of movement has been achieved.

Nonsurgical treatment of collateral ligament injury differs from surgical treatment only in the severity of the instability resulting from the injury and the effects of immobilization.* Haggmark and Eriksson[19] have shown that a hinged cast will protect the repair and cause less atrophy and less range of motion loss. Indelicato[28] demonstrated that immobilization with a cast brace will result in a shorter recuperation period. Several studies have shown that medial collateral ligament injuries can be treated without immobilization.[1,14,20,25,54] As a result, the therapist can advance the athlete from the starting phase to the final phase of rehabilitation as quickly as tolerated by the patient. This can be as short as 2 weeks or as long as 8 weeks.

Anterior cruciate ligament instability

The anterior cruciate ligament functions to prevent both excessive anterior movement of the tibia on the femur and abnormal tibial internal and external ro-

---

*Editors' note: See Chapter 30 for additional remarks.

Important goal in anterior cruciate ligament insufficiency ⟶ Hamstring rehabilitation

tation. Larson[32] feels that it functions to guide the knee through its arc of motion. This action allows the other ligaments of the joint to tighten, which in turn protects the menisci from excessive force. With these functions in mind, the primary goal in rehabilitation is the restoration of dynamic stability by training the muscles that act to prevent excessive tibial rotation in anterior glide on the femur. The muscle group mainly responsible for these functions is the hamstrings.

Giove and Miller[16] stated that the most valuable finding in *conservative* anterior cruciate ligament rehabilitation was the quadriceps-hamstrings ratio and the level of sports participation. The basic principle is to strengthen the hamstrings until they are *at least* of equal strength with the quadriceps on the involved side. This allows the athlete to perform at a higher level of activity. The usual ratio of quadriceps to hamstrings on Cybex equipment[51] at a speed of 180 degrees per second is 60:40 (Fig. 33-21). Our goal is to make the hamstring of the involved leg dominant. The optimal ratio of 55:45 can be achieved by emphasizing knee flexion throughout rehabilitation (Fig. 33-21, *A* and *B*).

In the nonsurgical patient, the acute therapy is designed to control swelling and pain. After this goal is attained, the program consists of isometric exercise alone or in combination with isotonic exercise, based on the patient's comfort level. The protocol begins with isometric hamstring sets and isometric quadriceps sets while the knee is resting on a rolled towel. The patient is instructed to obtain co-contraction of the quadriceps and the hamstrings used as hip extensors by pushing the back of the knee into the towel.* Straight leg raises are *not* per-

formed, because they may increase the anterior subluxation of the tibia on the femur. Further, we have demonstrated more electromyographic activity with isometric contractions.[35,47]

Isometric internal and external tibial rotation exercises, which are added once the patient has 90 degrees of knee flexion, have been shown to decrease the abnormal tibial rotation that is present.[49] These exercises progress to rubber band resistance. Then both tibial rotations are increased in 5-pound increments on the Universal Gym with the patient seated in a chair and the knee flexed to 90 degrees. Special emphasis is placed on the hamstrings, and the patient may do as many as six sets of 10 repetitions. The foot is placed in the loop of the cuff, and the tibia is rotated internally against the weight (Fig. 33-22). The chair position is then reversed to work external rotation. The patient is then advanced through the last phase of therapy and placed in a maintenance program that also emphasizes the hamstrings.

The most commonly used surgical procedures for anterior cruciate ligament instability are either intraarticular or extraarticular reconstructions. It has been shown by several authors that the tension on the anterior cruciate ligament is greatest from 30 degrees of flexion to full extension.[24] For this reason, we use postoperative casting with knee flexion of 35 to 40 degrees, followed at 6 weeks by bracing with an extension stop of 40 degrees. In intraarticular procedures, the site has to undergo revascularization followed by reorganization of collagen.[6,8,39] This necessitates a slower and longer process of therapy for patients who undergo these procedures,[5,40,42] and they are held for 15 weeks before the brace is brought into extension. Our studies have indicated that a gradual reduction in the flexion contracture, starting at 12 weeks, provides

---

*Editors' note: Steindler first pointed out the importance of phasic contraction to prevent instability in his marvelous book, *Kinesiology of the Human Body under Normal and Pathologic Conditions,* in 1955.

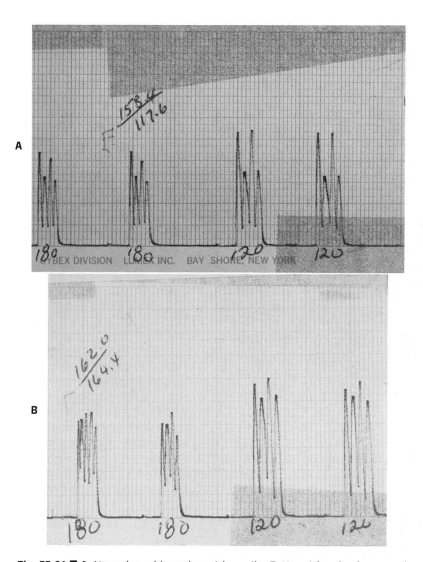

Fig. 33-21 ■ **A,** Normal quadriceps-hamstring ratio. **B,** Hamstring dominance ratio.

greater stability for the extraarticular repairs.[*2,56]

There are some variations during the starting phase for the surgical patients. For example, hip abduction exercises are performed with hip flexion of 45 degrees with the knee in 45 degrees of flexion, and weights are placed above the knee to pre-

vent excess varus load on the knee. Hip extension exercises can have weight added at the ankle. The flexed posture of the knee should be slightly increased beyond that permitted by the brace, thus decreasing any tendency of the exercise to result in passive extension. The quadriceps exercises are kept **isometric,** but the hamstrings are advanced to **isotonic resisted exercises.**

The intermediate phase features a decrease in the extension stop to 15 degrees. Short arc quadriceps exercises are initi-

---

*Editors' note: We too believe in stops and restricted motion to protect ligaments in a long rehabilitation effort rather than a quick program with little protection, as some authors advocate today.

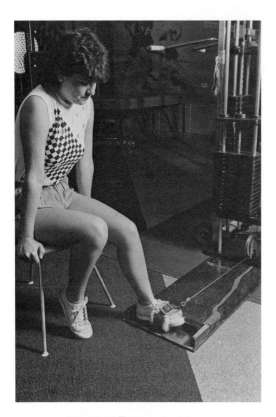

Fig. 33-22 ■ Internal rotators.

ated when the hamstrings can handle 15 pounds, and again the patient is instructed to generate a co-contraction of the quadriceps and hamstrings by hip extension.

The advanced phase features eccentric quadriceps exercise and removal of the extension stop. This allows the thigh girth to increase, because the quadriceps can produce full knee extension. Rehabilitation of the anterior cruciate ligament reconstruction is a very lengthy procedure. An athlete with such an injury will usually require a year before returning to full activity.

Posterior cruciate ligament instability

The posterior cruciate ligament's major function is to prevent excessive posterior displacement of the tibia on the femur.

Hughston et al.[26] consider the ligament to be the primary stabilizer of the knee in flexion, extension, and rotation. He states that in knee motion the tibial plateaus move anteriorly and posteriorly by rotating around the axis of the posterior cruciate ligament. A contraction of the quadriceps muscle pulls the tibia anteriorly, thus compensating for the posterior sagging of the tibia. Therefore the focus of this rehabilitation for both surgical and nonsurgical patients is on the quadriceps. Electromyographic studies have shown that patients can learn to activate knee extension earlier when running, thus providing stability.[*7]

In the conservative rehabilitation, the hamstring sets are omitted in the starting phase, since they may accentuate the posterior subluxation. Also, eccentric quadriceps exercises are started as soon as the patient can tolerate them. Along with step-ups, straight leg raises and short arc quadriceps exercises are used early. The intermediate phase eliminates both the internal and external tibial rotation exercises, because they accentuate the posterior subluxation of the tibia.

A common surgical procedure for posterior cruciate ligament reconstruction is repositioning of the origin of the medial head of the gastrocnemius muscle.[31] This transfer acts dynamically during the weight-acceptance and push-off phases of gait.[29] This can be demonstrated by having the patient maximally contract the gastrocnemius during active plantar flexion of the foot and watching the tibia move forward from the resting position.

In surgical patients, both the quadriceps and the gastrocnemius muscles are of primary importance. During immobilization, the patient is instructed to

---

*Editors' note: Nothing at this time is as definite and important in the management of posterior instability as the authors' thoughts in this section.

Important goal in posterior cruciate ligament insufficiency ⟶ Quadriceps rehabilitation